Third Edition

Pharmacy Practice
for technicians

Don A. Ballington, MS

Midlands Technical College
Columbia, South Carolina

Robert J. Anderson, PharmD

Mercer University Southern School of Pharmacy
Atlanta, Georgia

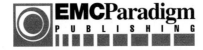

EMCParadigm
PUBLISHING

Senior Editor	Christine Hurney
Editorial Assistants	Susan Capecchi, Cheryl Drivdahl
Copy Editor	Rich Cronin
Cover and Text Designer	Leslie Anderson
Desktop Production	Petrina Nyhan, Jack Ross
Proofreader	Judy Peacock
Indexer	Terry Casey
Photos	Credits follow Index

Publishing Management Team

Bob Cassel, Publisher; Jeanne Allison, Senior Acquisitions Editor; Janice Johnson, Vice President of Marketing; Shelley Clubb, Electronic Design and Production Manager

Text and Encore CD	ISBN 0-7638-2223-X
Product Number	01659
Text-only ISBN	0-7638-2224-8
Text-only Product Number	04659

Care has been taken to verify the accuracy of information presented in this book. The authors, editors, and publisher, however, cannot accept responsibility for errors or omissions or for consequences from application of the information in this book and make no warranty, expressed or implied, with respect to its content.

Some of the product names used in this book have been used for identification purposes only and may be trademarks or registered trademarks of their respective manufacturers.

Printed in the United States of America.

10 9 8 7 6 5 4 3 2

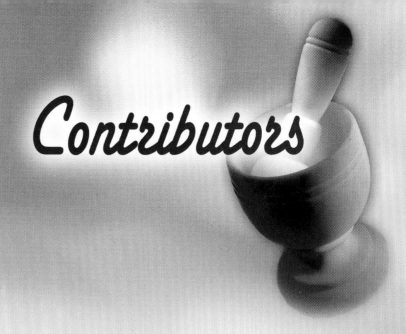

Contributors

Reneé Acosta, RPh, MS
Austin Community College
Austin, Texas

Cheryl Aiken, BS Pharm, PharmD, RPh
Brattleboro Retreat
Brattleboro, Vermont
Vermont Technical College
Randolph Center, Vermont

Betty Carpenter, BS Pharm
Pikes Peak Community College
Colorado Springs, Colorado

Nora Chan, PharmD
City College of San Francisco
San Francisco, California

Jennifer Danielson, BS Pharm, RPh,
    MBA, CDE
Pikes Peak Community College
Colorado Springs, Colorado

Tova Wiegand Green, BS Pharm
Ivy Tech Community College of Indiana
    Northeast
Fort Wayne, Indiana

Jeff Gricar, MEd, CPhT
Houston Community College
Houston, Texas

Barbara Lacher, BS, RPhTech, CPhT
North Dakota State College of Science
Wahpeton, North Dakota

Nancy Lim, PhD, RPh, CPhT
North Harris Community College
Houston, Texas

James Mizner, BS, MBA, RPh
ACT College
Arlington, Virginia

Candace Montgomery, CPhT
Ivy Tech Community College of Indiana
    Northeast
Fort Wayne, Indiana

Andrea Redman, PharmD, BCPS
Rockdale Medical Center
Conyers, Georgia
Mercer University Southern School of
    Pharmacy
Atlanta, Georgia

Phil Rushing, BS Pharm
Community Care College
Tulsa, Oklahoma

Bobbi Steelman, CPhT
Draughons Junior College
Bowling Green, Kentucky

Jason Sparks, CPhT
Austin Community College
Austin, Texas

Mary Ann Stuhan, RPh
Cuyahoga Community College
Cleveland, Ohio

Kimberly Vernachio, PharmD, RPh
Vernachio Managed Care Consultants
CVS Pharmacies
Canton, Georgia

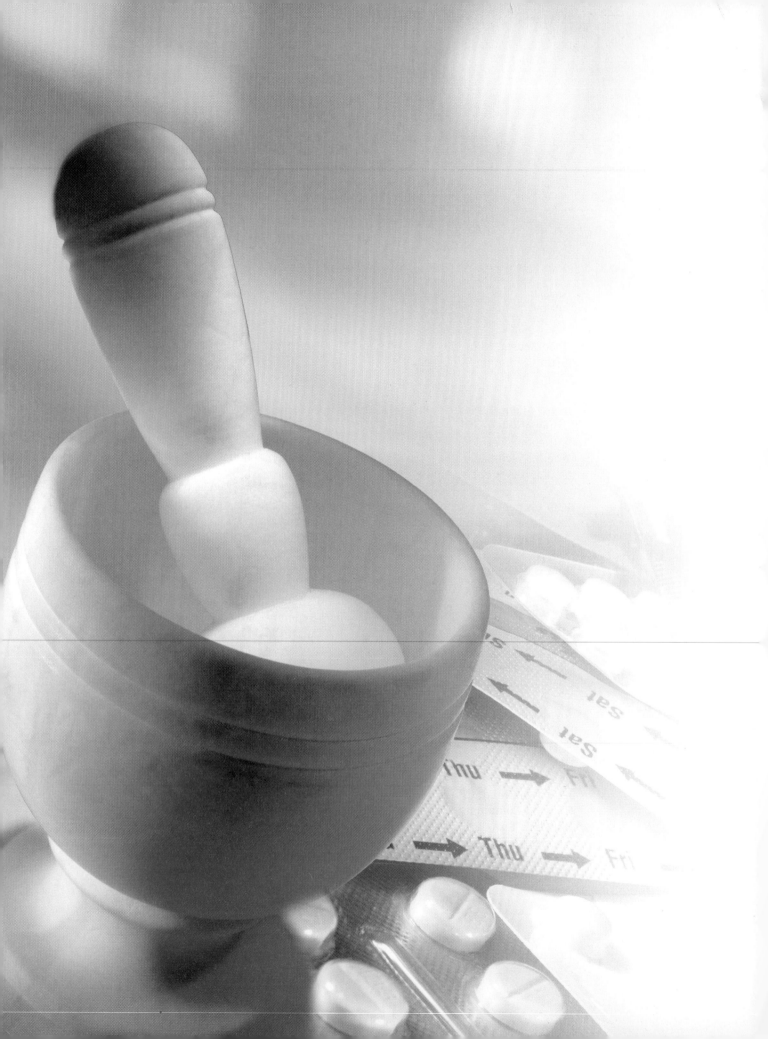

Contents

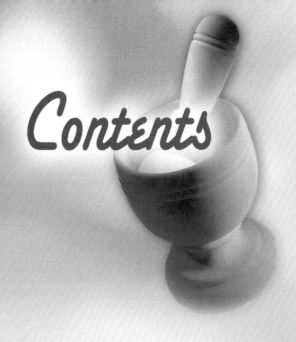

Chapter 5
Basic Pharmaceutical
Measurements and Calculations....95

UNIT 2
COMMUNITY PHARMACY..125

Chapter 6
Dispensing Medications in the
Community Pharmacy.................127

Chapter 7
The Business of Community
Pharmacy 151

UNIT 4
PROFESSIONALISM IN
THE PHARMACY 275

Chapter 12
Medication Safety 277

Chapter 13
Human Relations and
Communications 303

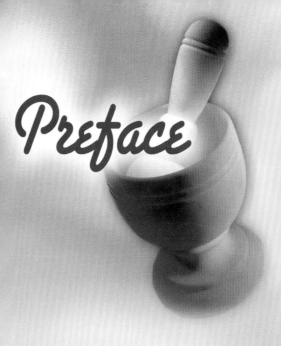

Preface

Pharmacy Practice for Technicians, Third Edition provides the pharmacy technician student with the necessary techniques and procedures to prepare and dispense medications in both the community and institutional pharmacy settings. Preparing medications involves using sterile and nonsterile techniques to count, measure, and compound drugs. The text covers reading the prescription in the community pharmacy or medication order in the hospital pharmacy; preparing, packaging, and labeling the medication; and maintaining the patient profile. It also introduces other medication and nonmedication activities related to pharmacy, including billing and inventory management. The activities of the pharmacy technician are very important to the level of quality of care the patient receives as the support provided by the technicians allows the pharmacist to spend more time counseling patients and monitoring drug therapy. The concepts taught in the text are reinforced by the new interactive, multimedia Encore CD.

This text and Encore CD offer the pharmacy technician educator and student the tools to achieve the competencies needed to obtain certification. The text supports the following goals under the categories of general operations, drug dose and knowledge, accurate drug calculations and measurement, and administrative and customer relations.

General Operations
- Perform pharmacy technician duties within the scope of the position and ethics of the industry.
- Perform the roles and responsibilities of the pharmacy technician and comply with performance and safety standards established for the community and hospital pharmacy settings.
- Perform record-keeping functions associated with dispensing pharmaceuticals, processing insurance claims, and maintaining drug inventory while protecting patient confidentiality.

Drug Knowledge
- Demonstrate a working knowledge of drug doses, routes of administration, and interactions within the scope of the pharmacy technician responsibilities.
- Read and understand drug labeling, packaging, and dose information, and dispense drugs as prescribed.
- Use drug references to accurately identify generic and brand equivalents and other information requested by the pharmacist.
- Use the medical terms, abbreviations, and symbols essential to prescribing, dispensing, administering, and charting medications correctly and precisely.

Accurate Drug Calculations and Measurement
- Follow the correct procedures and techniques related to compounding and admixture operations.
- Perform accurate calculations required for usual doses and solution preparations.
- Perform basic calculations to determine inventory and purchasing needs, profit margins, and inventory control.
- Perform accurate conversions between measurement systems.

Administrative and Customer Relations
- Translate prescribed dose and administration instructions to ensure patient understanding.
- Assist the pharmacist in all matters of customer relations and support.

Features of the Third Edition

Features of the third edition include these:
- New, interactive, multimedia CD with matching exercises, glossary, and concept reviews to reinforce learning of pharmacy practice.
- Addition of end-of-chapter key terms list and glossary to reinforce learning of pharmacy terminology.
- Expanded coverage of safety issues and ways pharmacy technicians can help the medical team avoid medication errors, including a new chapter focusing on medication safety and Safety Note sidebars throughout the text.
- Expanded coverage of skills needed by pharmacy technicians working in a hospital setting, as well as a comprehensive study of pharmacy technician responsibilities in community, hospital, and other pharmacy settings.
- Full-color design features and a rich art and photo program.
- Web Link sidebars and Internet research assignments as avenues for continually expanding and updating chapter material.
- Communication skills and role-playing exercises for authentic communication practice.
- Expanded coverage of pharmacy calculations, including business math.
- Expanded coverage of law and ethics, including federal, state, court, and voluntary standards.
- A workbook with exercises for each chapter, including crossword puzzles on medical terminology, pharmacy calculations, prescription practice, in-the-lab activities, and Web activities.

How This Text Is Organized

Pharmacy Practice for Technicians, Third Edition is divided into four units.
- Unit 1 Principles of Pharmacy Practice
- Unit 2 Community Pharmacy
- Unit 3 Institutional Pharmacy
- Unit 4 Professionalism in the Pharmacy

Each chapter begins with Learning Objectives and concludes with a Chapter Summary. These pedagogical tools will help students study and remember the important points raised in the chapter. In addition, new to this edition, Chapter Terms are provided for each chapter. End-of-chapter questions reinforce the information presented in the chapter, and provide opportunity for discussion and practice of communication skills. Pharmacy in Practice exercises require students to apply the theory to hands-on pharmacy scenarios. Internet Research exercises invite students to do further topic investigation on the Internet.

The appendixes provide valuable reference material, including a list of common prescription abbreviations for student reference (Appendix A), a review of Greek and Latin word parts (Appendix B), a list of the most commonly prescribed drugs and their drug categories (Appendix C), a list of common drugs that cannot be crushed (Appendix D), and a list of look-alike and sound-alike medications and recommendations from the Institute for Safe Medication Practices (ISMP) (Appendix E).

Resources for the Student

In addition to the textbook, three valuable resources are provided to help students master skills needed for pharmacy practice.

Encore CD The Encore CD included with each textbook is an exciting new feature of the third edition of *Pharmacy Practice for Technicians*. The Encore CD includes interactive review questions that students can use to test their knowledge of concepts presented in the book. There are two levels of tests—book and chapter— and each level functions in two different modes. In the Review mode, the student receives immediate feedback on each test item and a report of his or her total score. In the reportable Practice Test mode, the results are e-mailed to both the student and the instructor.

The Encore CD also includes Tech Check interactive matching activities that require the student to manipulate concepts from the chapter content. The Encore CD includes chapter-specific glossaries as well as a complete glossary and image bank with key illustrations from the textbooks in the pharmacy technician series published by EMC Corporation. To reinforce drug name recognition, the Encore CD also includes interactive flash cards of the top prescribed drugs.

Student Workbook Students are encouraged to use the workbook, in addition to the Encore CD, to reinforce the information taught in the text. The workbook that accompanies *Pharmacy Practice for Technicians, Third Edition* includes new crossword puzzles to reinforce chapter vocabulary and concepts, communication and application exercises to help students apply chapter instruction, Web activities to encourage research, and in-the-lab activities for Units 2 and 3.

Internet Resource Center The Internet Resource Center for this title at www.emcp.com provides additional resources, including chapter study notes, PowerPoint slide shows, interactive flash cards for learning the generic and brand names of the top-prescribed drugs, and other valuable resources.

Resources for the Instructor

Pharmacy Practice for Technicians, Third Edition is supported by several tools to help instructors plan their course and assess student learning.

Instructor's Guide The Instructor's Guide that accompanies *Pharmacy Practice, Third Edition* contains suggested course syllabus information as well as answers for all end-of-chapter and workbook exercises. It also provides teaching hints for each chapter, ready-to-use chapter tests, and midterm and final examinations.

Internet Resource Center All the resources from the print Instructor's Guide are available in electronic format on the password-protected section of the Internet Resource Center for this title at www.emcp.com. In addition, the site provides PowerPoint slide shows to enhance class presentations.

ExamView Computerized Test Generator A full-featured computerized test generator on CD offers instructors a wide variety of options for generating both print and on-line tests. The testbank offers 50 questions for each chapter. Instructors can create custom tests using questions from the testbank, edit existing questions, or add questions of their own design.

WebCT and Blackboard WebCT and Blackboard Web course management systems are available to support this product. Each system comes preloaded with course information, chapter outlines, and quizzes.

Resources for the Pharmacy Technician Series

In addition to *Pharmacy Practice for Technicians, Third Edition*, EMC Corporation publishes several other titles designed specifically for the pharmacy technician curriculum.

- *Pharmacology for Technicians, Third Edition:* includes an Encore CD with every textbook, a workbook, the Internet Resource Center, and for the instructor, a guide, PowerPoint presentations, a testbank, and Web course management systems.
- *Pharmacy Calculations for Technicians, Third Edition:* includes an Encore CD with every textbook, the Internet Resource Center, and, for the instructor, a guide, PowerPoint presentations, a testbank, and Web course management systems.
- *Pharmacy Technician Certification Exam Review:* includes two practice exams with answer feedback, study tips, and an Encore CD with over 1900 exam questions is also available.

About the Authors

Don A. Ballington, MS, is the program coordinator of the pharmacy technician training program at Midlands Technical College, in Columbia, South Carolina. He has served as president of the Pharmacy Technician Educators Council and in 2005 received the council's Educator of the Year award. Mr. Ballington has conducted site visits for pharmacy technician accreditation and helped develop the American Society of Health-System Pharmacists model curriculum. He has also been a consulting editor for the *Journal of Pharmacy Technology.* Over the course of his career at Midlands Technical College, he has developed a set of high-quality training materials for pharmacy technicians. These materials have been made available in three national textbooks: *Pharmacology for Technicians, Pharmacy Calculations for*

Technicians, and *Pharmacy Practice for Technicians*. All are now available in third editions.

Robert J. Anderson, PharmD, is an adjunct professor at the Southern School of Pharmacy at Mercer University in Atlanta, Georgia, with over 30 years of experience in academia and practice. He is also a part-time community pharmacist at Ball Ground Pharmacy and is president of RJA Consultants. Anderson has been a clinical pharmacy specialist at Kaiser Permanente, Southeast Region, in Atlanta. He has also been a director and associate director for the Department of Pharmaceutical Services at the University of Nebraska Medical Center in Omaha, Nebraska. He wrote chapters in *Clinical Pharmacology and Therapeutics* and *Handbook of Nonprescription Drugs*, and has served on the editorial boards of *Family Practice Recertification* and *American Journal of Managed Care Pharmacy*.

Acknowledgments

The authors and editorial staff would like to offer a special thank-you to Kimberly Vernachio for writing Chapter 12, *Medication Safety,* and to Jennifer Danielson for updating Chapter 14, *Your Future in Pharmacy Practice.* We appreciate your contributions to this title. In addition, we would like to thank Cheryl Aiken for writing the review and practice test questions for the Encore CD included with this textbook. We also would like to recognize Andrea Redman for writing testbank questions and for her valuable insights and input on the student workbook.

Finally, the quality of this body of work is a testament to the feedback we have received from the many contributors to this text (see page iii).

The author and editorial staff invite your feedback on the text and its supplements. Please reach us by clicking the "Contact us" button at www.emcp.com.

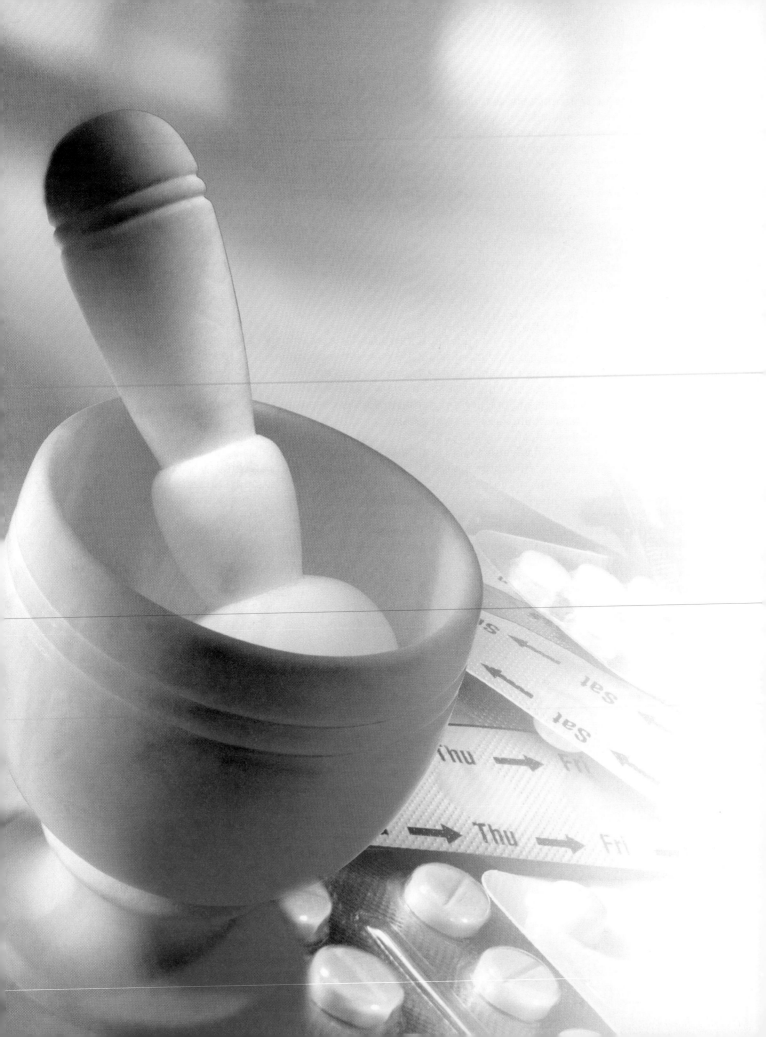

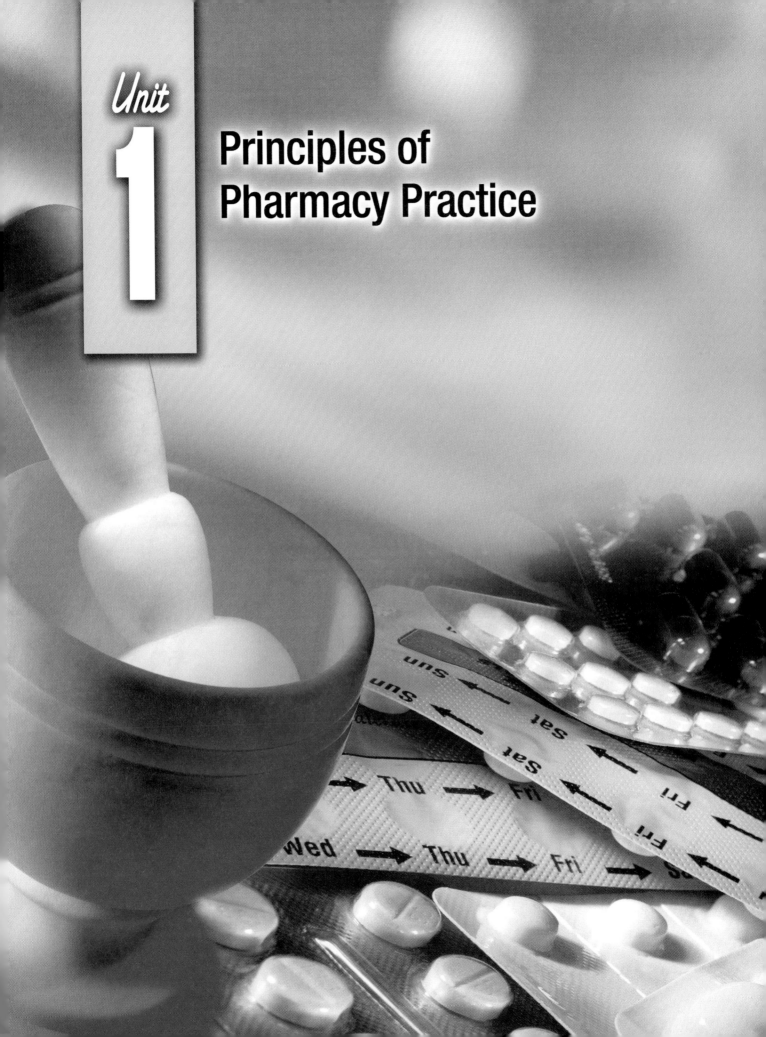

Unit

1

Principles of
Pharmacy Practice

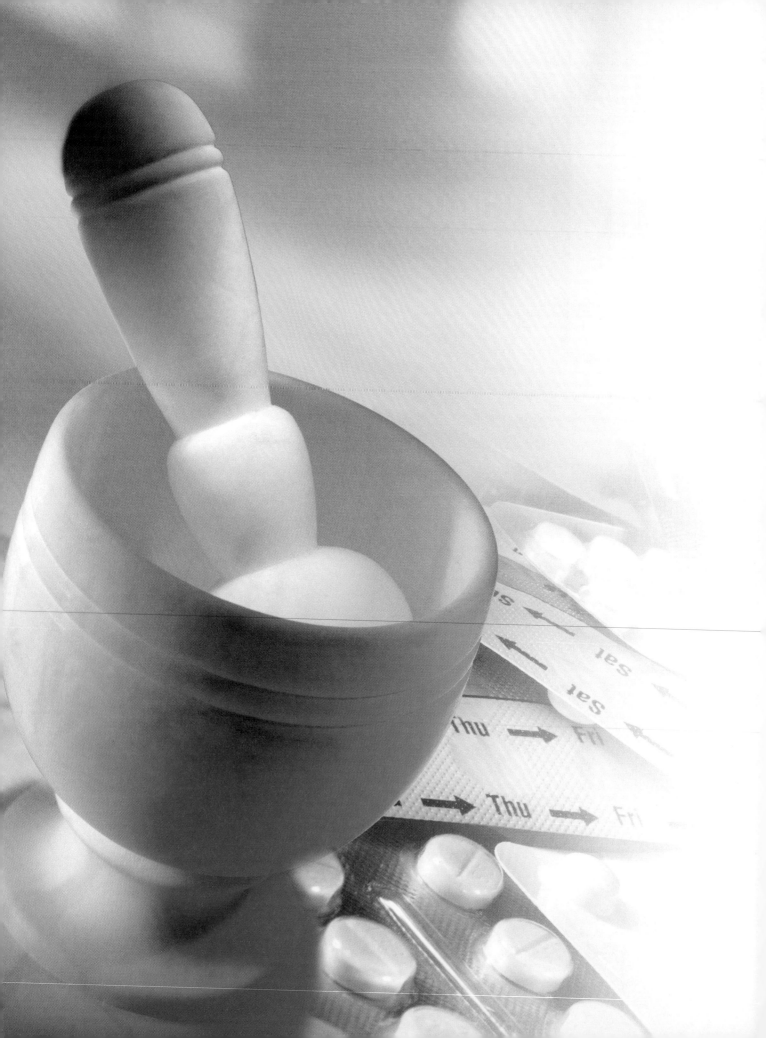

The Profession of Pharmacy

Learning Objectives

- Describe the origins of pharmacy.
- Describe four stages of development of the pharmacy profession in the twentieth century.
- Enumerate the functions of the pharmacist.
- Discuss the educational curriculum for today's pharmacy student.
- Explain the licensing requirements for pharmacists.
- Identify the duties and work environments of the pharmacy technician.
- Differentiate among the various kinds of pharmacies.

From its ancient origins in spiritualism and magic, pharmacy has evolved into a scientific pursuit involving not only the compounding and dispensing of medications but also the provision of accurate information and counseling about a wide range of medication-related issues. The contemporary pharmacy technician provides a wide variety of essential services to pharmacy customers, to supervising pharmacists, and to such healthcare professionals as physicians and nurses.

ANCIENT ORIGINS

In early civilization, disease was thought to be caused by evil spirits, demons, or evil forces. The medicine man had to identify the evil spirit and determine the appropriate remedy. Predictably, early recipes for drug preparation were freely mixed with incantations, rituals, and imitative magic. The word *pharmacy* comes from the ancient Greek word *pharmakon,* meaning *drug.* The use of drugs in the healing arts by all cultures is as old as civilization. Modern archaeologists, exploring the five-thousand-year-old remains of the ancient city-states of Mesopotamia, have unearthed clay tablets listing hundreds of medicinal preparations from various sources, including plants, animals, and minerals. The ancient Egyptians compiled lists of drugs, known as *formularies, dispensatories*, or *pharmacopoeias*. The most famous list was the Ebers papyrus, which was written about 1500 B.C. and included a collection of recipes.

In the Far East a similar mixture of natural sources of medicine and magic existed. To this day the people of China rely on natural herbs to treat common ailments. An example of a common herb that is widely used in Western culture today is ginseng for energy. The peoples of ancient India attributed the miraculous and curative powers of the gods and of their priestly shamans to an intoxicating drug, still unidentified but possibly derived from a mushroom. Many remedies were discovered by trial and error over many centuries.

To the ancient Greeks we owe the beginnings of a more scientific approach to the practice of medicine. Hippocrates believed that illness had a rational and physical

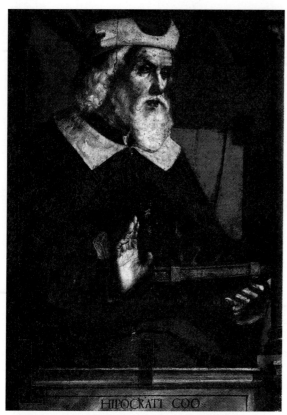

To Hippocrates, traditionally viewed as "the father of medicine," the ancients ascribed the creation of approximately 70 works dealing with the identification and treatment of disease. Today, Hippocrates is remembered for the Hippocratic oath, by which physicians pledge, among other requirements, "to do no harm."

explanation and was not the result of possession by evil spirits or disfavor with the gods. He established the *theory of humors*, which was to dominate medicine for almost two thousand years. According to this now long-discredited theory, health involved harmony among four fundamental bodily fluids, known as *humors*. Each humor was associated with particular personality characteristics. The humors were blood, phlegm, yellow bile, and black bile, and were associated, respectively, with cheerfulness, sluggishness, irritability, and melancholy.

Another ancient Greek physician, Galen, expanded on the theory of humors, brought together six centuries of knowledge and observation since Hippocrates, and conducted animal experiments to further his knowledge of the human body. He is best known for producing a systematic classification of drugs for the treatment of various pathologies that was unchallenged for nearly a century. The term *galenical pharmacy* was used to describe the process of creating extracts of active medicinals from plants (once a major activity of the pharmacist).

The greatest of the ancient pharmaceutical texts, however, was *De Materia Medica (On Medical Matters)*, written by Dioscorides in the first century A.D. Although a Greek physician, he served in the Roman army during the rule of Nero and traveled widely, gathering knowledge of medicinal herbs and minerals from Persia, Africa, Egypt, Greece, and Rome. His book served as the standard text on drugs, primarily herbal remedies, for fifteen hundred years.

Although drugs from herbal and mineral sources have been used for millennia, *pharmacy* as a distinct professional discipline is a relatively young field, starting in Europe in the Middle Ages. Around the time of the American Revolution, Dr. John Morgan voiced support for the separation of the professions of pharmacy and medicine. Until the nineteenth century, a physician usually owned the dispensary that distributed drugs to patients. However, gradually it became an independent entity owned and operated by the pharmacist. With the development of new synthetic drugs and an explosion of new research and access to information on drugs, the profession of pharmacy has grown concurrently with that medicine.

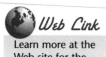

Web Link

Learn more at the Web site for the American Institute of the History of Pharmacy at **www.pharmacy .wisc.edu/aihp**

PHARMACIST

The profession of pharmacy exists today to safeguard the health of the public. Prescription medications can cure illness and prevent and control disease. However, side effects, adverse reactions, and interactions with other medications and foods can occur. The role of the modern **pharmacist** has evolved from the compounder and dispenser of natural and synthetic medicines to more of one involved in the dispensing of medication information and the early identification and prevention of medication-related problems such as appropriate dose, side effects, and safe combinations of drugs.

Evolution of the Pharmacist's Role

During the twentieth century the pharmacy profession evolved through four stages:

1. traditional era (dominated by the formulation and dispensing of drugs from natural sources)
2. scientific era (dominated by development of drugs and scientific testing of the effects of drugs on the body and mass production of synthetic drugs; started after World War II)
3. clinical era (evolved in the 1960s and combined traditional roles of the pharmacist with a new role as dispenser of drug information)
4. pharmaceutical-care era (a philosophy of care that expanded the mission statements of the profession to include responsibility for ensuring positive outcomes for drug therapy)

Before the 1940s the job of the pharmacist or apothecary consisted almost entirely of preparing and dispensing drugs. Important aspects of the traditional profession included **pharmacognosy**, knowledge of the medicinal functions of natural products of animal, plant, or mineral origins, and galenical pharmacy, knowledge of the techniques for preparing medications from such sources. A nineteenth-century apothecary not only sold drugs but also often gathered and manufactured them.

The emergence of the pharmaceutical industry in the twentieth century created a crisis for the profession. As the manufacturing of drugs moved from the apothecary shop to the factories of the pharmaceutical manufacturers, the pharmacist increasingly became more a retail merchant selling commodity products. This situation soon changed as educational institutions increased the emphasis on the sciences and expanded the curriculum. **Pharmacology**, the scientific study of drugs and their mechanism of action including side effects, became part of the pharmacy curriculum, along with physics, medicinal chemistry, and physiology.

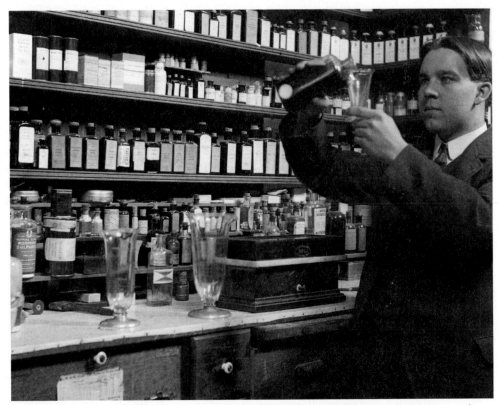

Dr. Emil King prepares medicine in his pharmacy in Fulda, Minnesota, 1905. Many physicians owned a pharmacy in the early nineteenth century and prepared their medications from natural sources.

By the 1960s additional basic science courses were developed including **pharmaceutics**, which studied the release characteristics of the drug dose form. By this time many pharmacists began to feel that their training had shifted too far in the direction of basic scientific knowledge and had strayed too far from actual pharmacy practice. Pharmacists constituted a highly knowledgeable, scientifically trained professional class with vast knowledge of drugs; yet they were underused and devoted the bulk of their energies to routine tasks and running a business rather than sharing information on drugs and interacting with patients and other professionals. In fact, up until the 1960s it was not ethical for a pharmacist to label the vials with the drug name or discuss potential side effects with the patient.

In 1973 the American Association of Colleges of Pharmacy established a study commission under Dr. John S. Millis to re-evaluate the mission of the pharmacy profession. The 1975 Millis Report, titled *Pharmacists for the Future,* defined pharmacy as a primarily knowledge-based profession and emphasized the role of the pharmacist in sharing knowledge about drug use.

This report led to a new emphasis in the profession on what is known as *clinical* or *patient-oriented pharmacy*. Curriculums were changed, and more colleges of pharmacy adopted Doctor of Pharmacy (PharmD) programs. New courses were developed, such as **pharmacokinetics** (individualizing doses of drugs based on absorption, distribution, metabolism and elimination from the body) and therapeutics and **pathophysiology** (applying pharmacology to disease). In addition, laboratories were moved from the university to more patient-oriented pharmacy practice settings, such as the hospital. Interdisciplinary experiences with physicians, residents, and interns in the university hospital became a standard practice.

In 1990 Drs. Charles Hepler and Linda Strand built on the Millis Report with a new framework defined as **pharmaceutical care**, which expanded the role of the pharmacist to include appropriate medication use to achieve positive outcomes with the prescribed drug therapy. The mission statements of many pharmacy organizations now reflect this new philosophy. Thus the modern pharmacist carries out the important role of monitoring response to therapy, as well as educating patients and dispensing prescription drugs.

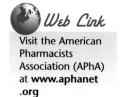

Web Link

Visit the American Pharmacists Association (APhA) at **www.aphanet .org**

Role of the Pharmacist

Historically, the primary duty of the pharmacist was the mixing of herbs and chemicals to create tablets, capsules, ointments, and solutions; however, "compounding" is nearly a lost art and a small part of the pharmacist's practice. Today the pharmacist still compounds and dispenses drugs but increasingly spends time doing the following:

- gathering information and inquiring about the medical, medication, and allergy histories of patients
- counseling on possible side effects and adverse reactions
- checking computer screens to monitor for drug interactions with other prescription drugs, over-the-counter (OTC) drugs, and diet supplements
- screening patients for minor illnesses that can be self-medicated
- providing information and making recommendations about OTC medications, as well as vitamins, minerals, and herbs
- providing drug information to physicians, physician assistants, nurse practitioners, and nurses
- providing advice about home healthcare supplies (e.g., home test kits, insulin needles, support hose) and medical equipment (e.g., home monitors to check blood sugar, wheelchairs, crutches, walkers, canes)

The specific responsibilities of the pharmacist will vary somewhat depending on the work environment; however, considerable overlap exists. For example, the community pharmacist may now be responsible for preparing intravenous (IV) medications for the home healthcare patient or sending medications to a nursing home. On the other hand, a hospital pharmacist may be involved in dispensing and counseling patients upon their discharge from the hospital.

The community pharmacist now has a broader scope of practice that includes not only drugs for existing disease but also patient care initiatives to prevent or identify disease. Because of their accessibility, many pharmacists are now trained to administer immunizations such as influenza (i.e., "flu") and pneumonia shots to the high-risk older adult population. Other pharmacists are active in screening for and educating their patients about high blood pressure, diabetes, cholesterol, or osteoporosis before damage to the body is done. Pharmacists also can be trained to assist and support motivated patients to quit smoking. Other educational trends for the pharmacist include assisting patients to take better care of themselves with healthier life-style choices and advising them about the selection of vitamins, minerals, herbs, and diet supplements.

The community pharmacist, whether an owner of the store or employed by one of the large pharmacy chains, still commonly functions as a small businessperson. Pharmacists in the community setting hire and supervise employees, evaluate insurance contracts, reconcile unpaid claims, maintain and order sufficient inventory, sell merchandise not directly related to health, and otherwise manage the retail operation. The successful pharmacist of today must be an entrepreneur, a clinician, and a good communicator.

In the hospital, in addition to dispensing oral medications (often individually labeled or "unit dose"), the pharmacist prepares and dispenses parenteral medications including IV solutions mixed with medications. (For more information on IV infusions, see the chapters in Unit 3, *Institutional Pharmacy*.) In larger university hospitals, more specialization exists among advanced-trained pharmacists (i.e., pediatrics, neonatal, internal medicine, critical care, cancer, transplant, nutrition, surgery), who often accompany physicians on their morning rounds, advise them on appropriate medication use, and monitor patients for adverse effects or drug interactions. These pharmacists are often responsible for educating and counseling patients about their drugs and diseases when they are discharged from the hospital. Other typical tasks for the hospital pharmacist include drug information, developing policies and procedures, purchasing drugs and medical supplies, monitoring narcotic and antibiotic use, and providing medications to each unit of the hospital, including emergency or "crash" carts. Many hospitals provide sufficient staffing to cover these services 7 days per week, 24 hours per day (similar to nursing provisions).

Treating patients at home is generally less costly than "round-the-clock" care in the hospital. The pharmacist who works in a **home healthcare pharmacy** may prepare medications and IVs for home use for patients of all ages including IV nutrition and antibiotics, as well as chemotherapy and pain medications for cancer patients. These medications are delivered to the patient's home by a pharmacist or nurse who is responsible for educating the patient or caregiver on the appropriate and safe use of medications and equipment, as well as monitoring the patient's response to the prescribed drug therapies.

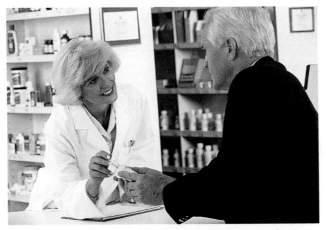

The pharmacist plays an important role in dispensing medications, as well as instructing patients about side effects of medications, food and drug interactions, and dosing schedules.

Pharmacists practice in many other health settings such as clinics and managed-care organizations that are also called **health maintenance organizations (HMOs)**, nuclear pharmacies, and long-term care facilities. In clinics and HMOs the pharmacist may be more involved in monitoring the response of drugs to better control chronic diseases such as high blood pressure, diabetes, asthma, high cholesterol, and patients with clotting disorders. Other pharmacists serve as specialists in psychiatry and drug abuse. In nursing homes the pharmacist specializing in "geriatrics" is responsible for both dispensing medication and conducting monthly drug chart reviews.

Nuclear pharmacy is another example for a potential area of specialization for pharmacists. A **nuclear pharmacist** is a board-certified and recognized specialty. The nuclear pharmacist is involved with procuring, storing, compounding, dispensing, and providing information about radioactive pharmaceuticals, which are used for diagnostic and therapeutic purposes.

Regardless of practice setting, the pharmacist typically dispenses medications and monitors their response, in part to prevent costly hospitalization from preventable adverse reactions and interactions. In addition, the pharmacist serves as a reliable source of drug information for the healthcare professional.

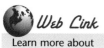

Web Link

Learn more about nuclear pharmacy at the Cardinal Health Web site at **nps.cardinal.com**

Education and Licensing Requirements

One indication of the professional status of pharmacy is the stringent licensing and educational requirements placed on practitioners. Over the past 50 years the curriculum in pharmacy has expanded from 4 to 6 years because of the complexity of new drugs and expanded roles for the pharmacist. With billions of prescriptions filled each year and more expected with our aging population, a number of new pharmacy schools have opened in the past decade to address expected pharmacist shortages.

All colleges of pharmacy now offer the Doctor of Pharmacy (PharmD) degree, which is usually a 6-year program. Most colleges of pharmacy require 2 years of prepharmacy education, including calculus, chemistry, physics, and biology. Many colleges require applicants to take the Pharmacy College Admission Test (PCAT), and some require an on-site interview. Acceptance into a pharmacy school has become extremely competitive in recent years. The typical successful applicant has a prior degree, grade point average (GPA) of 3.5/4.0, experience in pharmacy and community service projects, and excellent communication skills and self-motivation. Many pharmacy students started out working as a pharmacy technician in a community or hospital pharmacy and gained valuable experience that helped shaped their career goals.

Web Link

For a listing of accredited schools of pharmacy, visit the Web site for the American Association of Colleges of Pharmacy (AACP) at **www.aacp.org**

Once accepted, pharmacy students find that the coursework is extremely challenging. Basic science courses include anatomy and physiology, pathology of disease, biochemistry, pharmaceutics, pharmacology, and therapeutics. Practice or internship time in community and hospital pharmacies is interspersed throughout the curriculum. The last year in the PharmD program is spent in various practice settings such as hospitals, clinics, community pharmacies, home healthcare, or nursing homes to better prepare the student to practice all functions of pharmacy. Some schools of pharmacy have master's and doctoral programs in pharmacy that prepare pharmacists for a teaching or research career. Some pharmacy students pursue specialty residencies and fellowships after graduation.

In the United States, all states require pharmacists to be licensed. Obtaining a license involves graduating from an accredited college of pharmacy, passing a state board certification examination, and serving an internship under a licensed pharmacist either during or after formal schooling. In addition, in most states, pharmacists must meet continuing education requirements to renew their licenses. Most states have reciprocal agreements recognizing licenses granted to pharmacists in other states. Licensing and professional oversight are carried out by pharmacy boards in each state.

PHARMACY TECHNICIAN

The modern-day role of the pharmacist would not be possible without the assistance of trained and well-educated pharmacy technicians. A **pharmacy technician**, also called the *pharmacy tech*, is an individual working in a pharmacy who, under the supervision of a licensed pharmacist, assists in pharmacy activities that do not require the professional judgment of a pharmacist. The number of prescriptions filled increases more each year as our population ages and lives longer. The pharmacy technician can assume routine functions that allow the pharmacist to spend more time reviewing the computerized profile, counseling the patient, or communicating with the physician. Regardless of practice setting, the pharmacy tech can assist with workload by entering patient and prescription information into the computer, preparing a label, and retrieving and counting the medication. The pharmacist provides the final check on the original prescription with the medication bottle and label before counseling the patient.

Evolution of the Pharmacy Technician's Role

With the growth, interest, and expansion of the pharmacist role, there has been an increasing need in the workforce for educated, well-trained pharmacy technicians. Without pharmacy technicians, pharmacists do not have sufficient time to counsel patients, review medication profiles, monitor for side effects and adverse reactions, screen patients for disease, and discuss cost-effective drug therapy options with the prescriber. Without pharmacy techs, the risk of preventable and costly medication errors may increase.

Safety Note

Pharmacy technicians play a valuable role in reducing the risk of medication errors.

The role of the pharmacy technician has evolved over the past three decades. Originally, many pharmacy techs were trained as medics in the military and returned after service to our country to take positions in hospitals where they could better use their training and experience. In community pharmacy the role of the pharmacy tech has slowly evolved from that of a part-time clerk or cashier to more of a pharmacist's assistant.

A pharmacy technician assists the pharmacist with routine functions but leaves professional decision making and judgment calls to the pharmacist. Technician activities may range from ordering, stocking, and inventorying drugs to preparing the IV order to assisting in the dispensing process (e.g., gathering and entering patient and prescription information in the computer, retrieving the medication, dispensing and preparing a label for the medication). Although the technician carries out many of the duties traditionally performed by pharmacists, the pharmacist must always check his or her work. In addition to providing the final check on the medication order, the pharmacist is also responsible for patient counseling or giving specific advice to the patient on prescription or nonprescription medications. The technician functions in strict accordance with standard written procedures and guidelines, especially in the hospital setting with multiple employees.

A central defining feature of the technician's job is accountability to the pharmacist for the quality and accuracy of his or her work. Medication errors such as selecting the wrong drug or dose form can cause serious and sometimes life-threatening reactions if not detected. As a paraprofessional (i.e., skilled assistant to a professional person), the pharmacy technician bears a relationship to the pharmacist similar to that of an x-ray technician to a radiologist or a medical technologist to a pathologist. The pharmacist, in turn, takes final responsibility (and liability) for the technician's actions. It is important to note that the essential differences in the duties of a pharmacist and a technician involve accountability and making decisions about the patient's healthcare.

Education and Licensing Requirements

Most state boards of pharmacy now recognize the existence and importance of the pharmacy technician. Each state board of pharmacy regulates the activities and even the ratio of pharmacy techs to pharmacists within the pharmacies in each state.

In the past, on-the-job training was sufficient for the tech working in a pharmacy. To better assist the pharmacist in providing patient care, formal technician training programs have been developed in order to better train pharmacy technicians for their expanded roles in the pharmacy. Initially these programs were centered in the hospitals to better train their staff in the necessary functions of the hospital pharmacy. Today, some programs remain hospital based, but many more are being developed in community colleges and technical schools to meet the increasing personnel needs, especially in the community pharmacy setting.

The American Society of Health-System Pharmacists has developed a model curriculum as a guide to meet the needs of technicians in all practice settings. Academic-based programs vary in curriculum and length. In some states pharmacy technicians must be certified to practice. (See more on certification in Chapter 14, *Your Future in Pharmacy Practice*.) These academic programs help to prepare the student to pass the certification exam and start a challenging career as a certified pharmacy technician.

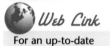

Work Environments and Conditions

Pharmacy technicians are employed in most of the same settings as pharmacists, including community pharmacies (i.e., drugstores), hospital pharmacies, home healthcare, and long-term care facilities (these will be discussed in more detail later in this chapter). Pharmacy technicians, like pharmacists, usually work in clean, well-lighted, and well-ventilated environments. To ensure a sterile environment and minimize infectious disease, many techs in the hospital and other practice settings work either in a "clean room" or under specialized ventilation cabinets called *laminar flow hoods* when they prepare infusions, total parenteral nutrition, or cancer chemotherapy. Gowns, masks, hairnets, foot booties, and gloves are often needed in this environment. In a specialized area of practice such as nuclear pharmacy, the pharmacy technician requires additional training.

For the most part, their work requires standing, often for long hours. Because people's health needs know no clock, both pharmacists and pharmacy technicians may be on call or work days, nights, weekends, and holidays. At any time, 24 hours a day, some number of the estimated 250,000 pharmacy technicians currently employed are on the job.

Characteristics of the Pharmacy Technician

A successful pharmacy technician must possess a wide range of skills, knowledge, and aptitudes. He or she must have a broad knowledge of pharmacy practice and a dedication to providing a critical healthcare service to customers and patients. In addition, the pharmacy technician must have high ethical standards, eagerness to learn, a sense of responsibility toward patients and toward the healthcare professionals with whom he or she interacts, willingness to follow instructions, an eye for detail, manual dexterity, facility in basic mathematics, excellent communication skills, good research skills, and the ability to perform accurately and calmly in hectic or stressful situations. The ability to "multi-task," or work on several projects at the same time, is a skill that will be useful in every pharmacy environment.

PHARMACY WORKPLACE OF TODAY

Pharmacists work primarily in community and hospital pharmacies after graduating from pharmacy school. Some will go on to pursue further education and higher degrees, residencies, or fellowships; others will enter fields such as managed care, or work in mail-order pharmacies, home healthcare, long-term care, nuclear pharmacy, or academia, as well as in drug information, sales, marketing, or research positions. With the ongoing approval of life-saving drugs and an increase in the aging population in the United States, the need for both pharmacists and pharmacy technicians is expected to continue.

Community Pharmacies

Three fifths of all pharmacists in the United States work in a **community pharmacy**, also called a *retail pharmacy*. Most community pharmacies are divided into a back prescription area offering prescription merchandise and related items and a front area offering over-the-counter (OTC) drugs, toiletries, cosmetics, and greeting cards. Some of these pharmacies are independently owned small businesses, others are part of large retail chains, and still others are franchise operations. However, the recent trend is toward fewer and fewer independent pharmacies, especially in metropolitan areas, because it is difficult to compete with the large-scale operations of chain pharmacies. The successful independent pharmacist must be an entrepreneur, offering needed but as yet unmet services to his or her community.

A **chain pharmacy** may be national or regional, and this type of pharmacy is found in department stores (e.g., Wal-Mart, Target), grocery stores (e.g., Kroger, Publix), or typical corner drugstores (e.g., Walgreens, Eckerds, CVS, Rite-Aid). Most chain pharmacies are located to allow for large-volume dispensing with heavy use of both pharmacy techs and automation. Many of the administrative decisions in chains are made at the corporate level.

An **independent pharmacy** is a community pharmacy that is owned and usually operated by a group of pharmacists rather than a corporation as in the case of a chain pharmacy. A pharmacist owner of an independent pharmacy makes his or her own decisions regarding the practice of pharmacy, with more attention and time spent to keep customers. Most compounding of prescriptions is done in this type of pharmacy.

A **franchise pharmacy** combines characteristics of an independent business and a large retail chain. Franchise agreements vary, but typically they involve a large retail company, the franchiser, that grants exclusive use of the company name and rights to sell company products to an owner/operator of a drugstore, the franchisee. Most franchise pharmacies sell only medication and health-related products and services and are also known as *apothecaries*. An example of such a franchise operation is The Medicine Shoppe.

Pharmacy technicians employed in a community pharmacy typically do the following:
- aid the pharmacist in the filling, labeling, and recording of prescriptions

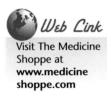

Web Link

Visit The Medicine Shoppe at **www.medicine shoppe.com**

- operate and are responsible for the pharmacy cash register
- stock and inventory prescription and over-the-counter (OTC) medications (those not needing a prescription)
- maintain computerized patient records
- prepare insurance claim forms
- order and maintain parts of the front-end stock

Somewhat related to retail pharmacy is the **mail-order pharmacy**, which is run by a centralized operation using both automation and pharmacy techs to dispense and mail large volumes of prescriptions every day. Each year more and more prescriptions are being filled by such mail-order pharmacies. Because of economies of scale, mail-order pharmacies can acquire drugs at lower cost and pass on savings to insurers and customers. Many health insurance companies encourage enrollees to use mail-order pharmacies to save money.

In spite of the cost savings of mail-order pharmacies, they have certain limitations. For example, most prescriptions for chronic disease must be filled with a three-month supply. If the patient experiences a side effect or adverse reaction, or the physician changes the medication, then the drug savings could be offset by drug wastage. The trade-off for lower cost is also more impersonal counseling, which is limited to a drug printout or calling a toll-free number. Concerns also exist about the time delay patients experience when waiting for needed mail-order medication(s) such as antibiotics, which typically should be taken immediately upon prescribing, as well as the safety of delivery of pain medications through the mail.

Institutional Pharmacies

Broadly defined, an **institutional pharmacy** is a pharmacy associated with any organized healthcare delivery system. Traditionally, a hospital pharmacy is the most common example. However, home healthcare, long-term care facilities, and managed-care organizations are more recent examples of places where institutional pharmacies can be found.

Hospital Pharmacy One fourth of all pharmacists work in a hospital setting. According to the American Hospital Association definition, a hospital is an institution that offers 24-hour healthcare service; that has six or more beds, a governing authority, and an organized medical staff; and that offers nursing and pharmacy services.

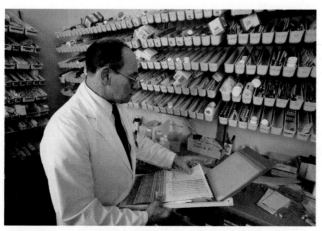

The pharmacy provides an important service to the hospital. Here, a pharmacist reviews a patient's medication administration record (MAR).

Similar to a community pharmacy, the **hospital pharmacy** carries out the functions of maintaining drug treatment records and ordering, stocking, compounding, repackaging, and dispensing medications and other supplies. The hospital pharmacist prepares, or supervises the preparation of, a unit dose system, which is a 24-hour supply of medication for a patient, as well as sterile IV medications. Typically this system makes use of a storage bin in a mobile medication cart that is delivered to the nursing station caring for the patient.

The pharmacy technician in a hospital setting may take part in these and other functions involving delivery, stocking, or inventorying of medications anywhere in the hospital. In addition, he or she may operate manual or computerized robotic dispensing machinery.

The staff of the typical hospital pharmacy may include administrators with master's degrees (e.g., Master of Business Administration [MBA] degrees) or PharmD degrees, staff pharmacists with Bachelor of Science (BS) degrees, staff and clinical pharmacists with PharmD degrees, and pharmacy technicians. Hospital pharmacies and drugstore chains are more likely than community pharmacies to require that pharmacy technicians be certified. Some pharmacy employers encourage technicians to become certified by paying for the certification exam and giving raises to those who pass it.

Home Healthcare Systems *Home healthcare* is defined as the delivery of medical, nursing, and pharmaceutical services and supplies to patients who remain at home. In recent years, spiraling hospitalization costs, regulatory changes, and advances in parenteral therapies (those involving the administration of nutrients and medications through subcutaneous [SQ, or SC] and IV injection) have created an explosion in this field. The home healthcare market continues to grow because of our aging society and as an alternative to the higher cost of hospitalizations. Many hospitalized patients are discharged as soon as possible to continue their recovery at home with IV solutions.

Pharmacists and pharmacy technicians working in home healthcare—through a hospital, community pharmacy chain, HMO, or private home healthcare provider— provide educational materials, carry out traditional compounding and delivery functions, prepare and provide infusions and infusion equipment, and often must be available for emergencies on a 24-hour basis.

Long-Term Care Facilities A **long-term care facility** such as an extended-care facility (ECF) provides institutional services predominantly to older adults or disabled "residents" who can no longer provide for routine or medical care for themselves, including adults who suffer from chronic (long-lasting) diseases or such debilitating illnesses as stroke or Alzheimer's disease. Both medical and residential care is provided with very few discharges. Skilled-care facilities (SCF) are limited to patients requiring more round-the-clock nursing care (such as IV infusions) or recovery after a recent hospitalization (most patients are discharged from SCF to home when they have adequately recovered). Other examples of long-term care facilities include patients with acute or chronic psychiatric disorders or rehabilitation facilities for those with serious traumatic brain or spinal cord injuries. Some long-term care facilities have an "in-house" pharmacy on their premises, whereas others either contract with a community pharmacy or allow each resident to choose his or her pharmacy.

Licensed pharmacists, who can be either employees of the facility or outside consultants, often provide the following services:

- establish record-keeping systems related to controlled substances
- review the drug regimens of residents, reporting irregularities related to drug treatments or controlled substances
- monitor the on-site repackaging and storage of pharmaceuticals

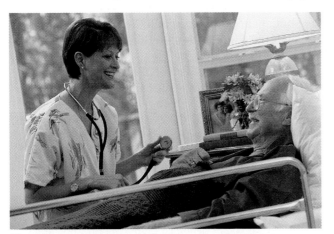

Pharmacists and pharmacy technicians will work with home healthcare workers who provide services to patients who remain at home.

- ensure that medications are uncontaminated and have not expired
- call attention to medication errors and possible adverse reactions or interactions
- educate residents and sometimes their family members regarding drug therapies and self-medication
- provide medications to outpatients or residents on weekend leave

In many of these areas the pharmacist may play a crucial role in ensuring regulatory compliance by the long-term care facility. For example, a licensed pharmacist must do a monthly check of each patient profile in a long-term care facility. The professional organization for "geriatric" pharmacists is the American Society of Consultant Pharmacists (ASCP).

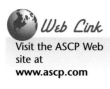

Web Link

Visit the ASCP Web site at **www.ascp.com**

Under supervision by the pharmacist, the pharmacy technician in a long-term care facility may do the following:
- log prescriptions and refill orders via computer
- prepare billings
- maintain drug boxes or trays for emergencies
- package and label medications
- deliver medications to the nursing home
- maintain records, retrieve patient charts, and organize them for the pharmacist's review
- conduct regularly scheduled inspections of drugs in inventory and in nursing stations to remove expired or recalled medications
- repackage drugs in unit doses labeled for each patient

In-house pharmacies may provide a 7-day supply of medication for the long-term care residents in "blister packs." Other community pharmacies that provide medications to nursing homes will generally fill medication carts or trays with a 30-day supply of medication, because medication orders rarely change in this environment.

Managed-Care Pharmacy Services **Managed care** is a relatively new form of healthcare that has grown dramatically over the past 35 years. One of the first managed-care organizations was Kaiser Permanente, a nonprofit private venture started in California in the 1930s. Another more familiar name for managed care is *health maintenance organization (HMO)*.

The philosophy guiding the care provided by an HMO is that by keeping patients of all ages healthy or their disease(s) controlled, the rate of cost of expensive hospitalizations and emergency room visits can be controlled. HMOs encourage their patients to take an active role in their own healthcare by eating right, exercising often, and avoiding negative life-style choices such as smoking and alcohol abuse. HMOs encourage patients to have annual checkups, to get all their immunizations on schedule, and to get necessary laboratory (like a cholesterol or sugar test) and diagnostic tests (like a pap smear or mammogram) to detect early diseases, which may be surgically correctible. Most HMOs have their own staff physicians who are on salary; if patients would like to see a specialist, they must first get a referral from their HMO physician. HMOs have been successful in slowing the pace of the inflationary increases in healthcare without compromising the quality of care. As a result, many employers now include an HMO option on their health plan.

Most HMOs are centralized primary-care clinics (i.e., they serve adult, pediatric, and obstetric-gynecology [ob-gyn] patients with pharmacy, x-ray, and laboratory departments under one roof). An HMO, like a hospital, usually has an approved drug list or **formulary** that has been recommended by a drug information pharmacist and approved by the medical staff. The formulary plus the use of low-cost generic drugs allows the organization to volume-purchase select drugs to lower operational and patient cost. Unlike a community pharmacy, an HMO pharmacy does not stock every brand of drug available. Many HMO pharmacies have a tiered pricing plan so that patients pay one price for a generic drug, a higher price for a "preferred" brand name drug, and an even higher price for a "nonpreferred" brand name product. Needless to say, most patients and physicians use the lower-cost alternatives whenever possible.

After the patient sees the physician, the patient may go to the HMO pharmacy to fill a prescription. As with many community pharmacies, patients with refills of prescription medication may call an automated telephone number to expedite processing and reduce waiting times. This "time savings" also allows the pharmacist to spend more time reviewing the computerized medication profile and counseling the patient. The pharmacy technician is readily used in such settings and performs functions similar to those in the community pharmacy, with the exception that insurance billing and cashiering are minimal. Many advanced-trained clinical pharmacists work closely with primary-care physicians to better control chronic disease by educating, monitoring, and, if necessary, adjusting the doses of medications per physician-approved protocols.

Chapter Terms

chain pharmacy a community pharmacy that consists of several similar pharmacies in the region (or nation) that are corporately owned

community pharmacy any independent or chain pharmacy that dispenses prescription medications to outpatients; also called a *retail pharmacy*

formulary a list of drugs that have been preapproved for use by a committee of health professionals; used in hospitals, in managed care, and by many insurance providers

franchise pharmacy a member of a small chain of professional community pharmacies that dispense and prepare medications but are independently owned; sometimes called an *apothecary*

health maintenance organizations (HMOs) organizations synonymous with managed care

home healthcare pharmacy a pharmacy that dispenses, prepares, and delivers drugs and medical supplies directly to the home of the patient

hospital pharmacy an institutional pharmacy that dispenses and prepares drugs and provides clinical services in a hospital setting

independent pharmacy a community pharmacy that is privately owned by the pharmacist

institutional pharmacy pharmacies that are organized under a corporate structure, following specific rules and regulations for accreditation

long-term care facility an institution that provides care for geriatric and disabled patients; includes extended-care facility (ECF) and skilled-care facility (SCF)

mail-order pharmacy a large-volume centralized pharmacy operation that uses automation to fill and mail prescriptions to the patient

managed care a type of health insurance system that emphasizes keeping the patient healthy or diseases controlled to reduce healthcare costs

nuclear pharmacist certified pharmacist specializing in procuring, storing, compounding, dispensing, and providing information about radioactive pharmaceuticals used for diagnostic and therapeutic purposes

nuclear pharmacy a pharmacy that prepares and distributes radioactive pharmaceuticals to treat and diagnose disease

pathophysiology the study of disease and illnesses affecting the normal function of the body

pharmaceutical care a philosophy of care that expanded the pharmacist's role to include appropriate medication use to achieve positive outcomes with prescribed drug therapy

pharmaceutics the study of the release characteristics of specific drug dose forms

pharmacist one who is licensed to prepare and dispense medications, counsel patients, and monitor outcomes pursuant to a prescription from a licensed health professional

pharmacognosy the study of medicinal functions of natural products of animal, plant, or mineral origins

pharmacokinetics the activity of a drug within the body over a period of time; includes absorption, distribution, metabolism, and elimination

pharmacology the science of drugs and their interactions with the systems of living animals

pharmacy technician an individual working in a pharmacy who, under the supervision of a licensed pharmacist, assists in activities not requiring the professional judgment of a pharmacist; also called the *pharmacy tech* or *tech*

Chapter Summary

- The profession of pharmacy has ancient roots, dating to the use of drugs for magical and curative purposes.
- Pharmacy has evolved over the past 50 years from preparing natural medications to dispensing synthetic medications.
- Today, pharmacists are highly educated professionals who are licensed to practice in a wide variety of practice settings.
- The pharmacist is responsible for dispensing the medication to patients, as well as the necessary information to appropriately use the products.
- The primary mission of pharmacy is to safeguard the public and help patients achieve favorable outcomes with their prescribed medication(s).
- Pharmacists in all settings provide a readily available resource to patients and healthcare professionals on information related to drug therapy.
- The pharmacy technician is a paraprofessional who, under the direct supervision of a pharmacist, carries out a wide range of duties in order for the pharmacist to effectively carry out his or her professional responsibilities.
- Because of our aging population and the subsequent need for prescription mediations required for many people to live longer and better lives, pharmacists and pharmacy technicians are in great demand.

Chapter Review

Choose the best answer from those provided.

1. A list of *approved* drugs is also known as a
   a. formulary.
   b. dispensatory.
   c. pharmacopoeia.
   d. All of the above

2. The profession of pharmacy exists today to
   a. distribute prescription drugs to the public.
   b. control narcotic drug use by the public.
   c. provide necessary OTC and herbal medications to the public.
   d. safeguard the health of the public.

3. Knowledge of the medicinal functions of natural products of animal, plant, or mineral origins is known as
   a. pharmacognosy.
   b. pharmacology.
   c. nuclear pharmacy.
   d. clinical pharmacy.

4. The emergence of the pharmaceutical industry threatened to reduce the role of the pharmacist to that of a
   a. compounder of medications.
   b. pharmaceutical scientist.
   c. drugstore operator.
   d. toxicologist.

5. The work that heralded the emergence of modern clinical pharmacy was the
   a. Ebers Report.
   b. Millis Commission Report.
   c. Report of the President's Commission on Controlled Substances.
   d. Kefauver-Harris Amendment to the Food, Drug, and Cosmetic (FDC) Act of 1938.

6. Another name for a community pharmacy is a
   a. retail pharmacy.
   b. long-term care facility.
   c. home healthcare pharmacy.
   d. health maintenance organization (HMO).

7. The primary role of a clinical pharmacist is to
   a. dispense medications.
   b. compound medications.
   c. develop a drug formulary.
   d. provide information about medications and monitor drug therapy to ensure optimal patient outcomes.

8. Licensing and professional oversight of pharmacists and pharmacies is carried out by the
   a. colleges of pharmacy.
   b. American Pharmacists Association.
   c. United States Pharmacopeial Convention (USP).
   d. state pharmacy boards.

9. A pharmacy technician can do all the following *except*
   a. counsel a patient.
   b. enter information into the computer.
   c. prepare a label.
   d. return drug stock to the shelf.

10. The final responsibility for the accuracy of the pharmacy technician's work is the
    a. pharmacy technician himself or herself.
    b. another pharmacy technician.
    c. supervising pharmacist.
    d. store manager.

Pharmacy in Practice

1. Go to the library and find a copy of the latest edition of the federal government's *Occupational Outlook Handbook.* Using information from this handbook, prepare a short report on the work conditions, duties, training, salaries, and job outlook for pharmacy technicians.

2. Call a local drugstore and hospital pharmacy and arrange to interview two practicing pharmacy technicians about their job duties. Compare your findings with the description you researched in Exercise 1. Prepare an oral report for your class.

3. Contact the program director of a pharmacy technician training program in another state. (Visit www.ashp.org and search for Technician Directory.) Request a copy of the program's curriculum. Based upon the information that you receive, contrast this curriculum with your current program.

Improving Communication Skills

1. Explain why you think it is important for patients to play an active role in their own healthcare. How can the pharmacist's role be adapted to meet this need?

2. The pharmacist has been at or near the top of many surveys that rank the public's trust. Pharmacists and those who work in a pharmacy strive to behave in a professional manner and communicate effectively with the patients they serve. Make a list of five things that you have noticed about the profession of pharmacy and/or a particular pharmacist that make you feel the trust is warranted.

3. Review the most recent National Association of Boards of Pharmacy (NABP) *Survey of Pharmacy Law* (www.nabp.net), and discuss the status of pharmacy technicians in your state. Where else might you find this information?

Internet Research

Exercises in this section focus on Web research and information retrieval. The information you access on the Internet needs to be thoughtfully reviewed and evaluated. As you complete the Internet questions in this and later chapters, use the following questions to help determine the reliability and validity of information:

- Who created this site, and who are the sponsors of the site? From whose perspective is the material written?
- Who is the intended audience of the site?
- What special knowledge do the site authors and contributors have?
- Is the material factual, or does it seem biased? Can the information be validated by a secondary source?
- When and how often is the Web site updated?
- Is this site easy to navigate? Can you find new information quickly and efficiently?
- Will you bookmark this site and use it regularly?

1. Visit one of the many on-line news services such as Microsoft Network (MSN), Cable News Network (CNN), American Broadcasting Company (ABC), Reuters, or medical on-line news services such as Medscape, WebMD, or Mayohealth. Search these sites and find at least three news items about a medical treatment or new drugs. Print and summarize the articles and present them to the class.

2. Visit a healthcare organization (e.g., American Heart Association, American Cancer Society, American Diabetes Association), and list five life-style changes that can prevent or minimize disease.

3. Visit http://bmj.com and enter 313 under "Volume" and 926 under "Page." Make a list of five ways the pharmacist and pharmacy technician can assist the older patient to be more compliant with his or her medications.

4. Visit www.ascp.com and review the guidelines on the various roles of pharmacy technicians in long-term care.

Pharmacy Law, Regulations, and Standards for Technicians

Chapter **2**

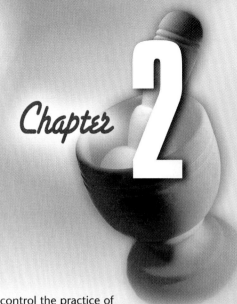

Learning Objectives

- Distinguish among common law, statutory law, regulatory or administrative law, ethics, and professional standards.
- Explain the potential for tort actions under the common law related to negligence and other forms of malpractice.
- List and describe the major effects on pharmacy of the major pieces of statutory federal drug law in the twentieth century.
- Discuss the role of the Food and Drug Administration, Drug Enforcement Administration, the United States Pharmacopeial Convention, and state boards of pharmacy.
- Enumerate the duties that may legally be performed by pharmacy technicians in most states.

A variety of mechanisms control the practice of pharmacy. These include common law—the system of precedents established by decisions in cases throughout legal history; statutory law—laws passed by legislative bodies at the federal, state, and local levels; regulatory law—the system of rules and regulations established by governmental bodies such as the **Food and Drug Administration (FDA)** and state boards of pharmacy; and professional standards—guidelines established by professional associations. The complex system of interrelated laws, regulations, and standards helps to ensure that drug therapies and merchandising are carried out safely and in the public interest.

NEED FOR DRUG CONTROL

Not until 1951, with the passage of the Durham-Humphrey Amendment to the Food, Drug, and Cosmetic (FDC) Act of 1938, was the distinction made under U.S. federal law between drugs that can and cannot be purchased without a prescription from a physician. In some countries, however, any drug can still be dispensed or sold without legal restriction. To persons working in pharmacy in the United States today, such laxity of control over drugs seems astonishing when one considers the possibility of inappropriate use, adverse reactions, and interactions with other drugs. The contemporary pharmacy is subject to many kinds of control at the federal, state, and local levels. Various groups and organizations, including the following, exercise controls on contemporary pharmacy:

- courts
- federal, state, and local legislative bodies such as the United States Congress, state legislatures, and municipal governing councils
- federal and state regulatory agencies
  - Food and Drug Administration (FDA), with general authority to regulate the manufacture and sale of drugs
  - Drug Enforcement Administration (DEA), with enforcement authority over controlled substances
  - Occupational Safety and Health Administration (OSHA), with authority over workplace safety

- Federal Trade Commission (FTC), with authority over business practices
- Health Care Financing Administration (HCFA) of the Department of Health and Human Services (DHHS) and Center for Medicare Services (CMS), with authority over reimbursement under the Medicare and Medicaid programs
- state health and welfare agencies
- state boards of pharmacy, with licensure and regulatory authority over pharmacy practice at the state level
- United States Pharmacopeia (USP), which publishes the compendia setting standards for drug formulation and dose forms
- professional organizations
  - American Pharmacists Association (APhA)
  - American Association of Colleges of Pharmacy (AACP)
  - National Association of Boards of Pharmacy (NABP)
  - Joint Commission on Accreditation of Healthcare Organizations (JCAHO)
  - American Society of Health-System Pharmacists (ASHP)
  - Academy of Managed Care Pharmacy (AMCP)
- individual institutions such as community pharmacies, hospitals, long-term care facilities, and home healthcare organizations

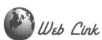

Web Link

APhA
www.aphanet.org
AACP
www.aacp.org
NABP
www.nabp.org
JCAHO
www.jcaho.org
ASHP
www.ashp.org
AMCP
www.amcp.org

The law offers a minimum level of acceptable standards, and ethics offer guidelines for personal conduct within a profession. State boards of pharmacy and professional organizations have established standards regarding many aspects for the provision of healthcare. Some organizations, such as the Joint Commission on Accreditation of Healthcare Organizations (JCAHO), offer additional levels of accreditation beyond what the minimum level of the law requires. Most hospitals and some outpatient facilities undergo a rigorous inspection process with JCAHO on a regular basis to maintain their current accredited status. Receiving JCAHO accreditation is the healthcare equivalent of getting the *Good Housekeeping* Seal of Approval. Although accreditation is voluntary under the law, many insurance carriers require it for reimbursement when providing services to members.

BRIEF HISTORY OF STATUTORY PHARMACY LAW

During the nineteenth century, drugs in the United States were unregulated. Medicines did not have to prove to be either safe or effective to be marketed. The highly addictive drug opium was popularized by the Chinese laborers working on the transcontinental railroad and was widely available and abused. In the West boisterous charlatans would take their traveling medicine shows from town to town to proclaim the latest "miracle cure." There were no regulations on labeling these so-called medicines and no research to support any of the claims. Most of these potions contained a high content of alcohol that usually made the customer "feel better." Occasionally, some of these potions were not so innocuous and caused injury or death to those who consumed them. To combat real-life abuses of this kind—abuses in both formulation and labeling—the United States Congress passed, in 1906, the first of a series of landmark twentieth-century laws to regulate the development, compounding, distribution, storage, and dispensing of drugs.

Pure Food and Drug Act of 1906

The purpose of the Pure Food and Drug Act of 1906 was to prohibit the interstate transportation or sale of adulterated and misbranded food and drugs. The act did not require that drugs be labeled, only that the labels not contain false information about the drugs' strength and purity. The act, although amended, proved unenforceable,

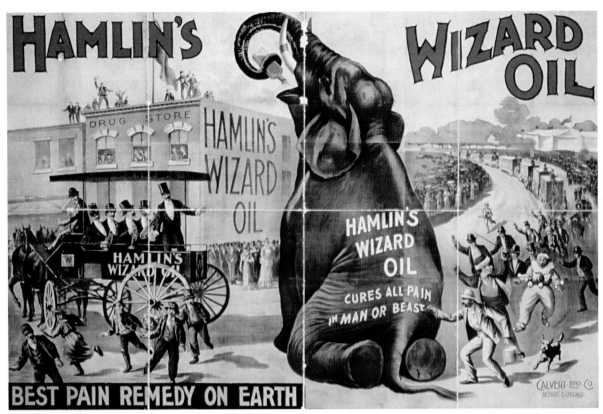

In the late 1800s there was no control on the sale of pharmaceutical products. Thus consumers were not protected.

and new legislation was required. In 1937 the need for new legislation was tragically demonstrated by 107 deaths resulting from the sale of a sulfa drug product that contained diethylene glycol, used today as antifreeze for automobile radiators.

Food, Drug, and Cosmetic Act of 1938

The Food, Drug, and Cosmetic (FDC) Act of 1938 is the most important piece of legislation in pharmaceutical history. It created the FDA and required pharmaceutical manufacturers to file a **new drug application (NDA)** with each new drug before marketing. Manufacturers must prove that the product is *safe for use* by humans. They must conduct and submit the results of toxicological studies on animals followed by clinical trials with human beings to determine degree of toxicity and the effect of the drug in humans respectively. The NDA must detail the chemical composition of the drug and the processes used to manufacture it. The FDC Act of 1938 also extended and clarified the definitions of adulterated and misbranded drugs. These definitions are provided in Table 2.1. This act also defined the relevant "official compendia" as the *United States Pharmacopeia* and the *National Formulary*.

Under this act, the FDA has the power not only to approve or deny new drug applications (NDAs) but also to conduct inspections of manufacturing plants to ensure compliance. The Supreme Court later held that the act applied to interstate transactions, as well as to intrastate transactions, including those within pharmacies. Unfortunately, the act required only that drugs be safe for human consumption, not that they be effective, or useful for the purpose for which they were sold.

Table 2.1 Definitions of Adulterated and Misbranded Drugs

Adulterated Drugs	• consisting "in whole or in part of any filthy, putrid, or decomposed substance," ones "prepared, packed, or held under unsanitary conditions"
	• prepared in containers "composed, in whole or in part, of any poisonous or deleterious substance"
	• containing unsafe color additives
	• purporting to be or represented as drugs recognized "in an official compendium" but differing in strength, quality, or purity from said drugs
Misbranded Drugs	• containing labeling that is "false or misleading in any particular"
	• in packaging that does not bear "a label containing (1) the name and place of business of the manufacturer, packer, or distributor and (2) an accurate statement of the quantity of the contents in terms of weight, measure, or numerical count"
	• not conspicuously and clearly labeled with the information required by the act
	• that are habit forming but do not carry the label "Warning—May Be Habit Forming"
	• that do not contain a label that "bears (1) the established name of the drug, if any, and (2) in case it contains two or more ingredients, the established name and quantity of each active ingredient, including the quantity, kind, and proportion of any alcohol, and also including, whether active or not, the established name and quantity" [of certain other substances listed in the act]
	• that do not contain labeling with "adequate directions for use" and "adequate warnings against use in those pathological conditions or by children where its use may be dangerous to health, or against unsafe dose or methods or duration of administration or application"
	• that are "dangerous to health when used in the dose or manner, or with the frequency or duration prescribed, recommended, or suggested in the labeling"

Durham-Humphrey Amendment of 1951

The Durham-Humphrey Amendment of 1951 states that drug containers do not have to include "adequate directions for use" as long as they bear the legend "Caution: Federal Law Prohibits Dispensing Without Prescription." The dispensing of the drug by a pharmacist with a label giving directions from the prescriber meets the law's requirements. The amendment thus established the distinction between so-called legend, or prescription, drugs and over-the-counter (OTC), or nonprescription, drugs. (These types of drugs will be explained in more detail in Chapter 3, *Drugs, Dose Forms, and Delivery Systems*.) It also authorized the taking of prescriptions verbally, rather than in writing, and the refilling of prescriptions. However, the refilling of prescriptions subject to abuse was limited. Under the amendment, prescriptions for such substances could not be refilled without the expressed consent of the prescriber.

Kefauver-Harris Amendment of 1962

The Kefauver-Harris Amendment of 1962 was passed in response to the birth of thousands of infants—mostly in Europe—with severe congenital abnormalities whose mothers had taken a new tranquilizer called *thalidomide*. It extended the FDC Act of 1938 to *require that drugs not only be safe for humans but also be effective.* The amendment requires drug manufacturers to file with the FDA an investigational new drug application (INDA) before initiating a clinical trial in humans. After extensive trials in which a product is proved both safe and effective, the manufacturer may then submit an NDA that seeks approval to market the product.

Comprehensive Drug Abuse Prevention and Control Act of 1970

The Comprehensive Drug Abuse Prevention and Control Act of 1970, commonly referred to as the *Controlled Substances Act (CSA)*, was created to combat and control drug abuse and to supersede previous federal drug abuse laws. The act classified drugs with potential for abuse as **controlled substances**, and ranked them into five categories, or schedules, ranging from those with great potential for abuse to those with little such potential. The agency made primarily responsible under this act is the **Drug Enforcement Administration (DEA)**, an arm of the Department of Justice. The DEA is charged with enforcement and prevention related to the abuse of controlled substances such as many narcotic pain medications.

A description of the five schedules of drugs is outlined in Table 2.2. Schedule II narcotics are most highly regulated, and sudden increases in usage in a particular pharmacy may cause the DEA to investigate. Often upon recommendation from the manufacturer and the FDA, the DEA classifies new drugs into a schedule and will even re-evaluate drugs that have been on the market for some time to determine whether they warrant being changed to a scheduled drug.

Poison Prevention Packaging Act of 1970

To prevent accidental childhood poisonings from prescription and nonprescription products, the Poison Prevention Packaging Act was passed in 1970. It is enforced by the Consumer Product Safety Commission and requires that most over-the-counter

Table 2.2   Drug Schedules Under the Controlled Substances Act of 1970

Schedule	Manufacturer's Label	Abuse Potential	Accepted Medical Use	Examples
Schedule I	C-I	highest potential for abuse	for research only; must have license to obtain; no accepted medical use in the United States	heroin, lysergic acid diethylamide (LSD)
Schedule II	C-II	high possibility of abuse, which can lead to severe psychological or physical dependence	dispensing severely restricted; cannot be prescribed by telephone except in an emergency; no refills on prescriptions	morphine, oxycodone, meperidine, hydromorphone, fentanyl, methylphenidate
Schedule III	C-III	less potential for abuse and addiction than C-II	prescriptions can be refilled up to five times within six months if authorized by physician	codeine with aspirin, codeine with acetaminophen, anabolic steroids
Schedule IV	C-IV	lower abuse potential than C-II and C-III; associated with limited physical or psychological dependence	same as for Schedule III	benzodiazepines, meprobamate, phenobarbital
Schedule V	C-V	lowest abuse potential	some sold without a prescription depending on state law; purchaser must be over 18 and is required to sign log and show driver's license	liquid codeine combination preparations

(OTC) and legend drugs be packaged in **child-resistant containers** that cannot be opened by 80% of children under 5 but can be opened by 90% of adults. The law provides that on request by the prescriber or by the patient or customer, the pharmacist may dispense a drug in a non–child-resistant container. The patient or customer, but not the prescriber, may make a blanket request that all drugs dispensed to him or her be in noncompliant containers. Many older patients and those with severe rheumatoid arthritis will request a non-child-resistant container. It is important to remind such patients to childproof their home when the grandchildren come to visit. Other exceptions provided for by the law are detailed in Table 2.3.

Drug Listing Act of 1972

The Drug Listing Act of 1972 gives the FDA the authority to compile a list of currently marketed drugs. Under the act, each new drug is assigned a unique and permanent product code, known as a *National Drug Code (NDC)*, consisting of 10 characters that identify the manufacturer or distributor, the drug formulation, and the size and type of its packaging. The FDA requests, but does not require, that the NDC appear on all drug labels, including labels of prescription containers. Using this code, the FDA is able to maintain a database of drugs by use, manufacturer, and active ingredients and of newly marketed, discontinued, and remarketed drugs. The bar coded information is also used to double-check the accuracy of prescriptions filled by automation. The NDC will be described more thoroughly in Chapter 3.

Table 2.3   Exceptions to the Requirement for Child-Resistant Containers Pursuant to the Poison Prevention Packaging Act of 1970

- single-time dispensing of product in noncompliant container as ordered by prescriber
- single-time or blanket dispensing of product in noncompliant container as requested by the patient or customer in a signed statement
- one noncompliant size of an OTC product for older adults or handicapped users, provided that the label carry the warning "This Package for Households without Young Children" or, if the label is too small, "Package Not Child Resistant"
- drugs dispensed to institutionalized patients, provided that these are to be administered by employees of the institution
- certain drugs and packaging exempt
- the following specific drugs:
  - betamethasone tablets with no more than 12.6 mg per package
  - erythromycin ethylsuccinate tablets in packages containing no more than 16 g
  - inhalation aerosols
  - mebendazole tablets with no more than 600 mg per package
  - methylprednisolone tablets with no more than 85 mg per package
  - oral contraceptives to be taken cyclically, in manufacturer's dispensing packages
  - pancrelipase preparations
  - potassium supplements in unit dose form, including unit dose vials of liquid potassium, effervescent tablets, and unit dose powdered potassium packets with no more than 830 mEq per unit dose
  - powdered anhydrous cholestyramine
  - powdered colestipol up to 5 g per packet
  - prednisone tablets with no more than 105 mg per package
  - sodium fluoride products with no more than 264 mg of sodium fluoride per package
  - sublingual and chewable isosorbide dinitrate in strengths of 10 mg or less
  - sublingual nitroglycerin (tablets to be taken by dissolving beneath the tongue)

Orphan Drug Act of 1983

An **orphan drug** is one that is intended for use in a few patients with a rare disease or condition. Developing and marketing such a drug would be prohibitively expensive. The Orphan Drug Act of 1983 encourages the development of orphan drugs by providing tax incentives and allowing manufacturers to be granted exclusive licenses to market such drugs. Over 250 orphan drugs have been approved by the FDA for marketing.

Drug Price Competition and Patent-Term Restoration Act of 1984

A given drug typically has several names, including its chemical name and its official **generic name** or nonproprietary name (e.g., ibuprofen), both of which are given in official compendia, and one or more brand or proprietary name (e.g., Advil, Motrin) given by manufacturers. A generic drug is one with the same chemical composition as a brand name drug that can be substituted (under regulations now existing in every state) for the **brand name** drug in prescriptions. Once the original patent expires, any manufacturer is allowed to market a generic drug, which usually is less costly than the brand name.

The Drug Price Competition and Patent-Term Restoration Act encouraged the creation of both generic drugs and innovative new drugs by streamlining the process for generic drug approval and by extending patent licenses as a function of the time required for the NDA approval process. The patent license was extended to allow the manufacturer of the brand name drug who completed the NDA to recoup research and development costs, as well as to provide an incentive to research new drugs for the marketplace.

Prescription Drug Marketing Act of 1987

Passed in response to concern over safety and competition issues raised by secondary markets for drugs, the Prescription Drug Marketing Act of 1987 prohibits the reimportation of a drug into the United States by anyone except the manufacturer. This has become a major political and economic issue as many seniors travel across the border or receive their prescriptions through the mail at presumed substantial savings. Pharmaceutical manufacturers have threatened to reduce the supply of drugs to Canada if illegal reimportation continues. Canada is concerned that reimportation may create a shortage of medications for its own citizens. The United States has elected not to enforce the private contraband of individuals but clearly discourages its practice and hopes that the new Medicare Modernization Act of 2003 will minimize reimportation.

The act also prohibits the sale or trading of drug samples, the distribution of samples to persons other than those licensed to prescribe them, and the distribution of samples except by mail or by common carrier. This action was taken in response to prescription drug samples being illegally diverted and distributed.

Omnibus Budget Reconciliation Act of 1990

The Omnibus Budget Reconciliation Act of 1990 (OBRA-90) requires that, as a condition of participating in the Medicaid program, states must establish standards of practice for drug use review (DUR) by the pharmacist. Among other provisions, the act requires "a review of drug therapy before each prescription is filled or delivered to an individual . . . typically at the point of sale . . . The review shall include screening for potential drug therapy problems due to therapeutic duplication, drug-disease contraindications, drug-drug interactions (including serious interactions with nonprescription over-the-counter drugs), incorrect drug dosage or duration of treatment, drug-allergy interactions, and clinical abuse/misuse."

Under the law a pharmacist must make an offer to counsel the patient or customer, but this person may refuse such counseling. The pharmacy technician usually has the patient sign a book or registry, which documents that the offer to counsel was made and refused. Otherwise, the pharmacist must offer to discuss with the patient all matters of significance, including the following:

- name and description of medication
- dose form
- dose
- route of administration
- duration of drug therapy
- action to take after a missed dose
- common severe side effects or adverse effects
- interactions and therapeutic contraindications, ways to prevent the same, and actions to be taken if they occur
- methods for self-monitoring of the drug therapy
- prescription refill information
- proper storage of the drug
- special directions and precautions for preparation, administration, and use by the patient

OBRA-90 uses the possibility of loss of Medicaid participation to enforce the clinical practices of screening prescriptions and counseling patients and caregivers. It also requires state boards of pharmacy or other state regulatory agencies to provide for the creation of DUR boards for prospective and retrospective review of drug therapies and educational programs for training physicians and pharmacists with regard to the use of medications. The law also requires that manufacturers rebate to state Medicaid programs the difference between the manufacturer's best price for a drug (typically the wholesale price) and the average billed price. Although initially required for patients eligible for Medicaid benefits, most state boards of pharmacy have required such counseling for all patients. Unfortunately, no additional reimbursement is provided for mandatory counseling, and dispensing fees have not kept pace with inflationary increases in healthcare.

Dietary Supplement Health and Education Act of 1994

One area in which the FDA is permitted limited oversight is in the diet supplement market, which includes vitamins, minerals, herbs, and nutritional supplements. The Dietary Supplement Health and Education Act (better known as *DSHEA*) was passed in 1994 and provided definitions and guidelines on diet supplements. Manufacturers are not required by this law to prove safety, efficacy, or standardization to the FDA as they are with prescription and nonprescription drugs. Because diet supplements are sold with nonprescription products, many consumers are unaware of the subtle difference in diet supplements.

Safety Note

The FDA does not regulate diet supplements.

The FDA may only review "false claims" advertisements and monitor safety. Manufacturers of these dietary supplements are not permitted to make claims of curing or treating ailments; they may only state that the products are supplements to support health. If health claims are made, the FDA can then require manufacturers to provide the research and proof to back up those claims similar to prescription and nonprescription drugs.

If the FDA wants to remove a dietary supplement from the market, it may do so; however, it must then hold public hearings, and the burden of proof is shifted to the FDA to prove that the dietary supplement is unsafe. For example, the drug ephedra, or its herbal equivalent ma huang, contained in many weight-loss products was removed from the market in 2004 by the FDA as a result of multiple reports of serious adverse reactions and some deaths; however, the courts overruled the FDA's action in 2005, allowing ephedra products to return to the market.

Health Insurance Portability and Accountability Act of 1996

The Health Insurance Portability and Accountability Act (HIPAA) of 1996 had many provisions that have affected all healthcare facilities, including pharmacies. One provision was the "portability" of moving health insurance from one employer to another without denial or restrictions. In the past, an employer could refuse to provide a new employee with health insurance or restrict coverage. For example, if the employee had a pre-existing medical condition similar to diabetes, then the employer could exclude any expenses related to that condition for 6 months or a year or more. In addition, if an employee leaves his or her current employment, then the former employer must offer COBRA (Consolidated Omnibus Budget Reconciliation Act of 1985) benefits. These benefits allow the employee to continue current medical coverage for up to 18 months but at his or her own expense.

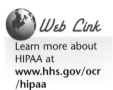

Web Link

Learn more about HIPAA at www.hhs.gov/ocr /hipaa

HIPAA mostly affects the confidentiality of patient medical records. With more and more electronic submission of personal data to health professionals, insurance companies, and pharmaceutical manufacturers, HIPAA has placed safeguards to protect patient confidentiality. All healthcare facilities must provide information to the patient on how they protect the patient's health information. In pharmacy, this may include any transmission of prescription data to anyone other than the patient and the healthcare professional, or it may include an area designed for private counseling. Every pharmacy must have a training program in place for its employees with annual renewals. For pharmacy technicians, this means they must, under penalty of law, not reveal any information on any patient outside the pharmacy. Violations would also be grounds for immediate termination. The ramifications of HIPAA are covered in more detail in Chapter 13, *Human Relations and Communications.*

Food and Drug Administration Modernization Act

The Food and Drug Administration Modernization Act was passed to update the labeling on prescription medications. Products labeled "legend" changed to read "℞ only." As mentioned earlier, legend is the term used in the past to indicate whether a drug was available by prescription or over-the-counter (OTC). The new labeling requirements were implemented in 2004. The law

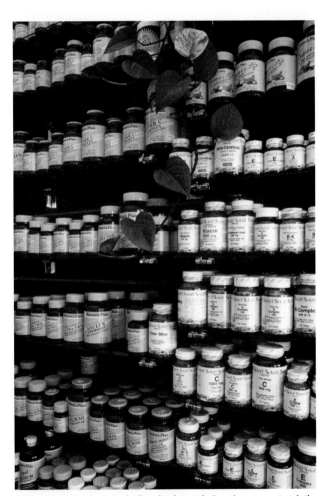

Dietary supplements including herbs and vitamins are not strictly regulated like prescription and OTC medications.

also authorizes fees to be added to a new drug application (NDA) process to accelerate the review and approval of new drugs.

Medicare Prescription Drug, Improvement, and Modernization Act of 2003

The Medicare Modernization Act (MMA), also called Medicare Part D, which became effective January 1, 2006, provides prescription drug coverage to patients eligible for Medicare benefits. This is a voluntary insurance program, not an automatic government benefit. This program provides some drug coverage, especially for those patients with economic hardships or those on high-cost medications. Patients are required to pay an extra premium (with their Medicare insurance) and are subject to a $250 deductible before benefits are realized. Patients may be penalized if they elect not to join when they are healthy and are taking no or few medications.

For patients on high-cost medications, a pharmacist may provide (and get reimbursed for) medication management therapy services (MMTS) or an annual in-depth review of the patient's medication profile. This review is to add a safety feature to prevent adverse reactions and drug interactions and to look at ways to reduce the patient cost. The details of this insurance program are further discussed in Chapter 7, *The Business of Community Pharmacy*.

A lesser-known provision of the MMA includes the development of health/savings accounts (HSAs). This act provides a health insurance option for patients under 65 years of age. Under an HSA the patient or his or her family agree to pay a monthly premium and carry a high deductible. In return the premium is fully tax deductible, and whatever amount is not used during that calendar year carries over to the next year. This is an example of a consumer-driven health insurance program that will become more popular in the near future. The individual decides (rather than the insurance representative) which physician to see, which prescriptions to fill, and which surgical procedures to accept from his or her premiums. If the person should have a serious illness with catastrophic healthcare costs, then insurance would be provided after the deductible is met.

REGULATORY LAW—ROLE OF NATIONAL OVERSIGHT AGENCIES

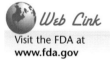
Web Link
Visit the FDA at
www.fda.gov

The acts and amendments provide the minimum level of acceptable standards. The FDA and DEA have used the acts and amendments passed in the twentieth century to address a broad scope of issues and provide a basic structure for the safe use of drug products and for the practice of pharmacy.

Food and Drug Administration

The FDA has the primary responsibility and authority to enforce the law and the ability to create and enforce regulations that will assist in providing the public with safe drug products. The FDA requires all manufacturers to file applications for investigation studies and approval of new drugs, provides guidelines for packaging and advertisement, and oversees the recall of products that are deemed dangerous. It has no legal authority over the practice of pharmacy in each state.

The FDA has regulations for manufacturers to follow while researching new chemical entities and developing those chemicals into drug products. Scientists conduct three phases of drug testing before the approval process. Occasionally when a medication appears to be very promising early on in the testing, the FDA may opt to "fast track" the drug and grant early approval. A recent example includes the quick approval of drugs to control the human immunodeficiency virus (HIV).

Once a drug is approved, the FDA oversight will continue. A manufacturer has very strict guidelines as to how the product may be packaged, labeled, advertised, and marketed to physicians (and now the public). A manufacturer may not make speculative or false claims about the potential of the product, and it must also disclose the side effects, adverse reactions, and contraindications. The FDA has been known to ask a manufacturer to cancel advertising campaigns and even to instruct the manufacturer to present a new advertising campaign to clear up any misconceptions. Even the OTC-marketed medications undergo this scrutiny from the FDA, and the label of OTC products must conform to a preferred format to make all of the information understandable to the layperson.

The FDA has the authority to obtain an injunction from the court and force the manufacturer to recall the drug product if it is contaminated, is of poor quality, or causes serious adverse reactions. Most companies voluntarily recall products when a problem occurs because it is in their best interest to do so, such as when Merck recalled the popular anti-inflammatory drug Vioxx after research studies that indicated it may cause a higher incidence of heart attacks. Three classes of recalls exist, and staff at the FDA determine which class recall is issued based on reports from the particular manufacturer and from healthcare providers. Table 2.4 describes the three types of recalls.

MedWatch MedWatch is a voluntary program that allows any healthcare professional to report a serious adverse event, product problem, or medication error that the professional suspects to be associated with the use of an FDA-regulated drug, biologic device, or dietary supplement. It serves as a clearinghouse to provide all information on safety alerts for drugs, biologics, diet supplements, and medical devices including drug recalls. It also provides information on all safety-labeling changes to the product package insert. These changes include contraindications, warnings, boxed warnings, precautions, and adverse reactions.

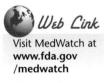

Web Link

Visit MedWatch at **www.fda.gov /medwatch**

If an adverse drug reaction is reported to a pharmaceutical company, then the company is required to file a report with the FDA. The FDA is increasingly interested in improving its postmarketing surveillance program to detect serious side effects not identified from research studies in the original NDA. The occurrence of some side effects may be so rare that it can only be detected in a large population after the drug comes to market. This report can be made on-line, via an 800 number (1-800-FDA-0178), or by mail on a downloaded form. (See Chapter 12, *Medication Safety*.)

Web Link

Visit the VAERS site at **vaers.hhs.gov**

Vaccine Adverse Event Reporting System A separate system called **Vaccine Adverse Event Reporting System (VAERS)** is a postmarketing surveillance system operated by the FDA and the Centers for Disease Control (CDC). The main purpose

Table 2.4 Recall Classes for Drugs

Class	Risk
Class I (C-I)	A reasonable probability exists that use of the product will cause or lead to serious adverse health events or death.
Class II (C-II)	The probability exists that use of the product will cause adverse health events that are temporary or medically reversible.
Class III (C-III)	The use of the product will probably not cause an adverse health event.

is to collect information on adverse events that occur after an immunization. This report can be made on-line, via an 800 number (1-800-822-7967), or by mail on a downloaded form.

Drug Enforcement Administration

The DEA is the primary agency responsible for enforcing the laws regarding both legal and illegal addictive substances. Although this agency directs most of its funds and personnel toward the illegal trafficking of drugs, it also has the responsibility to supervise the legal use of narcotics and other controlled substances.

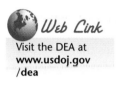

Web Link

Visit the DEA at **www.usdoj.gov /dea**

The DEA issues a license to medical practitioners that enables them to write prescriptions for scheduled drugs and to pharmacies to order scheduled drugs from wholesalers. Inspection of all medical facilities, including pharmacies, is a function of the DEA and is usually limited to facilities where suspicious activity has been detected. The DEA is able to track narcotics from manufacturer to warehouse to pharmacy, and it can determine which physicians prescribe scheduled drugs. Most pharmacies use a "perpetual inventory" (or tablet-by-tablet records) for complete accountability of narcotic drugs. Special forms and procedures must be completed and documented in all medical facilities for the disposal of expired narcotic drugs.

Registration with the Drug Enforcement Administration Through the Controlled Substances Act (CSA) every individual, institution, or business involved with manufacturing, distribution, dispensing, research, instructional activities, detoxification programs, importing, exporting, or compounding of controlled substances must be registered with the DEA. An individual pharmacy registers with the DEA, and a pharmacy employee in that pharmacy is not required to register. A separate registration is required for each pharmacy owned or operated by the same firm. A hospital will register with coverage for both inpatient and outpatient dispensing. Registrations will vary from 1 to 3 years in length. Most pharmacies are issued a 3-year registration.

It must be remembered that laws vary from state to state. Portions of some state laws are more stringent than the federal CSA. In these states if the state law is more stringent, it will be followed. If federal law is more stringent, then it will be followed.

Prescriber The CSA defines who may prescribe controlled substances. Practitioners are authorized to prescribe controlled substances by the jurisdiction in which they are licensed. Examples of practitioners include physicians, dentists, veterinarians, and podiatrists. The prescription must be written for a legitimate medical purpose in the course of professional practice activities. For example, a dentist may write a narcotic prescription for dental pain but not for back or cancer-related pain. Physician assistants cannot write Schedule II prescriptions, because they are not licensed with the DEA; in these cases the physician must write the prescription. Except in emergencies, the prescription must be written to minimize fraudulent use and maintain a record-tracking system if necessary.

Emergency Dispensing of Schedule II Drugs Occasions may arise in which the usual and customary procedures for filling and dispensing a Schedule II drug will result in the delay of an urgent medication needed for a patient. Pursuant to a valid medical reason, an emergency supply of a drug can be provided to a patient in most states. The prescriber may provide an oral or facsimile prescription. An emergency procedure is described as follows:

- A controlled substance administration is to be immediate if the patient is to receive proper treatment.

- The pharmacist will immediately convert an oral order into writing.
- If the pharmacist does not know the prescriber, then good faith efforts will be made by the pharmacy to verify that the prescriber is authentic.
- Within 7 days the prescriber must deliver a written version of the emergency oral order to the pharmacy that includes "authorization for emergency dispensing" written on its face.

Right to Refuse a Controlled-Substance Prescription A pharmacist has the right to refuse to fill a controlled-substance prescription. If a legitimate concern exists that a prescription was not written in good faith, then the pharmacist's duty is to determine the reason for issuing the prescription from the prescriber. If forgery is suspected, then the prescription should be retained for evidence, the "patient" detained, and the police notified. The pharmacist can detain the person presenting the prescription by saying, "This may take some time to fill. Can you come back in one hour?"

Safety Note

A pharmacist has the right to refuse to fill a prescription for a controlled substance.

DRUG AND PROFESSIONAL STANDARDS

The **United States Pharmacopeia (USP)** is an independent scientific organization that is responsible for setting official quality standards for all prescription drugs, OTC drugs, and dietary supplements sold in the United States. Although the USP develops standards for drug products, the **National Association of Boards of Pharmacy (NABP)**, in addition to state and national professional pharmacy organizations, helps set professional standards for pharmacists. NABP is an organization that meets regularly to establish general consensus among the member states and to develop and implement model regulations for those states.

United States Pharmacopeia

The mission of the USP is to promote the public health by developing and disseminating quality drug standards and information for medicines, healthcare delivery, and related products and practices. The USP develops authoritative, unbiased information on drug use and disseminates this information to healthcare professionals. The FDC Act of 1938 designated the USP to develop the official compendia for drugs marketed in the United States. The USP publishes the ***United States Pharmacopeia–National Formulary (USP–NF)***, a book that contains standards for medicines, dose forms, drug substances, excipients or inactive substances, medical devices, and dietary supplements. A manufactured drug product must conform to these standards to avoid possible charges of adulteration and misbranding.

USP Chapter 797 sets standards that involve the storage, packaging, and preparation of sterile compounded products when they deviate from manufacturer product package inserts. The Sterile Compounding Committee, which is a council of experts of the USP, developed these standards. They have been adopted by many accrediting agencies, including the state boards of pharmacy and the Joint Commission on Accreditation of Healthcare Organizations (JCAHO). Examples of standards that may affect the practice of pharmacy include the following:

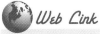 *Web Link*

For a summary of USP Chapter 797, visit **www.usp.org /healthcareInfo /pharmInfo/** and look at the proposed *USP–NF* chapters.

- specifications for "clean room" and filters to prepare sterile preparations
- recommendations for personnel cleansing and gowning
- expiration dates and storage conditions for IV nutrition, single and multidose vials, and ampules

- safety precautions and practices for handling hazardous drugs including radio-active pharmaceuticals that are compounded sterile products
- sterility and pyrogen or bacterial testing for all at-risk sterile products such as sterile compounded ophthalmic solutions

These guidelines will be discussed further in Unit 3, *Institutional Pharmacy*.

National Association of Boards of Pharmacy

The NABP is the only professional organization that represents all 50 of the state boards of pharmacy. The NABP meets several times each year to discuss national trends and issues of importance with regard to pharmacy law. For example, it provides guidance to the state boards of pharmacy on drug importation. In addition, NABP verifies the licensure of on-line pharmacies via its Internet VIPPS® program (Verified Internet Pharmacy Practice Sites), which assists the state board and consumer in identifying legitimate on-line pharmacies.

NABP has no regulatory authority like the FDA or DEA. It also helps to coordinate the issuing of an "NCPDP Provider ID" number that is administered by the National Council for Prescription Drug Programs (NCPDP). This provides over 70,000 pharmacies with a unique identifying number for interactions with the FDA, DEA, and many third-party processors of prescription claims.

Individual states have differing laws regarding the practice of pharmacy. Because many of the states developed laws pertaining to pharmacy over many years as acts and then amendments, the laws seem to have been put together in an unorganized fashion. A need for a common model developed, and the NABP developed the Model State Pharmacy Practice Act (MSPPA). Individual states can then model their practice acts on the MSPPA and individualize certain aspects of the regulation as needed within the given state. The MSPPA, along with various other recommendations is often used as the "backbone" for the state regulation that the state board of pharmacy puts into place.

STATE BOARDS OF PHARMACY AND LEGAL DUTIES OF PHARMACY PERSONNEL

State boards of pharmacy consist of leaders from the pharmacy community that are appointed by the governor. The activities of the board vary from state to state but generally oversee existing laws and regulations or make necessary amendments when appropriate to ensure that pharmacies and pharmacists are practicing according to the state practice guidelines. The board has the authority to suspend or revoke the license or registration of a pharmacist with evidence of violations of state or federal laws.

State boards of pharmacy provide regulations regarding refilling of prescriptions, both scheduled and nonscheduled drugs. Although most states have similar laws regarding prescription refills, each state must provide its own regulation because a national "law" does not exist. Typically, nonscheduled drug prescriptions are refillable for up to 1 year from the date written. Medications categorized as Schedule III, IV, and V drugs are refillable for up to 6 months from the date written. Although the law regarding refills on narcotics is covered by The Drug Abuse Control Amendments issued by the federal government, most states have a law that duplicates the federal law. For example, some states may not recognize "emergency prescriptions" of Schedule II narcotics or may require a written prescription for Schedule V–exempt narcotics like cough medicines.

7. Which of the following organizations has no legal authority over the practice of pharmacy?
   a. Drug Enforcement Agency (DEA)
   b. Food and Drug Administration (FDA)
   c. National Association of Boards of Pharmacy (NABP)
   d. state boards of pharmacy
   e. United States Congress

8. Who has the authority to remove a pharmacy license or registration?
   a. state boards of pharmacy
   b. Food and Drug Administration (FDA)
   c. federal court judge
   d. state court judge
   e. Drug Enforcement Agency (DEA)

9. If a patient sues a pharmacy, then who has the burden of proof in the case?
   a. pharmacy
   b. pharmacist and technician who filled the prescription
   c. patient
   d. state or local prosecutor
   e. judge overseeing the case

10. A pharmacist may be sued for _____ when he or she speaks falsely of a physician to a patient.
   a. libel
   b. slander
   c. battery
   d. negligence
   e. malpractice

Pharmacy in Practice

1. A pharmacy technician accidentally chooses the antidepressant drug Prozac instead of the prescribed medication, the antisecretory medication Prilosec, used for treatment of heartburn and gastroesophageal reflux disease. The pharmacist fails to check the medication, and the customer experiences no relief of the heartburn and a rare adverse reaction to the Prozac, rendering him temporarily impotent, a condition that causes the patient great psychological distress. The patient decides to sue the pharmacist and the pharmacy technician for negligence. To establish a valid case, what four claims must the patient prove, and to what degree must he prove them? Given the facts as stated, what arguments and/or evidence can the patient put forward to support each of these four claims?

2. In the case of *Baker vs. Arbor Drugs, Inc.,* which went to trial in 1996, the plaintiff, Baker, was taking the antidepressant drug tranylcypromine, under a prescription that he regularly filled at Arbor Drugs. The patient went to a physician with a cold, and the physician, despite having records indicating that

the patient was taking tranylcypromine, prescribed phenylpropanolamine. When Baker came to Arbor Drugs to have his prescription filled, the pharmacy's computer warned a pharmacy technician that a potential interaction existed between the new prescription and Baker's prescription for tranylcypromine that had been filled a few days earlier. The technician overrode the computer warning, and the pharmacist filled the prescription, unaware of the potential drug interaction. As a result of taking the phenylpropanolamine, Baker suffered a stroke. Baker brought suit, and on appeal received a judgment against the pharmacy. Discuss this case with other students. Consider the following questions, given the facts as stated:

    a. Were both the pharmacist and the pharmacy technician guilty of negligence? Consider all four criteria for negligence.

    b. In what ways did the physician, the pharmacy technician, and the pharmacist fail to carry out their duties properly?

    c. What requirement, under OBRA-90, did the pharmacist fail to meet? What relevance does this case have to the expanded clinical role of the pharmacist?

    d. Under what legal principle did Baker sue the pharmacy for the actions of its employees—the pharmacist and the technician?

    e. Under what legal principle could Baker not sue the manufacturer of the phenylpropanolamine product, given that the physician and the pharmacy had been warned of the dangerous drug interaction?

    f. What role do computers play, in contemporary pharmacy, in helping pharmacists and technicians to meet the counseling requirements of OBRA-90?

    g. Is this a case in which a court could conceivably make a finding of contributory negligence or comparative negligence? Explain.

    h. In what respect was the pharmacist guilty of nonfeasance, nonaction? In what respect was the pharmacy technician guilty of malfeasance, misconduct?

3. In the course of her normal duties, a pharmacy technician employed by Hometown Drugs, Inc., discovers from a patient profile that the young man who is dating her daughter is taking a regular prescription for a powerful antipsychotic drug. The technician keeps this information to herself but, in response to the information, attempts to dissuade her daughter from marrying the young man. Has the technician committed a breach of her ethical responsibilities? Explain in writing why you think this is or is not so.

4. Pharmacists with alcohol or substance abuse problems sometimes fail to seek help for fear that a state board of pharmacy might take some disciplinary action should the problem become known. What might professional associations and state boards do, in your opinion, to combat this problem?

5. New legislation or amendments are often passed in response to deficiencies in previous legislation. Give three examples from the text.

6. Under what conditions can a non-child-resistant lid be used on a prescription? What is an example of a drug that is dispensed without a child-resistant lid?

Improving Communication Skills

1. List three ways to protect patient confidentiality in the community pharmacy.

Internet Research

1. Visit www.fda.gov. Find the telephone number to report problems in your state. Research recent drug approvals. What are they, and for what disease conditions are they generally prescribed?

2. Go to www.fda.gov/medwatch and complete an adverse drug reaction form on an imaginary drug that you or a family member may have taken in the past. (Do not submit the form.) Find a recent Class I drug recall.

3. What are the legal requirements for dispensing insulin and insulin syringes in your state?

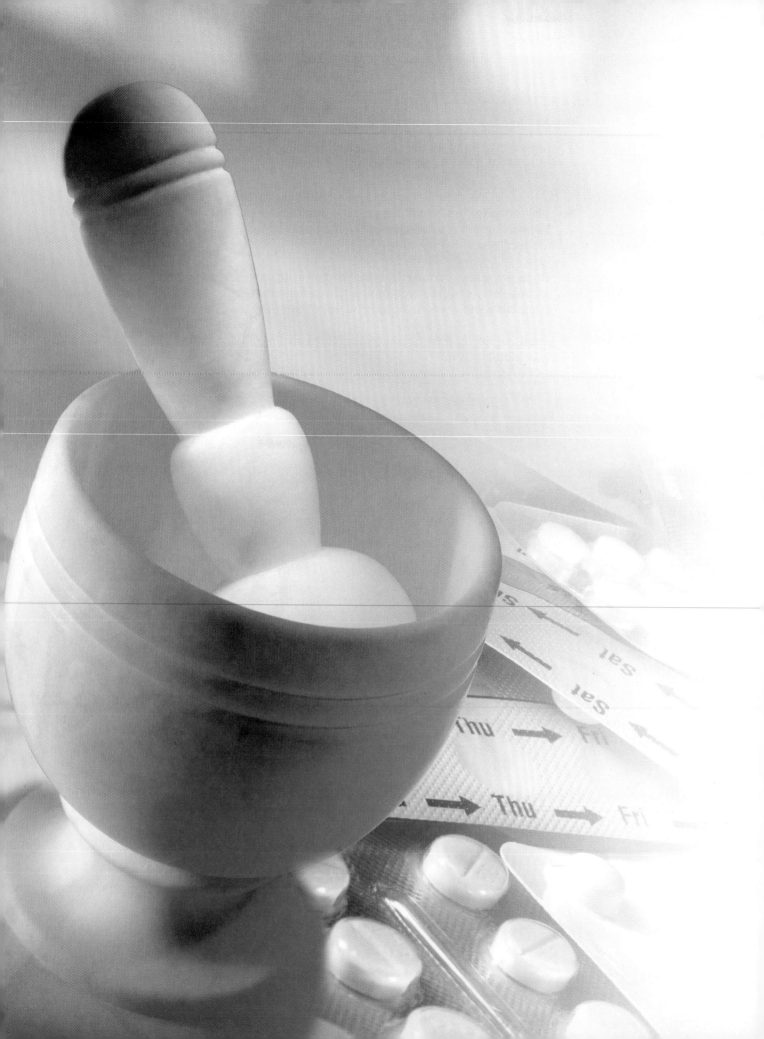

Drugs, Dose Forms, and Delivery Systems

Learning Objectives

- Define the term *drug* and distinguish between over-the-counter and legend drugs.
- Explain the parts of a National Drug Code number.
- Categorize drugs by source as natural, synthetic, synthesized, or semisynthetic.
- Explain the uses of drugs as therapeutic, pharmacodynamic, diagnostic, prophylactic, and destructive agents.
- Define and differentiate between the terms *dose form* and *delivery system.*
- Enumerate and explain the properties and identify advantages and disadvantages of the major dose forms and delivery systems for drugs.
- Identify the function of various commonly used pharmaceutical reference texts.

In the past five decades technological advances in the synthesis and delivery of pharmaceuticals have transformed everyday lives, providing improved antibiotics, vaccines, cancer chemotherapy, and medications to better control chronic diseases such as high blood pressure, high cholesterol, and diabetes. Modern pharmaceutical science has given us a vast array of medicines to be administered in an equally wide variety of forms. In this chapter, you learn the dose forms and delivery systems of the many pharmaceuticals scientists have created.

PHARMACEUTICALS

A **drug** is defined as any substance taken into or applied to the body for the purpose of altering the body's biochemical functions and thus its physiological processes. In years past, the pharmacist and the physician compounded drugs in a more crude state, often powders, extracts, and tinctures containing herbal remedies. Modern science has led to the development of highly researched and standardized medications that are more potent and toxic than the natural herbal remedies of the past.

Drugs are products designed with a specific use in mind and contain many other components besides the active ingredient. The **active ingredient** (or ingredients) is the biochemically reactive component (or components) of the drug. An active ingredient is rarely given in pure (i.e., undiluted, uncut) form. Instead, one or more active ingredients are combined with one or more **inert ingredients** or inactive ingredients that have little or no physiological effect. Most drugs contain one or more active ingredients commingled, dispersed, or in solution or suspension within an inert primary base, or vehicle, that may contain other ingredients, such as antimicrobial preservatives, colorings, and flavorings. These inactive ingredients are needed to stabilize the tablet or liquid formulation, provide the raw material for many topical creams and ointments, ensure sterility of injectable products, or assist in the masking of unpleasant tasting medications for pediatric patients.

Figure 3.1

NDC Number and Bar Code

For both of these labels for Vistaril, the first four digits of the NDC number (0069) indicate Pfizer Labs. The second four digits indicate the product code. The last two digits of the NDC numbers define the packaging size and type. (a) The product code (5420) identifies the drug as hydroxyzine pamoate, 50 mg. (b) The product code (5440) identifies the drug as hydroxyzine pamoate, 25 mg/5 mL.

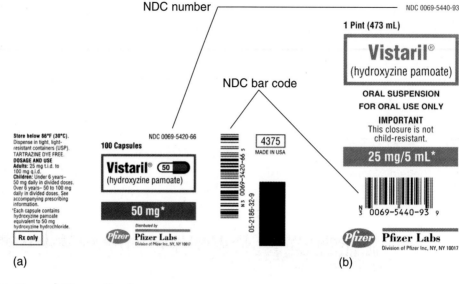

(a)　　　　　(b)

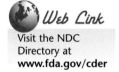

Web Link

Visit the NDC Directory at **www.fda.gov/cder**

National Drug Code

Under the Drug Listing Act of 1972, each medication must have a unique **National Drug Code (NDC) number** that appears on all drug labels, including labels of prescription containers. The 10-character NDC includes a four- or five- digit *labeler code*, identifying the manufacturer or distributor of the drug; a three- or four- digit *product code*, identifying the drug (active ingredient and its dose form); and a two-digit *package code*, identifying the packaging size and type. The NDC *bar code* number is commonly used by the Food and Drug Administration (FDA) for drug recalls and by pharmacies to compare medications dispensed in the filling process to minimize medication errors. Figure 3.1 shows NDC numbers and corresponding bar codes on labels for two different forms of hydroxyzine pamoate.

Classes of Drugs

Drugs are classified as **over-the-counter (OTC)** or *legend*. A legend drug can be dispensed only with a prescription from a healthcare professional licensed in that state to practice. Such drugs are labeled with the legend "Caution: Federal Law Prohibits Dispensing Without Prescription" or an equivalent symbol (Rx) (Figure 3.2). Therefore prescription drugs are also known as *legend drugs*. The new legend in the updated labeling law is "Rx only."

Drugs with potential for abuse are classified, under the Comprehensive Drug Abuse Prevention and Control Act of 1970, according to five drug schedules as presented in Chapter 2 (based on the potential for abuse and physical and psychological dependence). Schedule II drugs such as narcotics and amphetamines have a high potential for abuse and dependence, whereas Schedule V cough syrups have a low potential for abuse and limited potential for creating physical or psychological dependence.

Figure 3.2

Drug Caution Legends

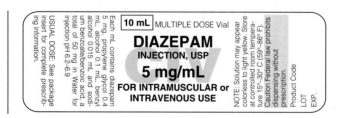

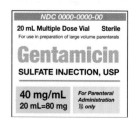

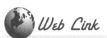

Web Link

To learn more about the Drug Facts label, visit the Consumer Healthcare Products Association Web site at **http://www .chpa-info.org** and select "For Consumer."

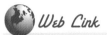

Web Link

To learn more about independent testing of diet supplements, visit **www .consumerlab.com**

Safety Note

Not all homeopathics are OTC.

An OTC drug is one that can be dispensed without a prescription. The FDA has approved many drugs that have come off patent and proven relatively safe over the years to be sold as OTC medications. Such examples include Advil (ibuprofen), Aleve (naproxen), Benadryl (diphenhydramine), Claritin (loratadine), and hydrocortisone. The label of an OTC drug must contain all the information necessary for a consumer to safely take the medication including indication, dose for various age groups, side effects, warnings, and expiration date.

Most pharmacies have an inventory of vitamins, minerals, herbs, and diet supplements. Diet supplements, especially herbs, should be considered weak drugs that can cause side effects, adverse reactions, and drug interactions. As discussed in Chapter 2, these medications do not have the same stringent controls as legend and OTC medications, and they are loosely regulated by the Dietary Supplement Health and Education Act (DSHEA) amendments of 1994. The quality of many of these products should be verified with an independent laboratory. Diet supplements are considered "food supplements" to maintain health, and a patient should not exceed the recommended daily dose without the knowledge of a physician or pharmacist. The pharmacy technician can assist the pharmacist by gathering information on the patient use of diet supplements and adding this data to the computer profile.

Another class of drugs is called **homeopathic medications**. The term *homeopathy* is derived from the Greek words *homos* (i.e., similar) and *pathos* (i.e., suffering or disease). Homeopathic practice uses subclinical doses of natural extracts or alcohol tinctures. In other words, the active ingredient is diluted from one part per ten (1:10) to more than one part per thousand (1:1000). The concept is that these small doses are sufficient to stimulate the body's own immune system to overcome the specifically targeted symptom. Most homeopathics are OTC, but some are prescription only. Homeopathy was popular in the United States in the early nineteenth century and remains popular in many areas of Europe today.

SOURCES OF DRUGS

Drugs come from various sources and can be classified as natural, synthetic (created artificially), synthesized (created artificially but in imitation of naturally occurring substances), and semisynthetic (containing both natural and synthetic components).

Drugs from Natural Sources

Some drugs are naturally occurring biological products, made or taken from single-celled organisms, plants, animals, and humans. Many herbal products come from natural sources. Examples of modern-day drugs from natural sources are listed:

- Penicillin was discovered in 1928 and is extracted from certain molds.
- Vitamin B_{12} and the antibiotic streptomycin are produced from cultures of the bacterium *Streptomyces griseus*.
- Opium, the narcotic, comes from the poppy plant and is a source for both legal drugs such as morphine and illegal drugs such as heroin.
- Quinine, used to treat malaria and colchicine, as well as acute gout, comes from the bark of the cinchona tree.
- Acetylsalicylic acid, more commonly known as *aspirin*, is derived from the bark of the white willow tree (which contains salicylic acid).
- Insulin, a life-saving drug for the treatment of diabetes mellitus, is extracted from the pancreas of various animals.
- Human growth hormone, or somatotropin, comes, as its name suggests, from human bodies (the anterior pituitary produces it).

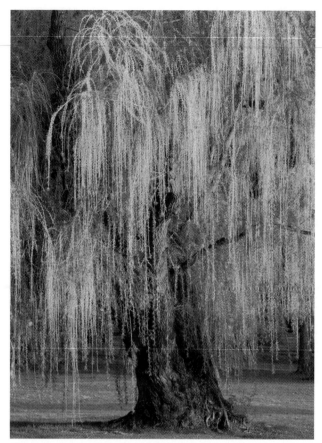

The bark of the willow tree, which contains salicylic acid, has been used for centuries to treat toothache.

- (Milk of) Magnesia is a combination of magnesium oxide or hydrated magnesium carbonate and is used as an antacid or laxative.

Synthetic, Synthesized, and Semisynthetic Drugs

In the modern era many naturally occurring chemicals have been synthesized. A **synthesized drug** is a drug created artificially in the laboratory but in imitation of naturally occurring drugs like adrenaline, which is used for heart and asthmatic attacks. A **synthetic drug** is one that is created artificially to exert a specific pharmacological effect. Barbiturates, sometimes prescribed as a sleep medication, are examples of synthetic drugs. A naturally occurring drug like a barbiturate does not exist. **Semisynthetic drugs** contain both natural and synthetic molecules. An example would be semisynthetic penicillins, which combine artificially created molecules with naturally occurring ones. These new penicillin derivatives are effective against different bacteria or bacteria that have developed resistance to the natural penicillins.

Biotechnology combines the science of biology, chemistry, and immunology to produce synthetic, unique drugs with specific therapeutic effects. These drugs can be created by means of the recombinant deoxyribonucleic acid (recombinant DNA) techniques of genetic engineering. **Deoxyribonucleic acid (DNA)** is the complex, helically shaped molecule that carries the genetic code (Figure 3.3). This molecule contains the instructions, or recipe, for creating messenger **ribonucleic acid (RNA)**, which in turn contains the recipe for arranging amino acids into proteins for living organisms. **Recombinant DNA** is DNA constructed of segments taken from different sources (e.g., from a human being and a sheep). By transferring a segment of recombined DNA into a host cell, scientists can change what proteins the cell produces. In effect, this converts the cell into a small-scale protein factory to produce chemical substances that can be used as drugs. For example, using the bacterium *Escherichia coli*, microbiologists and geneticists can induce the production of human insulin or human growth hormone. Human insulin has replaced animal-derived insulin; it is more active with fewer side effects.

Another biotechnological method of drug production is the use of cells from inoculated animals to produce, in the laboratory, hybrid cells that create substances known as **monoclonal antibodies (MAbs)**. **Antibodies** are created by the immune system in response to foreign substances in the body known as *antigens*. Laboratory-produced MAbs can be used to attack tumors and to diagnose a great variety of conditions, from pregnancy to anemia to syphilis. **Genetic engineering**, the hybridization techniques for creating MAbs, and other biotechnologies are already used to create a great variety of drugs, such as clotting factors for treating hemophiliacs and interferons for

Figure 3.3

Modeling DNA
(a) A single nucleotide. (b) A short section of a DNA molecule consisting of two rows of nucleotides connected by weak bonds between the bases adenine *(A)* and thymine *(T)*, guanine *(G)* and cytosine *(C)*. (c) Long strands of DNA twisted to form a double helix.

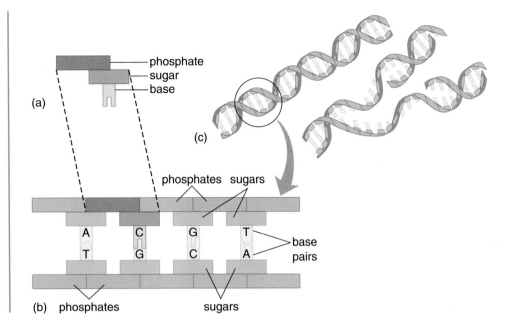

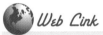

Web Link

Learn more about the Human Genome Project at **www.doe genomes.org**

combating viral infection and some cancers. Such technologies promise to bring many new drugs to the market.

Numerous drugs in various stages of research use technology involved with the mapping of the human genome. The Human Genome Project has been under way since the 1980s and is best described as the mapping of the biochemical instructions that make up the human body in health and disease. For example, a defective gene has been identified in many patients with breast cancer. As more of the genome is mapped and understood and more disease states are located, potential disease can be identified at an earlier date, and new treatments can be specifically designed to treat the identified biochemical errors located in the human genome.

USES OF DRUGS

Medications today are being used not just to treat and cure illnesses but also to aid in diagnosis and even prevent illnesses. Healthcare providers have numerous agents at their disposal and a wide variety of dose forms and drug delivery systems to customize treatment of a patient. It is essential to understand the inherent differences, as well as the advantages and disadvantages, of the different dose forms used today. The action of a medication cannot be taken into account without considering the dose form selected. The patient outcome may depend on selecting the most appropriate medication *and* dose form to meet the patient's needs.

Several classifications for uses of drugs exist, and most are not mutually exclusive. The following should assist the student in sorting out which classification best describes the various uses of drugs.

Therapeutic Agents

A **therapeutic agent** is any drug that helps to do the following:
- *Maintain Health*—Drugs with this purpose include vitamins and minerals to regulate metabolism and otherwise contribute to the maintenance of normal growth and functioning of the body. A specific example is the use of baby aspirin for patients identified as being at risk for heart attack.

- *Relieve Symptoms*—Drugs with this purpose include anti-inflammatory drugs like ibuprofen used to treat fever, pain, or inflammation; narcotics to treat and prevent severe pain in terminally ill patients with cancer; or a diuretic or water pill to control excess fluid.
- *Combat Illness*—Drugs with this purpose include antibiotics to cure pneumonia, strep throat, or a bladder infection. Although antiviral medications do not cure human immunodeficiency virus (HIV) or acquired immunodeficiency syndrome (AIDS), they may allow the immune system to remain intact so as to delay disease progression.
- *Reverse Disease Processes*—Drugs with this purpose include medications that control depression, blood pressure, cholesterol, or diabetes.

Pharmacodynamic Agents

A **pharmacodynamic agent** alters bodily functioning in a desired way. Drugs can be used, for example, to stimulate or relax muscles, to dilate or constrict pupils, or to increase or decrease blood sugar. Examples of pharmacodynamic agents include caffeine to forestall sleep, oral contraceptives that depress hormones to prevent pregnancy, expectorants to increase fluid in the respiratory tract, anesthetics to cause numbness or loss of consciousness, glucagon to increase blood sugar in diabetics, and digoxin to increase heart muscle contraction or slow heart conduction in patients with heart disease.

Diagnostic Agents

A **diagnostic agent** facilitates an examination (usually one conducted to arrive at a diagnosis) or conclusion as to the nature or extent of a disease condition. Chemicals containing radioactive isotopes, used diagnostically (and also therapeutically), are known as **radiopharmaceuticals**. Isotopes are forms of an element that contain the same number of protons but differing numbers of neutrons. Unstable, radioactive isotopes give off energy in the form of radiation, measured in rads. One rad is equal to 100 erg of energy absorbed by 1 g of body tissue. Nuclear medicine uses radioactive isotopes such as technetium (^{99m}Tc) and iodine (^{131}I) for imaging regional function and biochemistry in the body, as in positron emission tomography (PET) or single photon emission computed tomography (SPECT). Nuclear pharmacy involves the procuring, storage, compounding, dispensing, and provision of information about radiopharmaceuticals, and it is one possible area of specialization for both pharmacists and pharmacy technicians.

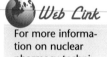

Web Link

For more information on nuclear pharmacy technician training programs, visit **www.aphanet.org**

Prophylactic Agents

A **prophylactic agent** prevents illness or disease from occurring. Examples of prophylactic agents include the antiseptic and germicidal liquid iodine used to prep skin preoperatively for the prevention of infection. Any vaccine is considered a prophylactic agent to prevent diseases such as influenza, pneumonia, measles, mumps, rubella, chicken pox, smallpox, poliomyelitis, and hepatitis.

Destructive Agents

A **destructive agent** has a *-cidal* action; that is, it kills bacteria, fungi, viruses, or even normal cells or abnormal cancer cells. Many antibiotics, especially given in high doses and **intravenous (IV) infusions**, are bactericidal (i.e., they kill [rather than just maim] the bacterium if it is sensitive to the drug). Another example of a destructive agent is radioactive iodine, which is used to destroy some of the thyroid gland in patients with hyperthyroidism.

Another common example of destructive agents are **antineoplastic drugs** used in cancer chemotherapy to destroy malignant tumors. Cancer is often caused by an unregulated growth of abnormal dysfunctional cells. Antineoplastics are used in combination to slow cancer cell growth. Unfortunately, most cancer drugs cannot distinguish cancer from normal cells, so side effects such as hair loss, further depression of the immune system, and ulcerations of the mouth or gastrointestinal (GI) tract commonly occur. These drugs require special storage, preparation, and monitoring (see Chapter 10, *Infection Control and Safe Handling of Hazardous Agents*). Research from drug studies and the development of unique drug delivery systems continue to improve our ability to dose and target cancer cells more specifically.

COMPARISON OF DOSE FORMS AND DELIVERY SYSTEMS

The term **dose form** refers to the physical manifestation of a drug as a solid, liquid, or gas that can be used in a particular way. Examples of common dose forms include tablets, capsules, creams, ointments, solutions, injections, and aerosols.

The term **delivery system** has several definitions in healthcare and may include any of the following:

- Device used to deliver the drug (e.g., teaspoon, syringe, nebulizer, IV fluid, infusion pump)
- Design feature of the dose form that affects the delivery of the drug, such as the coating on some capsules that resists breakdown by the gastric fluids in the stomach so that the capsule will release medication, instead, into the intestines
- Means for *transporting a drug to its site(s) of action within the body*

Delivery systems differ in their pharmacological properties; that is, their sites of action, rate of delivery, and quantities of active ingredient delivered differ. Consider, for example, the drug nitroglycerin, commonly used to treat angina pectoris (pain in the chest and left arm associated with a sudden decrease in blood supply to the heart). Nitroglycerin dilates blood vessels, thus increasing blood supply to the heart and decreasing blood pressure. Three common delivery systems for nitroglycerin are sublingual tablets, placed under the tongue; ointment measured and applied directly on the skin; and transdermal patches, worn on the skin. Sublingual nitroglycerin tablets are fast acting but deliver their active ingredient for only a short period of time, about 30 minutes. Transdermal patches, in contrast, act slowly, with a delivery onset of about 30 minutes, but they can deliver a steady amount of the drug for up to 24 hours. The ointment is much less costly than the patch; it has a similar onset but a shorter duration of effect (up to 12 hours).

The choice of delivery system depends on many factors, including the following:

- active ingredient to be delivered
- amount of active ingredient to be delivered
- means or route that ingredient is to be delivered
- to what sites
- at what rate
- over what period of time
- for what purpose

Currently drugs are administered in a wide variety of dose forms that are part of an even wider variety of delivery systems. Because of the variety and overlap of dose forms and delivery systems, it is impossible to create a rigid, mutually exclusive taxonomy, or classification. The following discussion reviews the characteristics of both dose forms and the delivery systems used.

SOLID DOSE FORMS

Solid dose forms are used more frequently than any other form and are safer for the patient to self-administer. Capsules and tablets are the two most common types and are very inexpensive to manufacture. A wide variety of capsule types and sizes exist. Other solid dose forms such as effervescent salts, implants, lozenges, plasters, powders, and suppositories are used less frequently but are still very important, because they enable the physician and pharmacist to meet the needs of an individual patient more adequately.

Tablets

Tablets are available in a wide variety of shapes, sizes, and surface markings. The **tablet** is a solid dose form produced by compression and contains one or more active ingredients and, commonly, other pharmacological ingredients. These ingredients include diluents, binders (to promote adhesion of the materials in the tablet), lubricating agents (to give the tablet a sheen and to aid in the manufacturing process), disintegrants (to help break up the ingredients), solubilizers (to maintain the ingredients in solution or to help the ingredients pass into solution in the body), colorings, and coatings. For obvious reasons, tablets also commonly contain flavorings. Coatings can be used to protect the stability of the ingredients in tablets; improve appearance, flavor, or ease of swallowing; or provide for controlled (sustained or delayed) release of medication.

Tablets are extremely convenient because of the ease with which various doses can be delivered. A patient can take one tablet, several tablets, or a portion of a tablet, as required. Some tablets are *scored* once or twice to facilitate breaking into portions for half or even quarter doses. Scoring of a tablet is designed to equally divide the dose in each section. If a tablet is not scored, then it is generally recommended that it should not be broken because the dose may not be equal in each piece. However, because of rising drug costs, it is not uncommon for patients, as well as managed-care organizations and Veterans Administration (VA) hospitals, to use a tablet splitter for unscored tablets to treat conditions such as high blood pressure and high cholesterol (providing up to 50% savings). Limited studies suggest that the practice does not appreciably affect the control of the disease state with select medications. Odd-shaped tablets are often difficult to cut, even with a tablet splitter.

Punch-and-die machines that compress the ingredients of each tablet in a single stroke create almost all tablets produced today. Compression tablets are the most inexpensive and common dose form used today. Some tablets are produced by multi-

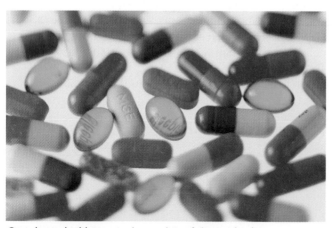

Capsules and tablets come in a variety of sizes and colors. Distinctive markings help patients identify the drugs.

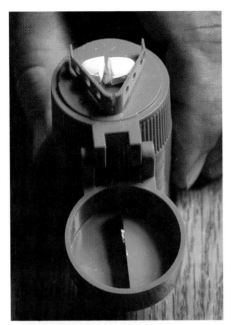

A tablet splitter can save money for the patient on high-cost medications.

Safety Note

Careful tablet splitting may be a way to reduce medication costs, but it is not recommended for all drugs. Patients must be warned not to take a full tablet if such action would result in an overdose of medication.

Safety Note

ECT tablets should not be split.

Figure 3.4

Multiple Compression Tablets (MCTs)
(a) Two layers or compressions. (b) Three layers or compressions.

(a)

(b)

ple compressions and are, in effect, either tablets on top of tablets or tablets within tablets. These are called *multiple compression tablets (MCTs)* (Figure 3.4). An MCT may contain a core and one or two outer shells (or two or three different layers), each containing a different medication and colored differently. MCTs are created for appearance alone, to combine incompatible substances into a single medication, or to provide for controlled release in successive events, or stages.

Some manufacturers have begun to manufacture an oblong tablet that is a hybrid of the capsule and tablet, called the *caplet*. The caplet is simply a tablet shaped like a capsule and sometimes coated to look like a capsule. The inside of the caplet is solid, whereas the inside of a capsule is often powder or granular material. The caplet offers the advantage of easier swallowing than a large tablet and more stability (and longer shelf life) than a capsule. Caplet formulations on the market include the OTC drug Tylenol and the antibiotic erythromycin.

Most tablets are uncoated; however, some contain a special outside layer that dissolves or ruptures at the site of application. These coatings may help mask the bitter taste of a tablet, prevent destruction in the stomach, or delay release of drug into the intestines. Common tablet coatings include sugar, film, or enteric.

- Sugar-coated tablets (SCTs) contain an outside layer of sugar that protects the medication and improves both appearance and flavor. The sugar coating of tablets tends to improve taste and increases the chance that the patient will be compliant and take the prescribed medication at the prescribed time. The major disadvantage of sugar coating is that it makes the tablets much larger and heavier, thus more difficult to swallow.
- Film-coated tablets (FCTs) contain a thin outer layer of a polymer (a substance containing very large molecules) that can be either soluble or insoluble in water. Film coatings are thinner, lighter in weight, and cheaper to manufacture than sugar coatings, and they are colored to provide an attractive appearance. The antibiotic erythromycin is an example of an FCT formulation designed to mask a bitter taste.
- Enteric-coated tablets (ECTs) are used for drugs that are destroyed by gastric acid, which might irritate the esophageal tract or stomach, or are better absorbed by the intestines if they bypass the stomach. The enteric coating is designed to resist destruction by the acidic pH of the gastric fluids and to release the active ingredient once it reaches the higher pH of the small or large intestine, such as in serious inflammatory diseases of the GI tract. For this reason, these tablets should not be split. Examples of ECTs are aspirin and potassium chloride, because both drugs can be irritating to the stomach.

A **controlled-release medication** is designed to regulate the rate at which a drug is released from the tablet and into the body. Such dose forms may vary the rate of dissolution or the release of the active drug and may offer a therapeutic advantage over conventional dose forms, thus cannot be split or crushed (see Appendix D). The major types of controlled-release medications are delayed, extended, and transdermal.

- A delayed-release dose form does not release the active drug immediately after administration. An example of delayed-release dose forms is an enteric-coated product.

- An extended-release form allows a reduced frequency of dosing compared with conventional forms; this term is synonymous with long-acting, timed-release, and sustained-release dose forms. Many medications for blood pressure use this type of dose form that allows once-daily dosing and better compliance to the prescribed regimen.

- The transdermal system dose form is also a delivery system designed to deliver drugs to the systemic circulation by passage *through the skin* (similar to how the extended-release tablets act by passage through the stomach and/or small intestine). A common example is the various commercially available nicotine patches. (See Chapter 4, *Routes of Drug Administration*, for additional discussion on the transdermal system.)

Most tablets are meant to be swallowed whole and to dissolve in the gastrointestinal (GI) tract. For example, some tablets are designed to be chewed or to be dissolved in liquid, in the mouth, under the tongue, or in the vagina.

- Chewable tablets contain a base that is flavored and/or colored. The dose form is designed to be masticated (or chewed), and it is preferred for antacids, antiflatulents, commercial vitamins, and tablets for children. Single chewable tablets, for example, can be dosed in small children in lieu of other dose formulations to control asthma symptoms.

- Effervescent tablets are granular salts that release gas and so disperse active ingredients into solution when placed in water or juice. Most people are familiar with effervescent tablets such as Alka-Seltzer to relieve headaches or hangovers.

- Buccal tablets (and gum) are placed in the buccal pouches (between the cheek and the gum) and dissolved and absorbed by the buccal mucosa. (For more information on this route of administration, see Chapter 4.)

- Sublingual tablets are designed to be dissolved under the tongue (*sub*, meaning *under*, and *lingua*, meaning tongue) and absorbed. Medication dissolved under the tongue (e.g., nitroglycerin) is absorbed very quickly and has the advantage of immediately entering the bloodstream.

- Vaginal tablets (or inserts) are designed to be placed into the vagina by means of an applicator and dissolved and absorbed through the vaginal mucosa; vaginal tablets may be less "messy" than equivalent cream formulations, although absorption of active drug is less predictable.

Capsules

The **capsule** is a solid dose form consisting of a gelatin shell that encloses the drug. Gelatin is a protein substance obtained from vegetable matter and from the skin, white connective tissue, and bones of animals. The gelatin shell of a capsule, which can be hard or soft, may be transparent, semitransparent, or opaque and may be colored or marked with a code to facilitate identification. In commercial manufacturing, the body and the cap may be sealed to protect the integrity of the drug within (a practice that has increased since the 1980s, when highly publicized incidents of capsule tampering occurred). In most cases the capsule is meant to be swallowed whole (patients often prefer capsules because they are tasteless and are often easier to swallow than tablets).

The capsule will contain powders, granules, liquids, or some combination with one or more active ingredients. In most cases these active ingredients will also contain one or more pharmacologically inert filler substance, or diluent. The capsule may also contain disintegrants, solubilizers, preservatives (which maintain the integrity of the ingredients), colorings, and other materials. Because a capsule is enclosed, flavorings are not common for this dose form.

As with tablets, capsules can be designed in a controlled-release dose form to deliver a drug over a particular period of time (i.e., sustained release) or at a particular site (i.e., delayed action). Names for controlled-release dose forms include constant release, continuous action, continuous release, controlled release, delayed absorption, depot, extended action, extended release, gradual release, long acting, long lasting, long-term release, programmed release, prolonged action, prolonged release, protracted release, rate controlled, repository, slow acting, slow release, sustained action, sustained release, sustained-release depot, timed coat, timed disintegration, and timed release.

The controlled-release capsules are taken less often, and patients are more likely to be compliant. It is much easier to remember to take medication once daily than to take several doses throughout the day. A long-acting form may also give the patient better control over the disease state such as high blood pressure. Although the units may be initially more expensive, fewer need to be purchased. In addition to cost, another drawback is the longer time it may take for side effects to subside.

Suppositories

Suppositories are solid dose forms designed for insertion into body orifices such as the rectum or the vagina or, less commonly, the urethra. Suppositories may be the preferred dose form in some cases when the patient has severe nausea and vomiting. However, many patients avoid the use of a suppository when possible because of their discomfort.

Suppositories vary in size and shape, depending on their site of administration and the age and gender of the patient for whom they are designed. Some are meant for local action, such as in the treatment of rectal hemorrhoids. Rectal suppositories, however, are often used as vehicles for systemic drugs because the rich supply of blood and lymphatic vessels in the rectum provides for exceptional absorption. They are often used in children or adults who cannot take oral medication to control symptoms of fever, nausea, or vomiting, as well as to treat those with severe symptoms of inflammatory bowel disease or pain.

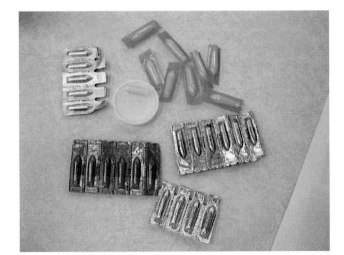

Its site of administration determines the size and shape of a suppository.

Effervescent Salts

Effervescent salts are granules or coarse powders containing one or more medicinal agents such as an analgesic, as well as some combination of sodium bicarbonate with citric acid, tartaric acid, or sodium biphosphate. When dissolved in water, effervescent salts release carbon dioxide gas, causing a distinctive bubbling. A common example of an effervescent salt is sodium phosphate, used as a cathartic for stimulating evacuation of the bowels before a procedure.

Implants or Pellets

Implants, or pellets, are dose forms that are placed under the skin by means of minor surgery. They are used for long-term, controlled release of medications, especially as long-term contraceptives. An example of an implant is Norplant, which contains levonorgestrel to prevent pregnancy. The advantages of such products include enhanced patient compliance and convenience, but complications at the site of insertion have limited their widespread use.

Lozenges, Troches, or Pastilles

Lozenges, also known as *troches* or *pastilles*, are dose forms containing active ingredients and flavorings, such as sweeteners, that are dissolved in the mouth. They generally have local effects. Commercial OTC lozenges for relief of sore throat are quite common, although many other drugs, including such prescription drugs as nystatin or clotrimazole, are also available in lozenge form.

Plasters

Plasters are solid or semisolid and medicated or nonmedicated preparations that adhere to the body and contain a backing material such as paper, cotton, linen, silk, moleskin, or plastic. An example is the salicylic acid plaster used to remove corns.

Powders and Granules

Commonly dispensed powders include antacids, brewer's yeast, laxatives, douche powders, dentifrices and dental adhesives, and powders for external application to the skin. These are usually ordered in bulk by the pharmacy and are dispensed as needed in the prescribed amount. In large-scale commercial manufacturing, powders are milled and pulverized by machines. An example of a medication in the powder dose form is polymyxin B sulfate and bacitracin zinc topical powder, which is used to prevent infection.

Granules are larger than powders and are formed by adding very small amounts of liquid to powders; then the mixture is passed through a screen or a granulating device. Tablets are often prepared by compressing granules, and capsules are often filled with granules. Granules are generally of irregular shape, have excellent flow characteristics, are more stable than powders, and are generally better suited than powders for use in solutions because they are not as likely simply to float on the surface of a liquid. They may contain colorings, flavorings, and coatings and may have controlled-release characteristics (Theo-Dur Sprinkles). The pharmacist combines some granular drug products with water before dispensing such as antibiotic suspensions, whereas others are dispensed as granules.

LIQUID DOSE FORMS

Liquid dose forms consist of one or more active ingredients in a liquid vehicle. These dose forms can be divided into two major categories: (1) solutions, in which active ingredients are dissolved in the liquid vehicle; and (2) dispersions, in which undissolved ingredients are dispersed throughout a liquid vehicle.

Liquid dose forms that are meant for oral consumption have several advantages over solid dose forms, including ease of swallowing and of adjusting the dose. A liquid dose can be easily adjusted, whereas tablets or capsules cannot always be divided as easily. For the patient, taste preference may be either an advantage or

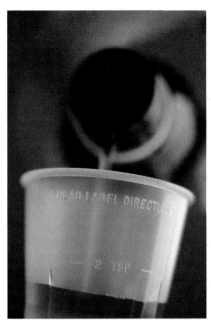

Liquid medications are easy to swallow, and the dose can be adjusted.

disadvantage. For adults this is not usually a concern; however, children's medication is often flavored in the most palatable way possible to improve compliance. Liquid dose forms are often less stable than their solid counterparts, and care should be taken to monitor storage conditions of the liquid dose forms, to rotate stock, and to check expiration dates often.

Liquid and semisolid dose forms meant for topical application are common examples of dispersions. **Creams** and lotions, for example, are easily absorbed (i.e., "vanishing") and can cover large areas of the skin. **Ointments**, however, are "sticky" and will leave the area feeling greasy. An ointment is especially good for extremely dry areas where moisture needs to be retained, as well as for areas prone to friction from clothing or other body parts. Ointments generally have a longer contact time with the skin and thus a longer duration of action. **Gels** are yet another product that may be designed with a specific indication in mind. They apply evenly and leave a dry coat of the medication in contact with the area.

Solutions

Solutions may be classified by vehicle as aqueous (i.e., water based), alcoholic (alcohol based), or hydroalcoholic (i.e., water and alcohol based). The vehicle that makes up the greater part of a solution is known as a **solvent**. An ingredient dissolved in a solution is known as a **solute**. An enema is usually a water-based solution administered rectally for cleansing the bowel before a GI procedure or for delivering active drug. An evacuation enema, like Fleet, is administered to clean the bowels. A retention enema, such as Cortenema, is administered to deliver medication locally or systemically.

Collodion is an example of a vehicle that is a liquid dissolved in a mixture of alcohol and ether and used for a variety of topical purposes. On application, the highly volatile alcohol and ether solvent vaporizes, leaving a film coating containing the medication on the skin. The OTC product, Compound W, is a collodion containing salicylic acid used to remove corns or warts.

Solutions may also be classified by their contents: aromatic waters, elixirs, syrups, extracts, fluidextracts, tinctures, spirits, or irrigating solutions. A low-alcohol or alcohol-free product is preferred for most pediatric products.

- Aromatic waters is a solution of water containing oils or other substances that have a pungent, and usually pleasing, smell and are volatile (i.e., easily released into the air). Rose water is an example.
- An elixir is a clear, sweetened, flavored solution containing water and ethanol (hydroalcoholic). An example of a drug in this dose form is phenobarbital elixir, containing phenobarbital, orange oil, propylene glycol, alcohol, sorbitol solution, color, and purified water.
- A syrup is an aqueous solution thickened with a large amount of sugar, generally sucrose, or a sugar substitute such as sorbitol or propylene glycol. Syrups may contain additional flavorings, colors, or aromatic agents. Syrups may be medicated, such as lithium citrate or ipecac, or nonmedicated such as cherry syrup or cocoa syrup. Syrups are often the preferred vehicle to mask the taste of pediatric medications, because they do not contain alcohol. Syrups are also sometimes used for older patients who cannot easily swallow the commonly available solid forms of certain drugs.

- An extract is a potent dose form derived from animal or plant sources from which most or all the solvent has been evaporated to produce a powder, an ointment-like form, or a solid. Extracts are produced from fluidextracts and used in the formulation or compounding of medications.
- A fluidextract is a liquid dose form prepared by extraction from plant sources and commonly used in the formulation of syrups. Vanilla extract is an example of a fluidextract.
- A tincture is an alcoholic or hydroalcoholic solution of extractions from plants. Examples include iodine tincture and belladonna tincture.
- Spirits are alcoholic or hydroalcoholic solutions containing volatile, aromatic ingredients. Examples include camphor and peppermint spirit, both of which can be used as medicines or flavorings.
- An irrigating solution is any solution for cleansing or bathing an area of the body. Some are used topically in the eye or ear or for irrigation of tissues exposed by wounds or surgical incisions. Examples of irrigating solutions used in surgical procedures are Neosporin-Polymyxin and 1% acetic acid. The term *douche* is most commonly used for irrigating solutions, often reconstituted from powders, administered into the vaginal cavity.

Solutions are sometimes classified by site or method of administration as topical (local), systemic (throughout the body), epicutaneous (on the skin), percutaneous (through the skin), oral (for or through the mouth), otic (for or through the ear), ophthalmic (for the eye), parenteral (for injection or intravenous [IV] infusion), rectal (for or through the rectum), urethral (for the urethra), or vaginal (for or through the vagina).

Parenteral solutions are sterile solutions, with or without medication, for administration by means of a hollow needle or catheter used to place the solution through one or more layers of the skin. Two major delivery systems for parenteral solutions exist: (1) IV infusions and (2) injections, which are commonly IV, intramuscular (IM) (into the muscle), subcutaneous (under the skin), or intradermal (ID) (into the skin). Parenteral solutions are discussed in greater detail later in this chapter and in Unit 3, *Institutional Pharmacy.*

Dispersions

Unlike a solution, a dispersion is not dissolved but simply distributed throughout the vehicle. A **suspension** is the dispersion of a solid in a liquid, whereas an **emulsion** is the dispersion of a liquid in another liquid. In either case an incomplete mixture of the solid or liquid exists. **Dispersions** are classified by the size of the dispersed ingredient(s) into suspensions and emulsions that both contain relatively large particles, as well as magmas, gels, and jellies, which contain fine particles. If a dispersion contains ultrafine particles, less than a micron in size, then it is said to be a **colloidal dispersion**. One type of colloidal dispersion is the microemulsion.

Some suspensions come already prepared, whereas others come in the form of dry powders that are reconstituted with purified water. Suspensions may be classified by route of administration into oral (taken by mouth), topical (lotions applied to the skin), and injectable suspensions. A well-prepared suspension settles slowly but can be redispersed easily by a gentle shake and pours easily. A suspension may be a preferred method for dispensing a solid to a young or older adult patient who would find it difficult to swallow a solid dose form. Examples of suspensions include antacids like the magnesia and alumina oral suspension with the brand name Maalox, the antifungal mycostatin oral suspension, and the injectable NPH insulin.

Emulsions vary in their viscosity, or rate of flow, from free-flowing liquids such as lotions to semisolid preparations such as ointments and creams. Common types of

Safety Note
Suspensions should always include a "Shake Well" label.

emulsions are **oil-in-water (O/W) emulsion** or **water-in-oil (W/O) emulsion**. For example, O/W emulsions contain a small amount of oil dispersed in water. Emulsions contain an emulsifying agent to render the emulsion stable and less prone to separation. A liniment is an oleaginous (hydrocarbon-containing) emulsion containing medications and meant for rubbing on the skin. The OTC pain medication Ben-Gay is an example of this type of dose form.

A **lotion** is a liquid for topical application containing insoluble dispersed solids or immiscible liquids. Examples include calamine lotion, used for relief of itching, and benzoyl peroxide lotion, used to control acne.

Like suspensions, gels contain solid particles in liquid, but the particles are ultra-fine, of colloidal dimensions, and sufficient in number (therefore linked to form a semi-solid). Examples of gels include lidocaine gel and the antacid aluminum hydroxide gel. The following are examples of ultrafine dispersion dose forms:

- A jelly is a gel that contains a higher proportion of water in combination with a drug substance, as well as a thickening agent. Jellies are present in many anti-septics, antifungals, contraceptives, and lubricants. Lubricants are commonly used in pelvic and rectal examination of body orifices or as an aid in sexual intercourse to postmenopausal women with vaginal dryness from a hormone deficiency. Because of their high water content, jellies are subject to contamination; therefore they usually contain preservatives.
- Glycerogelatins are topical preparations made with gelatin, glycerin, water, and medicinal substances. The hard substance is melted and brushed onto the skin, where it hardens again and is generally covered with a bandage. An example is zinc gelatin (Unna's Boot), used as a pressure bandage to treat varicose ulcers.
- A magma, or milk, is similar to a gel in that it contains colloidal particles in liquid, but the particles remain distinct, in a two-phase system. An example is Milk of Magnesia, containing magnesium hydroxide, used to neutralize gastric acid.
- A microemulsion, like other emulsions, contains one liquid dispersed in another; however, unlike other emulsions, it is clear because of the extremely fine size of the droplets of the dispersed phase. An example of a microemulsion is Haley's M-O.

Ointments are semisolid dose forms meant for topical application and are packaged in jars or tubes. Ointments may be medicated or nonmedicated and may contain various kinds of bases:

- oleaginous or greasy bases made from hydrocarbons such as mineral oil or petroleum jelly
- W/O emulsions such as anhydrous lanolin, lanolin, or cold cream
- O/W emulsions such as hydrophilic ointment
- water-soluble or greaseless bases such as polyethylene glycol ointment

Pastes are like ointments but contain more solid materials and consequently are stiffer and apply more thickly. Examples are zinc oxide paste (an astringent) and acetonide dental paste (an anti-inflammatory preparation).

Creams are considered O/W emulsions. They apply smoothly to the skin and leave a very thin film. Most creams are considered vanishing, which means they are invisible once applied and thus preferred by many patients. Like ointments, they are packaged in jars or tubes.

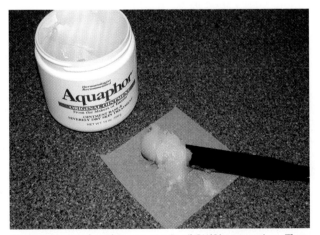

Ointments are referred to as *water-in-oil (W/O) preparations*. They contain a small amount of water dispersed throughout oil. They will apply smoothly to the skin but will often leave the skin with a greasy feeling. Ointments are often yellowish and opaque.

INHALATION DOSE FORMS

Gases, vapors, solutions, or suspensions intended to be inhaled via the nasal or oral respiratory routes are known as **inhalations**.

A **spray** is a dose form that consists of a container with a valve assembly that, when activated, emits a fine dispersion of liquid, solid, or gaseous material. An aerosol is a spray in a pressurized container that contains a propellant, an inert liquid or gas under pressure, meant to carry the active ingredient to its location of application. Depending on the formulation of the product and on the design of the valve, an aerosol may commonly emit a fine mist or a coarse liquid spray. Several inhalation products (e.g., Advair Diskus [fluticasone-salmeterol] and Spiriva [tiotropium]) are available as breath-activated devices of powders in place of aerosolized propellants.

Most sprays and aerosols are for topical application to the skin or to oral mucous membranes such as OTC local anesthetics, antiseptics, deodorants, and breath sprays. Other sprays are inhalation aerosols that the patient breathes in through the nose or mouth to deliver prescription drugs. Sprays and aerosols are often used for nasal decongestants and for inhalation of antiasthmatic drugs. Many anti-inflammatory medications are available both as a nasal spray for allergies and as an aerosol for inhalation for asthma.

DELIVERY SYSTEMS

Modern prescription drugs often are created using a high level of technology, and in some cases the technology is carrying over to the way a medication is delivered to the patient. Delivery systems used to deliver specific medications are often manufactured and packaged as a unit and then dispensed as a unit for the patient. They contain not only the medication but also a specialized delivery mechanism. The wide variety of delivery systems available offer patients a welcome alternative to traditional administration.

Inhalation Delivery Systems

This method of administration is one of the most rapid means (second only to the IV method) of administering any medication. Gases such as oxygen, nitrous oxide or "laughing gas," and ether are administered by inhalation. General anesthetics used during surgical procedures often use this delivery system. Pharmacists and pharmacy technicians in both community pharmacy and home healthcare settings are increasingly dealing with the delivery of oxygen tanks to the homes of patients with chronic lung disease.

Medicated inhalations intended for the lung are often administered via devices such as metered-dose inhalers (MDIs) or nebulizers. MDIs are handheld, breath-activated, propellant-driven inhalers that are commonly used for patients with asthma or chronic lung disease. (Proper technique and use of spacer devices is critical to proper use and is further discussed in Chapter 4.)

Nebulizers, also called *atomizing machines,* are effective for delivering mists or micronized powders to the lungs.

Nebulizers are atomizing machines that deliver the medication as a mist containing extremely small, or micronized, powder. Common vehicles for inhalation solutions include sterile water for injection (SWI) and sodium chloride, also called *normal saline (NS)*. The solution is placed in a device that will aerosolize both the medication and the vehicle. An example of a medication delivered by inhalation is albuterol for relief of bronchial spasms. A "nebulized" mist of medication may be more effective than an "aerosolized" spray in delivering medications into the deeper areas of the lung in infants and young children.

Vaporizers and humidifiers are other mechanical devices commonly used to deliver moisture to the air for relief of cold symptoms. Volatile medications can be used with some vaporizers. A good example of a volatile medication is Vicks Vaposteam.

Syringe, Injection, and Infusion Delivery Systems

Injections of medications act rapidly to control and treat symptoms. Some medications are only available in an injection form, such as insulin. Syringes are calibrated devices used to accurately draw up, measure, and deliver medication to a patient through a needle. Injections must be sterile because they introduce medication directly into the body. Only trained professionals and healthcare providers should give injections, and some risk to the patient is always present. In recent years patients have been taught how to self-administer injections or infusions at home by the home health nurse or pharmacist.

Two types of syringes are commonly used for injections: (1) glass and (2) plastic. Glass syringes are fairly expensive and must be sterilized between uses, whereas plastic syringes are easy to handle and disposable, and they come from the manufacturer in sterile packaging. Plastic is clearly preferred and used both within and outside the hospital setting. Different states have different regulations on the sale of syringes because of their potential diversion for injection of illegal drugs; some states (or insurance companies) may require a prescription or the placement of syringes behind the prescription counter to control their sales.

The larger hypodermic syringes have cannulas or barrels that range from 3 to 60 mL of liquid. The cannula is the bore area inside the syringe that correlates with the volume of solution. Common types of syringes (Figure 3.5) include the insulin syringe (which measures from 30 to 100 U) and the tuberculin syringe (with cannulas ranging from 0.01 to 1 mL [used for skin tests and drawing up very small volumes of solution]). The syringe and needle will be explained in more detail in Chapter 11, *Preparing Sterile Intravenous Products.*

Injections may be administered to almost any organ or part of the body. The advantages and disadvantages of the various routes of parenteral administration are discussed in the next chapter. Injectables come prefilled or are filled at the time of injection from single or multidose vials. Single-dose vials generally have no preservative and are dispensed as single use only. Multiple-dose vials, although they contain a preservative, should be dated and discarded (usually after 30 days) per policy and procedures of the pharmacy. Sometimes the medication comes in ampules, which are small glass containers that are opened by breaking off the neck of the container. Because of the danger of contaminating the medication with glass particles, medication that comes in ampules must be filtered before it is injected. (For more information on injections, see Chapter 11.)

In addition to syringes, devices available for injection include **patient-controlled analgesia (PCA) infusion devices**, which are programmable machines that deliver small doses of painkillers on patient demand; jet injectors, which use pressure rather than a needle to deliver the medication; and ambulatory injection devices, like insulin

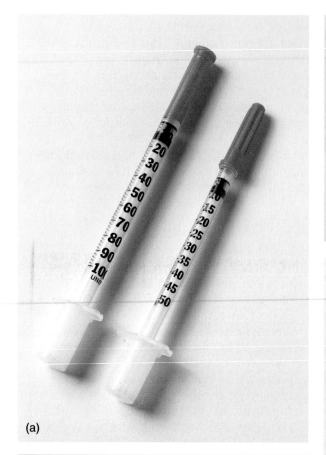

(a)

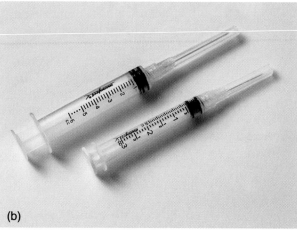

(b)

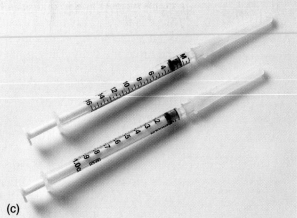

(c)

Figure 3.5

Typical Syringes
(a) Insulin syringes in 100-U and 50-U sizes. (b) Hypodermic syringes in 6-cc and 3-cc sizes. (c) Tuberculin syringes marked with both metric and apothecary measures.

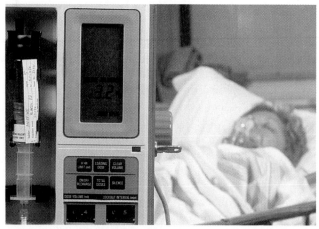

A patient-controlled analgesia (PCA) pump can allow the patient to regulate the amount of pain medication he or she receives. This results in better pain control with less drug used.

pumps, that the patient can wear while moving about. Some injection devices make use of pumps that regulate the amount, rate, and/or timing of injections.

IV infusion is a method for delivering a large amount of fluid over a prolonged period of time and at a slow, steady rate into the blood system. Infusions are used to deliver blood; water; other fluids; electrolytes; nutrients such as proteins, amino acids, lipids, and sugars; and drugs. When drugs are prepared and added to an IV solution line, they are *piggybacked*. Typical uses of IV infusions are to deliver pain-killing or blood-clot-buster medications, to replenish body fluids, and to deliver nutrients to patients who cannot or will not feed themselves.

Intrauterine and Cervical Delivery Systems

An **intrauterine delivery system** is a drug-releasing device placed into the uterus. Several such systems contain a progestin hormone that is used to prevent pregnancy on a long-term (1 to 5 years) basis. This system is not as effective a contraceptive as oral contraceptives. Devices also exist that remain in the vagina and are placed as a ring surrounding the cervix to slowly release medication. They are replaced monthly by the patient and used as contraceptive aids. Occasionally, the patient will expel these devices spontaneously and may experience a high risk of pelvic infection.

Transdermal Delivery Systems

A **transdermal delivery system (TDS)**, or patch, is a dose form meant for delivery percutaneously (through the skin). It consists of a backing, a drug reservoir, a control membrane, an adhesive layer, and a protective strip. The strip is removed, and the adhesive layer is attached to the skin. Drug movement is by osmosis through the control membrane, delivering medication systemically, rather than locally. In some patches, the membrane controls the rate of drug delivery, whereas in others the skin itself controls it. Medications given with this dose form can be controlled over 24 hours or longer. Patient convenience and compliance are improved with the use of transdermal patches. Examples will be discussed in Chapter 4, *Routes of Drug Administration.*

Other Delivery Systems

In the hospital, unit dose disposable syringes are prefilled syringes that contain a single premeasured dose of medication and are thrown away after use. These special syringes are used to deliver oral liquid medications to pediatric patients in the hospital setting. An **oral syringe** is a calibrated device consisting of a plunger and a cannula, or barrel, used without a needle for administration of precisely measured amounts of medication by mouth.

A **bulb syringe** consists of a bulb and a tapering funnel with a hollow end and is used to administer liquids topically, as for irrigation of the ears (to remove ear wax) or eyes (to flush out an irritant). The bulb is first depressed to expel the air that it contains, and the tip is then inserted into the liquid to be administered. The bulb is released while the end is in the liquid, and the liquid rises to fill the vacuum thus created. The end of the bulb is then removed from the liquid, and the liquid is administered by depressing the bulb again.

Like a bulb syringe, a dropper uses a bulb to create a vacuum for drawing up a liquid. A dropper contains a small, squeezable bulb at one end and a hollow glass or plastic tube with a tapering point. The dropper may be incorporated into the cap of a vial or other container. The abbreviation *gtt* is used as a unit of pharmaceutical measurement for droppers and IV infusions to indicate *drops.* Because of the differing viscosities (the thicknesses and flow characteristics) of differing fluids, the size of a drop varies considerably from medication to medication. Medication droppers are medication specific; that is, they cannot be used to measure other medications. Droppers are often used for otic or ophthalmic administration, as well as for oral medications. Droppers are critically important to deliver the correct dose of medication to infants.

Ocular inserts are small, transparent membranes containing medications that are placed between the eye and the lower conjunctiva (i.e., the mucous membrane on the inside of the eyelid). An example is the product with the brand name Ocusert, used to deliver pilocarpine for the treatment of glaucoma.

Some hospices (facilities caring for the terminally ill) and long-term care facilities make use of straws (long, hollow tubes) prefilled with pain medications. Another delivery system of a contraceptive is the recently reintroduced polyurethane sponge containing a spermicide, nonoxynol 9.

DRUG REFERENCES

Two reference works published by the United States Pharmacopeia (USP) establish the official legal standards for drugs in the United States: *United States Pharmacopeia* (which describes drug substances and dose forms) and the *National Formulary* (which describes pharmaceutical ingredients). Both are revised every 5 years, and supplements are published in the interim between revisions. They are also printed in a combined edition, *United States Pharmacopeia–National Formulary (USP–NF)*.

Several other reference books are also helpful to practitioners:

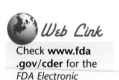

Web Link

Check **www.fda .gov/cder** for the *FDA Electronic Orange Book.*

- *Physician's Desk Reference* is published annually with reprints of package inserts from the pharmaceutical manufacturers of most drugs. It is also useful for identifying unknown drugs by color, shape, and coding.
- *Drug Facts and Comparisons* includes factual information on product availability, indications, administration and dose, pharmacological actions, contraindications, warnings, precautions, adverse reactions, overdose, and patient instructions. It is updated monthly with new inserts and is also available on CD-ROM.
- *USP Drug Information*, originally published by the USP, is a source of patient counseling information for the pharmacist.
- *American Hospital Formulary Service (AHFS)* is an excellent source of information, especially on parenteral drugs commonly used in the hospital.
- *Handbook of Nonprescription Drugs* is published by the American Pharmacists Association and provides a good reference for OTC drugs.
- *FDA Electronic Orange Book* (also called *Approved Drug Products with Therapeutic Equivalence Evaluations*) is available on-line and provides information on generic equivalency of drugs that may have many sources; for example, can a less-expensive blood pressure medication be "substituted" for a brand name of the same drug? Each state may vary in procedures for dispensing "generic equivalents."
- *Remington: The Science and Practice of Pharmacy* is an excellent text, especially for use in a compounding pharmacy where determinations of drug stability and compatibility are important.
- *Lawrence Review of Natural Products* provides scientific monographs on herbal medications.
- *Homeopathic Pharmacopeia of the United States* is a compilation of standards for the source, composition, and preparation of homeopathic medications that may be sold in the community pharmacy.

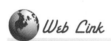

Web Link

Go to this book's Information Resources Center (IRC) at **www.emcp .com**, and visit the Resources page found in the Pharmacy Library for a list of these and other valuable resources.

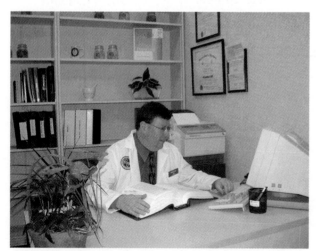

Pharmacists will use *Drug Facts and Comparisons* and computerized databases for up-to-date drug information.

active ingredient chemical in the drug product producing the desired therapeutic effect

antibodies part of the immune system to neutralize antigens or foreign substances in the body

antineoplastic drugs drugs used to kill cancer cells

biotechnology field of study that combines the science of biology, chemistry, and immunology to produce synthetic, unique drugs with specific therapeutic effects

bulb syringe device used to irrigate the eyes or ears with water

capsule dose form containing powder, liquid, or granules in a gelatin covering

colloidal dispersion dispersion of ultrafine particles

controlled-release medication dose form that is formulated to release medication over a long duration of time

creams cosmetically acceptable oil-in-water (O/W) emulsions for topical use on the skin

delivery system device used to deliver the drug; a design feature of the dose form that affects the delivery of the drug; how a medication is formulated to release the active ingredient

deoxyribonucleic acid (DNA) helix-shaped molecule that carries the genetic code

destructive agent drug that kills bacteria, fungi, viruses, or even normal or cancer cells

diagnostic agent drug used to diagnose other diseases

dispersions liquid dose forms in which undissolved ingredients are mixed throughout a liquid vehicle

dose form how a medication is manufactured (e.g., capsule, tablet)

drug medical substance or remedy used to change the way a living organism functions; also called a *medication*

effervescent salts granular salts that release gas and dispense active ingredients into solution when placed in water

emulsion dispersion of a liquid in another liquid

gels dispersions containing fine particles for topical use on the skin

genetic engineering hybridization technique for creating monoclonal antibodies (MAbs)

homeopathic medications very small dilutions of natural drugs claimed to stimulate the immune system

implants medications placed under the skin to deliver the active ingredient slowly

inert ingredients inactive chemicals that are added to active ingredients to improve drug formulations; also called inactive ingredients

inhalations gases, vapors, solutions, or suspensions intended to be inhaled via the nasal or oral respiratory routes

intrauterine delivery system way to deliver medication to prevent conception or treat cancer

intravenous (IV) infusions medications or fluids administered directly into a vein

lotion liquid for topical application containing insoluble dispersed solids or immiscible liquids

lozenges medications in a sweet-taste formulation that is absorbed in the mouth

monoclonal antibodies (MAbs) single-cell antibodies produced in a laboratory to produce a pure antibody against a known specific antigen; used in cancer immunotherapy

National Drug Code (NDC) number unique number assigned to a product to identify the manufacturer, drug, packaging size, and type

nebulizers devices used to deliver medication in a fine-mist form to the lung; often used in treating asthma

ocular inserts type of contact lens device with active medication for administration in the eye

oil-in-water (O/W) emulsion emulsions containing a small amount of oil dispersed in water; like a cream

ointments semisolid emulsions for topical use on the skin

oral syringe device without a needle to administer medication to pediatric or elderly patients unable to swallow tablets or capsules

over-the-counter (OTC) drug drug sold without a prescription

parenteral solutions products that are prepared in a sterile environment for administration by injection

pastes water-in-oil (W/O) emulsions containing more solid material than an ointment

patient-controlled analgesia (PCA) infusion devices devices used by a patient to deliver small doses of medication to the patient for chronic pain

pharmacodynamic agent drug that alters body functions in a desired way

plasters solid or semisolid, medicated or nonmedicated preparations that adhere to the skin

prophylactic agent drug used to prevent disease

radiopharmaceuticals drugs containing radioactive ingredients often used for diagnostic or therapeutic purposes

recombinant DNA technique that uses living organisms or parts of organisms for specific purposes such as creating a synthetic drug like insulin

ribonucleic acid (RNA) important component of genetic code that arranges amino acids into proteins

semisynthetic drugs drugs that contain both natural and synthetic components

solute an ingredient dissolved in a solution or dispersed in a suspension

solutions liquid dose forms commonly containing carbohydrates, proteins, electrolytes, minerals, or medications

solvent vehicle that makes up the greater part of a solution

spray dose form that consists of a container with a valve assembly that, when activated, emits a fine dispersion of liquid, solid, or gaseous material

suppositories solid formulations containing a drug for rectal or vaginal administration

suspension dispersion of a solid in a liquid

synthesized drug drug that is artificially created

synthetic drug drug that is artificially created but in imitation of natural-occurring substances

tablet solid dose form produced by compression and containing one or more active ingredients

therapeutic agent drug that prevents, cures, diagnoses, or relieves symptoms of a disease

transdermal delivery system (TDS) method of delivering medication via the skin; like a patch

water-in-oil (W/O) emulsion emulsion containing a small amount of water dispersed in an oil; like an ointment

Chapter Summary

- Drugs are natural, synthetic, synthesized, or semisynthetic substances taken into or applied to the body to alter biochemical functions and achieve a desired pharmacological effect.
- Uses of drug may include one or more of the following: therapeutic, pharmacodynamic, prophylactic, diagnostic, or destructive agents.
- Drugs can be classified as over-the-counter (OTC) or legend as regulated by the FDA.
- Diet supplements, which include vitamins, minerals, and herbals, are regulated under the DSHEA amendments.
- Drugs are administered in many dose forms and using many delivery systems. The choice of dose form and delivery system is based on what active ingredient is to be delivered, how much is to be delivered, by what means or route, to what sites, at what rate, over what period of time, and for what purpose.
- Solid dose forms commonly include tablets and capsules. Tablets may be coated, chewable, controlled release, effervescent, and/or specially formulated for buccal, sublingual, or vaginal use.
- Liquid dose forms include a wide variety of solutions, as well as dispersions such as suspensions and emulsions. Creams and ointments are special emulsions for application to the skin.
- Delivery systems commonly include syringe, injection, and infusion devices; metered dose inhalers (MDIs) or nebulizers for inhalation use; transdermal delivery systems (TDSs); and droppers and oral syringes for pediatric and infant use.
- A multitude of good reference texts and Internet Web sites exist that the practicing pharmacist and pharmacy technician can use to study various pharmaceutical products.

Chapter Review

Knowledge Inventory

Choose the best answer from those provided.

1. A biochemically reactive component in a drug is known as a(n)
   a. inert ingredient.
   b. active ingredient.
   c. diluent.
   d. vehicle.

2. A National Drug Code (NDC) number *does not* identify the
   a. product manufacturer.
   b. drug.
   c. packaging size and type.
   d. schedule of the drug.

3. A radiopharmaceutical used for imaging is an example of a
   a. therapeutic agent.
   b. pharmacodynamic agent.
   c. diagnostic agent.
   d. prophylactic agent.

4. When people use the term *delivery system*, they generally intend, in addition to the dose form, to refer to the
   a. physical characteristics of the dose form that determine the method of administration and the site of action of the drug.
   b. restrictions placed upon the ordering, storage, and dispensing of the drug because of its classification under the Comprehensive Drug Abuse Prevention and Control Act.
   c. chemical composition of the drug, including its active ingredients, inert ingredients, and any colorings, flavorings, preservatives, disintegrants, solubilizers, and emulsifying agents.
   d. use of the drug as a therapeutic, pharmacodynamic, diagnostic, prophylactic, or destructive agent.

5. A dose form used in the rectum, vagina, and urethra is a(n)
   a. inhalation aerosol.
   b. suppository.
   c. elixir.
   d. fluidextract.

6. Drugs with an enteric coating
   a. dissolve in the stomach.
   b. dissolve in the intestines.
   c. are comprised of sugar for palatability.
   d. are made of polymers, which form a protective film.

7. A solution containing water and ethanol would be described as
    a. hydroalcoholic.
    b. aqueous.
    c. magma.
    d. immiscible.

8. Some examples of dispersions are
    a. suspensions and emulsions.
    b. tinctures, fluidextracts, and extracts.
    c. aromatic waters.
    d. elixirs and syrups.

9. Dose forms that are often or always sweetened include
    a. parenteral solutions, spirits, and tinctures.
    b. medicated syrups and elixirs.
    c. collodions, microemulsions, and ointments.
    d. liniments and extracts.

10. To determine generic equivalency of a brand name product, which reference source would you use?
    a. *Drug Facts and Comparisons*
    b. *FDA Electronic Orange Book*
    c. *Physician's Desk Reference*
    d. *Homeopathic Pharmacopeia of the United States*

Pharmacy in Practice

1. Recombinant DNA will, in the future, play a great role in gene therapies, in which recombinant DNA is used to supply the body with genes to supplement or replace the action of the existing genes with which the body is endowed. Do some research on gene therapy for the treatment of cystic fibrosis, the most common of all fatal genetic diseases. Such therapy uses a cold virus containing recombinant DNA that carries a gene called the *cystic fibrosis transmembrane regulator*. Prepare a brief report explaining how such therapy works.

2. Determine the brand name, dose form, and primary indication for the following gene therapy or biotechnology-based medications:
    a. epoetin alpha
    b. efavirenz
    c. infliximab
    d. somatotropin
    e. trastuzumab
    f. becaplermin
    g. palivizumab

3. A tree diagram is a chart that shows a classification system. A single characteristic is used to differentiate the items classified under each node on the chart. For example, a tree chart might classify animals in this way:

Animals

Vertebrates *(With Backbones)*	*Invertebrates* *(Without Backbones)*
• mammals	• flatworms
• reptiles	• roundworms
• fish	• insects
• birds	• arachnids
• amphibians	• mollusks

Create tree charts to classify
   a. solid dose forms
   b. liquid dose forms
   c. solutions (by vehicle)
   d. solutions (by contents)
   e. solutions (by site or method of administration)
   f. dispersions (by size of the dispersed ingredients)

4. Go to a community or retail pharmacy and make a list of five over-the-counter (OTC) products of acetaminophen in as many different dose forms as you can identify. For each product on your list, give the manufacturer, the brand name, the active and inactive ingredient(s), and the dose form/delivery system.

5. Different dose forms have different pros and cons. For example, tablets and capsules are premeasured (pro) but may be difficult for some patients to swallow (con). Create a table comparing the ease of administration, dangers of contamination, duration of shelf life, ease of self-administration, suitability for patients of various ages or conditions, uniformity of dose size, control of dose rate, and site of application for each dose form.

Dose Form	Advantages	Disadvantages
a. tablets		
b. capsules		
c. injections (IM and SC)		
d. IV infusions		
e. syrup		
f. sublingual tablet		
g. transdermal patch		
h. suppository		

Improving Communication Skills

1. A prescription has been brought in for a steroid cream (0.25%) to be applied to an infant's eczema on the cheeks. The mother states that she has the same drug at home in an ointment (1%) and wants to know whether she should just use what she has at home, because the drug is expensive. Creams and ointments are very different, and in this case the strength is different as well. What will the pharmacist tell this mother about the differences between the two products?

2. A young man has come in to pick up some prescriptions for his asthma. His physician has just changed his prescription from oral prednisone to an inhaled steroid to control an exacerbation of his asthma. The physician told the patient that the inhaled product would be safer for him in the long run. Why? What are the advantages of the inhaled products over the oral tablets?

3. An older man has just picked up two prescriptions for nitroglycerin. One was for sublingual tablets and the other was for transdermal patches. Why is the patient using two different forms of the same drug? What are the advantages of each?

Internet Research

1. Go to the Web site of the Association of Natural Medicine Pharmacists (www.anmp.org) and locate the primary indication, dosage, and clinical efficacy of the following natural medicines:
   a. Gingko
   b. Saw Palmetto
   c. Ginger

2. Go to www.consumerlab.com and check laboratory testing results for gingko biloba and saw palmetto. Report your findings.

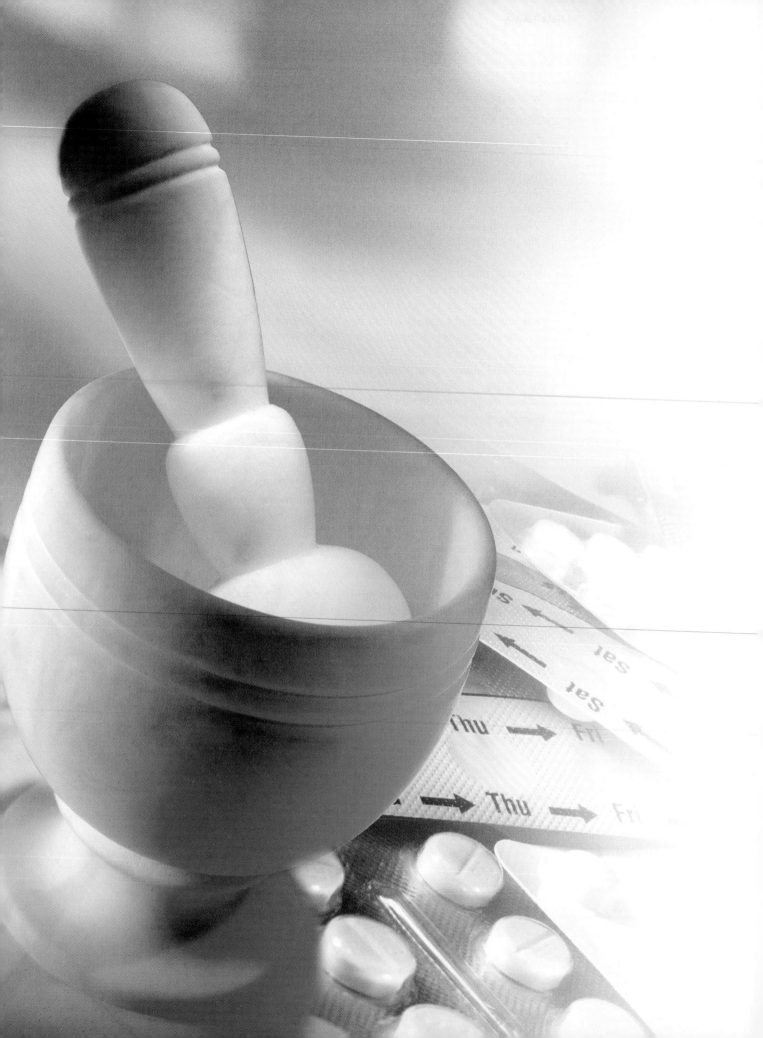

Routes of Drug Administration

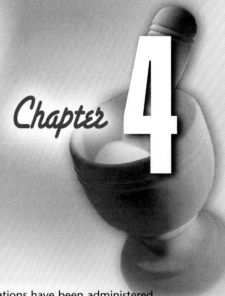

Chapter 4

Learning Objectives

- Define the phrase *route of administration*.
- Identify the factors that can influence the route of administration.
- Define the terms *local use* and *systemic use,* and explain how these uses are considered when a prescriber selects a drug for a particular patient.
- List the major routes of administration and the advantages and disadvantages associated with each dose form.
- Discuss correct techniques for administration of oral, topical, and parenteral dose forms including IV, IM, ID, and subcutaneous.

S ince ancient times, medications have been administered orally and topically. In the modern era, a wide variety of additional ways to get medications into the body have been developed. This chapter discusses the various routes of drug administration including dose forms, proper technique, advantages and disadvantages, and guidelines for appropriate use. Even though the pharmacy technician does not administer medications, it is important for the technician to understand methods related to administering drugs onto or into the body.

FACTORS INFLUENCING THE ROUTE OF ADMINISTRATION

As the previous chapter explained, drugs come in many different forms. These forms have been designed by pharmaceutical scientists for administration or application to the body in a wide variety of ways. Many factors determine the choice of **route of administration**, or way of getting a drug onto or into the body.

Ease of Administration

Prescribers will assess particular qualities or characteristics to determine the route of administration chosen for a particular patient. In some situations, patients are unable, because of lack of consciousness, to perform an action such as swallowing a tablet, capsule, or liquid. A very young or an older adult patient might have difficulty swallowing, and in such a case the healthcare provider might have to avoid solid, orally administered dose forms in favor of oral, liquid dose forms or nonoral routes of administration. An oral route of administration might also be inadvisable for a patient experiencing nausea and vomiting, which may expel the drug prematurely from the body.

Site of Action

One obvious factor affecting the choice of route of administration is the desired site of action of the drug. A major distinction can be drawn between drugs intended for local or systemic use. The term **local use** refers to site-specific applications of drugs, for example, when one applies an analgesic ointment to a minor burn or takes an antacid for local relief of excessive gastric acid. The term **systemic use** refers to the application of a drug to the site of action by means of absorption into the blood and subsequent transportation throughout the body. Even when a drug is meant for systemic administration, it still is usually targeted to a specific site of action. The nature of the disease state being treated and the drugs and dose forms available aid the physician in determining the route for which a medication is best suited.

Onset of Action

Different routes of administration have different onset rates. Oral medications for systemic use must proceed through a series of discrete steps such as dissolution in the stomach, absorption in the stomach or small intestine, biotransformation in the liver, and finally tissue distribution before they exert their **therapeutic effect**. Some medications have molecules that are too large to be absorbed, or they are broken down too rapidly in the stomach or in the liver and cannot be taken orally. Liquid solutions or suspensions will work faster than oral tablets or capsules because the medication is more readily available for absorption. Special formulations, such as tablets placed under the tongue or gum placed between the cheek and gums, will work quickly because the medication bypasses the stomach and liver and proceeds directly into the bloodstream.

In general, the fastest method of administration for action within the body is intravenously. The drug is injected or infused directly into the bloodstream and carried immediately throughout the body. Injections in the muscle or skin generally will work faster than swallowing tablets or capsules. Topical medications, especially those applied to the skin, instilled into the eye, or inhaled into the lungs, work quickly because of their localized therapeutic effects.

Duration of Action

A route of administration of a drug may be chosen on the basis of its action over a period of time, which is also known as its **duration of action**. A controlled- or extended-release tablet may last for 12 to 24 hours compared with 4 to 6 hours with the same drug in an immediate-release formulation. Many pharmaceutical companies develop long-acting drug formulations to extend the "patent life" of their brand name products. Another example, a transdermal patch, can be used to deliver small amounts of a drug steadily over many hours or even days; this route may be beneficial for patients who forget to take their dose at the scheduled time. A similar sustained-duration effect can be achieved by means of a continuous intravenous (IV) infusion. Injections into the muscle and skin will last longer than injections directly into the bloodstream, thus requiring less need for repeat doses.

Quantity of Drug

Sometimes a route of administration is chosen because of the amount of a drug that must be delivered. A tablet containing a lot of filler, or diluent, might be a preferred method for administering a drug containing a very small amount (e.g., 0.5 mg) of an active ingredient. IV infusion is an excellent method for systemic delivery of large quantities of material, such as blood or glucose, which are rapidly diluted in the bloodstream. IV injections and infusions can also deliver a higher dose of medication to the target site, which is important in the case of serious illnesses such as cancer treatments or severe bacterial infection.

Metabolism by the Liver or Excretion by the Kidney

The liver or kidney eliminates most drugs. Liver metabolism generally breaks down active drug to inactive *metabolites* for elimination and to prevent drug accumulation. The liver may prematurely break down some drugs before the active drug has a chance to work. This is called the **first-pass effect** and influences the activity of several drugs such as nitrates, including nitroglycerin. Such drugs have to be given in large oral doses or by another route of administration to bypass or overcome metabolism by the liver. This is often the reason that the dose of an oral drug is many times greater than the injectable dose of the same medication.

If patients have age-related or disease-related changes in liver or kidney function, then it is possible that the drug can accumulate and cause toxicity. This possible side effect is a major reason why older patients are often prescribed lower doses of medication (their kidneys are less efficient in eliminating the drug, especially if they have other diseases such as diabetes or high blood pressure that can adversely affect kidney function). If patients are on multiple potent prescription drugs, then the risk of a drug-drug interaction causing drug accumulation and toxic blood levels increases.

Toxicity

Toxicology is the study of toxic effects of drugs or other substances on the body. Drugs are potent substances, and the physician must often weigh the therapeutic benefit against the risk of toxicity. Some drugs, like the heart drug digoxin or the asthma drug theophylline, have a narrow therapeutic-toxic index called the "therapeutic window." This means very little difference exists in the therapeutic versus toxic blood level. These drugs require a high level of drug monitoring, and often laboratory drug levels are ordered if the physician suspects toxicity.

Sometimes the toxicity of a drug directly affects the route of administration chosen. For example, a caustic drug that might cause injury if delivered intravenously might be delivered orally instead. On the other hand, if a drug is too painful or the dose too large to give as an injection into the muscle or the skin, then it may be administered orally or even intravenously.

ORAL ROUTES OF ADMINISTRATION

Medication administration for absorption along the gastrointestinal (GI) tract into systemic circulation is referred to as *oral*. However, the term *oral* sometimes also refers to applying topically to the mouth (as in the local treatment of a cold sore). The abbreviation *po* (from the Latin *per os*) is used to indicate the oral route of medication administration. Other common abbreviations are listed in Appendix A.

Oral Dose Forms

Tablets, capsules, liquids, solutions, suspensions, syrups, and elixirs are common dose forms for **oral administration** of drugs. Sublingual and buccal tablets are unique oral dose forms. In **sublingual administration**, the drug is placed under the tongue, where it is rapidly absorbed by the sublingual mucosa. In **buccal administration**, the drug is placed between the gums and the inner lining of the cheek, in the so-called buccal pouch, where it is absorbed by the buccal mucosa. Dose forms for sublingual and buccal administration include tablets and lozenges or gum.

The oral route of drug administration is convenient, well tolerated, and easy to take or administer in most instances. Capsules are preferred over tablets for patients who have difficulty swallowing. For most medications, water is preferred over using coffee, tea, juices, or carbonated drinks to aid in the swallowing process. Some medication is suitable to be sprinkled on food when swallowing a solid is difficult for the patient. Liquid doses are generally swallowed more easily and are suitable for patients having swallowing difficulties or for small children.

Advantages and Disadvantages of the Oral Route

The oral route of administration is by far the most common because of the ease and safety of administration. In the case of capsules or tablets, the active ingredient is generally contained in powders or granules. These dissolve in the GI tract, and the active ingredient becomes available for absorption into the bloodstream.

Safety Note

The oral route is not appropriate for patients who are unable to swallow.

Disadvantages of the oral route include (1) delayed onset because the dose form must disintegrate before it is absorbed and (2) destruction or dilution of the drug by GI fluids and/or food or drink present in the stomach or intestines. The oral route is not indicated in patients who are experiencing nausea or vomiting or who are comatose, sedated, or otherwise unable to swallow. Unpleasant taste is another disadvantage of some liquid dose forms, requiring that the taste be masked by flavorings to promote compliance.

Sublingual (and to some extent the buccal route) administration of medications has a very rapid onset (less than 5 minutes) and is thus appropriate for immediate relief, as in the use of nitroglycerin sublingual tablets for treatment of chest pain as a result of angina pectoris. The rapid onset is the result of the medication entering the bloodstream directly without passage through the stomach or breakdown in the liver. A disadvantage of the sublingual tablets is their short duration of action (less than 30 to 60 minutes), making this route of administration inappropriate for routine delivery of medication. General disadvantages of the buccal route are medicinal taste and local mouth irritation.

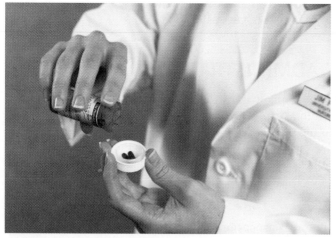

Capsules are a commonly used dose form because they are easy and safe to dispense.

Dispensing and Administering Oral Medications

Patients should be told not to crush tablets or open capsules intended to be swallowed whole, such as sustained-release, long-acting, and enteric-coated drugs. They should also be told what foods to take (and not take) the medication with, as well as what behaviors to avoid while taking the medication (e.g., sun exposure, driving). The dispensed drug will generally include colorful "auxiliary" labels to remind the patient what to do (or not do) while taking a particular medication.

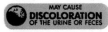
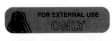
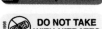
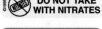
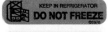
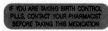
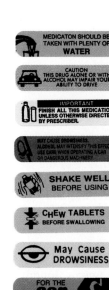
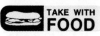
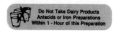
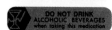

The pharmacist often adds additional labels to the prescription vial or container to further explain proper use to patients and inform them of certain precautions.

Safety Note

Always check the manufacturer recommendations for storage and expiration dating on reconstituted products.

Safety Note

If nicotine gum is chewed vigorously, then too much nicotine will be released, causing unpleasant side effects.

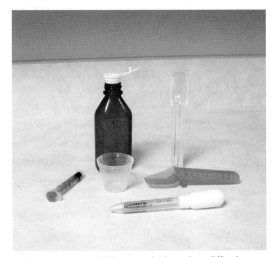

Infants or young children might have less difficulty taking liquid medication that is administered with one of these devices.

Patients who can swallow but have difficulty in swallowing solids should be instructed to place the dose on the back of the tongue and tilt the head forward. Tilting the head forward stimulates swallowing.

It is important to remind the patient or parent that the medication dose in liquid form should be accurately measured in a medication cup or medication measuring spoon. Common household utensils often are not accurate measurements of a "teaspoonful" or "tablespoonful." An oral syringe (without the needle) or measuring dropper may be used to administer an oral liquid medication slowly to patients who cannot open their mouths or for infants or small children. If the liquid medication is a suspension, then patients should be reminded to store properly and shake the bottle before dosing. The expiration date for most pediatric antibiotic suspensions "reconstituted" or mixed with water is 7 days at room temperature and 14 days if stored in the refrigerator.

Sublingual nitroglycerin tablets should be stored in their original container (brown bottle) with the lid screwed on tightly to prevent sunlight and air from causing a loss of potency. Patients should be given instructions on the proper storage of nitroglycerin. The use of pillboxes is not recommended for these tablets. Physicians usually advise patients to refill their nitroglycerin with a fresh bottle every 6 months.

An example of a buccally administered medication is nicotine gum or lozenge for smoking cessation. It is important that the patient understand the difference between chewing gum and taking nicotine gum. Counseling on the proper technique for administration of the nicotine gum is as follows:

1. Chew the gum slowly and stop chewing when you notice a tingling sensation in the mouth.
2. "Park" the gum between the cheek and gum, and leave it there until the taste or tingling sensation is almost gone.
3. Resume slowly chewing a few more times until the taste or sensation returns.
4. Park the gum again in a different place in the mouth.
5. Continue this chewing and parking process until the taste or tingle no longer returns when the gum is chewed (usually 30 minutes).

If the nicotine gum is chewed vigorously like chewing gum, too much nicotine will be released, causing unpleasant side effects. The proper administration allows the gum to release the nicotine slowly and decrease cravings.

The lozenge should be allowed to dissolve slowly over a 30-minute period without chewing or swallowing. A similar tingling sensation (from the release of nicotine) is expected. The patient should shift the lozenge to different areas of the mouth. It is important to remind the patient not to eat or drink for 15 minutes before or while using gum or lozenge dose forms.

TOPICAL ROUTES OF ADMINISTRATION

Topical administration is the application of a drug directly to the surface of the skin. However, a broader definition of topical includes the administration of drugs to any mucous membrane such as the eye, nose, ears, lungs, vagina, urethra, and colon.

Topical Dose Forms

Dose forms for topical administration commonly include creams, ointments, lotions, gels, transdermal patches, or disks for the skin; solutions, suspensions, or ointments for the eye or ear; aerosol and nonaerosol sprays and powders for the nose and lungs; tablets, creams, or ointments for the vagina; inserts for the urethra; and suppositories, creams, ointments, solutions, and foams for the rectum.

Transdermal administration is designed to deliver a drug to the bloodstream via absorption through the skin via a patch or disk. Although the skin presents a barrier, absorption does occur slowly; therapeutic effects may last for 24 hours up to 1 week. Chemicals in the patch or disk will force the drug across the membranes of the skin and into the layer of skin where optimal absorption into the bloodstream will occur.

Ocular administration is the application of a drug to the eye. Conjunctival administration is the application of a drug to the conjunctival mucosa, the lining of the inside of the eyelid. Nasal administration is the application of a drug into the passages of the nose. Otic administration is the application of a drug to the ear canal.

Rectal dose forms are usually suppositories. A suppository is a solid dose form that is formulated from a base such as cocoa butter or glycerin to melt in the rectum at body temperature and release the active drug. Creams, ointments, and foams are also used for their local effects. Rectal solutions, or enemas, are used for cleansing the bowel, for laxative or cathartic action, or for drug administration in colon disease.

Advantages and Disadvantages of the Topical Route

Drugs are administered topically primarily to take advantage of their local therapeutic effects. Most drugs applied topically are not designed to be well absorbed into the deeper layers of the skin or mucous membrane. For example, most mild cases of poison ivy may be treated with an over-the-counter (OTC) product like hydrocortisone cream; if the equivalent tablets were administered, then the risk of side effects would be much greater. Alternatively, an asthmatic may have faster relief and fewer side effects with an inhaled medication instead of a tablet or capsule. Drugs given topically for local effects include anesthetics, anti-inflammatories, antifungals, antiseptics, astringents, moisturizers, pediculicides (for killing lice), protectants (e.g., sunscreen), and scabicides (for killing mites).

The transdermal route offers a method of administering medications that will provide a steady level of drug in the system. Drugs such as nicotine, nitroglycerin, narcotic analgesics, clonidine, scopolamine, estrogen, and testosterone are administered topically for their systemic effects on smoking cessation, chest pain, chronic pain, blood pressure, motion sickness (on cruises), and hormone replacement therapy respectively. The main disadvantages of the patch are cost and occasional skin irritation at the site.

The ocular, conjunctival, nasal, and otic routes of administration are almost always prescribed for local effects, to treat conditions of the eye, the nose or sinuses, or the ear. Sprays for inhalation through the nose, however, may be used for either local or systemic effects. Some ophthalmic and nasal medications have systemic side effects and precautions are advised if the patient has selected medical conditions. For OTC medications the label should be consulted for appropriate use of the product.

The **intrarespiratory route** of administration is defined as the application of a drug through inhalation into the lungs, typically through the mouth. The usual dose form is an aerosol. "Environmentally friendly" propellants are now required by the government to replace chlorofluorocarbons (CFCs) because of concerns about adverse effect on the Earth's ozone layer. A **metered-dose inhaler (MDI)** is a common device used to administer an aerosolized drug into the lungs. A diskus is a newer dosage form to administer the drug as a micronized powder to the lungs.

The lungs are designed for the exchange of gases from the tissues into the bloodstream, and serve as an excellent site for the absorption of drugs. General anesthetic gases are also administered via inhalation for surgical or office procedures. Entry into the bloodstream is extremely rapid, second only to IV injections or infusions. This route is primarily used to deliver bronchodilators and anti-inflammatory drugs to asthma sufferers. An example would be the "rescue" medication albuterol, which is commonly prescribed for an asthmatic with acute onset of shortness of breath. The major disadvantage of MDIs is poor inhalation technique by the patient, thus decreasing the amount of drug reaching into the pulmonary circulation.

The **vaginal route** of administration is application of a drug within the vagina; common dose forms include emulsion foams, inserts, ointments, solutions, sponges, suppositories, and tablets. Generally speaking, this route of administration is for local effects such as cleansing (e.g., douches), contraception, or treatment of common bacterial or yeast infections. The major disadvantage is inconvenience and "messiness" of the creams and ointments.

The **urethral route** of administration is application of a drug to or within the urethra; common dose forms include solutions and suppositories. Drugs delivered by this route may be effective in treating incontinence or impotence in men. Inconvenience and localized pain would be considered disadvantages.

Rectal administration may be a preferred method of delivery for systemic drugs in four situations: (1) when an oral drug might be destroyed or diluted by acidic fluids in the stomach; (2) when an oral drug might be too readily metabolized by the liver and eliminated from the body; (3) when the patient is unconscious and needs medication; and (4) when the patient may be unable to take oral drugs because of nausea and vomiting or severe acute illness in the GI tract.

Rectal doses do not transverse the digestive system for absorption and can be used in both young children and adults. For example, a young child with a high fever who will not (or cannot) take an oral liquid may need an acetaminophen suppository; an adult with severe nausea and vomiting from a bad case of the flu, or perhaps cancer chemotherapy, may require a suppository to treat the acute symptoms and prevent dehydration.

A major disadvantage of the rectal route of administration is its inconvenience. Another disadvantage is erratic and irregular drug absorption. However, such a route is often preferable for its local effects in treating hemorrhoids, relieving constipation, cleansing the rectum over a short period of time, or relieving acute symptoms from a diseased intestinal tract.

Dispensing and Administering Topical Medications

Topical administration of drugs can provide a therapeutic effect at the desired part of the body while minimizing side effects and adverse reactions that may be more prevalent when a drug is systemically absorbed in the body. It is important for the patient to fully understand the appropriate use and administration of each topical drug at the time of dispensing. Improper technique or overuse of topical drugs can increase the risk of side effects or alter drug efficacy.

Ointments, Creams, Lotions, and Gels Topical dose forms are applied to the skin for local or systemic effects. The patient or healthcare giver should apply the dose form as directed. Ointments, lotions, creams, and gels are generally applied to the skin. Lotions, creams, and gels are worked into the skin, whereas ointments are skin protectants and do not work into the skin but stay on the surface.

Some topicals require special precautions and counseling for proper application. For example, with nitroglycerin ointment the patient or caregiver should wear gloves to avoid absorbing excessive amounts of drug, which could cause a headache. Many topical corticosteroids exist, from mild OTC hydrocortisone to very potent prescription agents. Most of these drugs are applied sparingly to affected areas of the body for short periods of time; some steroids cannot be applied to the face. Unless directed by the physician, the affected area should not be covered up with a bandage or other dressing (or, in the case of an infant, a diaper), because occlusive dressings can significantly increase drug absorption and the risk of side effects. The overuse of potent topical corticosteroids can lead to serious systemic side effects.

Transdermal Patches The site of administration for patches should be rotated and relatively hair free; patches should not be placed over a large area of scar tissue, which may decrease the release of the drug. Some patches are replaced every day, whereas others maintain their therapeutic effect for 3 to 7 days depending on the product. Most physicians advise their patients to remove the nitroglycerin patch at bedtime to prevent **drug tolerance** from developing. Drug tolerance occurs when the body requires higher doses of drug to produce the same therapeutic effect. Patients should be advised to carefully discard their used patches; the nicotine patch, for example, could cause serious side effects if ingested by young children or pets. Some forms of the testosterone patch give best results when applied to the skin of the scrotum in the male with a documented hormone deficiency.

Ophthalmic Medications Ophthalmics must be at room temperature or body temperature before application. All medications should be stored according to the package information (to reduce bacterial growth and ensure the drug's stability). Ophthalmic medications are considered sterile products. Only medications with preservatives can be repeatedly used.

Before application the patient should be advised to wash the hands to prevent contamination of the site of application or the medication. The opening of the container (i.e., tube or dropper) should not touch the application site, or the medication may become contaminated. The eye is prone to infection, and only sterile ophthalmic solutions or suspensions should be used. For example, an otic medication for the ear cannot be dispensed as an ophthalmic medication even if it contains the same drugs and concentration! Some products are *unit of use* (i.e., they are to be used for one administration only and then discarded).

Previously applied medications should be cleaned away, as should any drainage from the eye. Cotton balls work well for this purpose. The intended location is the conjunctiva. Poorly administered eyedrops could result in loss of medication through

Figure 4.1

Administering Ophthalmic Medication
(a) Drops.
(b) Ointment.

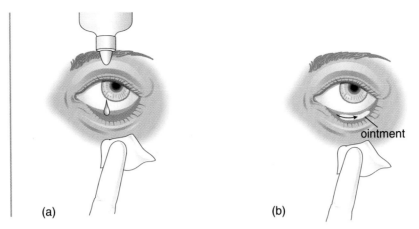

(a)   (b)

ointment

the tear duct, whereas poorly placed ointments may be distributed over the eyelids and lashes.

To apply either drops or ointment, the patient's head should be tilted back. Once the medication is administered, it is important for the patient to place a finger in the corner of the eye, next to the nose, to gently close the duct thus preventing loss of medication through the tear duct. The patient should also keep the eye closed for 1 or 2 minutes after application. Figure 4.1 shows the application of both ophthalmic drops and ointment.

When multiple drops of more than one medication are to be administered, the patient should be advised to wait 5 minutes between different medications or the first drop may be washed away. If an ointment and a drop are to be used together, the drop is used first; then the patient should wait 10 minutes before applying the ointment. Ointments are generally applied at night; they are the drug form of choice when extended contact with the medication is desired, because tears wash them out less easily. (The patient should be reminded that he or she might experience some temporary blurring of vision after application.)

Otic Medications Like ophthalmics, otics must be at room temperature or body temperature. Heated drops may cause rupturing of the eardrum. Cold drops can cause vertigo and discomfort. Alcohol causes pain and burning sensation and therefore should not be used if the patient has a ruptured tympanic membrane (eardrum). Alcohol may cause additional damage to the middle ear. If eardrum damage is suspected, then a low-alcohol content solution or suspension should be used.

The head is tilted to the side with the ear facing up (Figure 4.2). Anyone 3 years or older should have the lobes pulled up and back. Children under 3 years of age should have their ear lobes pulled down and back. The head should remain tilted for 2 to 5 minutes. Cotton swabs placed in the ear after administration of drops will prevent excess medication

Figure 4.2

Administering Otic Medications
(a) Children over 3 years of age and adults should have their lobes pulled up and back when otic medications are administered. (b) Children under 3 years old should have their lobes pulled down and back.

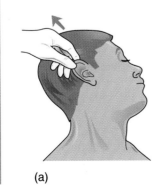

(a)

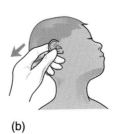

(b)

from dripping out of the ear. The swabs will not reduce the amount of drug that is absorbed.

Nasal Medications Nasal medications are applied by drops (instillation), sprays, or aerosol (i.e., spray under pressure). Application may be for relief of nasal congestion or allergy symptoms. Flu vaccine may also be administered via the nose. The patient should be instructed to tilt the head back, insert the dropper or spray or aerosol tip into the nostril, point it toward the eyes, and apply the prescribed number of drops or sprays (and repeat the process in the other nostril if indicated). Breathing should be through the mouth to avoid sniffing the medication into the sinuses. It is very important that the patient not overuse nasal decongestants and to follow label instructions carefully.

Inhaled Medications The metered-dose inhaler (MDI) provides medication with compressed gas. The MDI will deliver a specific, measured amount of medication each time the device is activated. If the MDI contains a steroid, then the patient should rinse the mouth thoroughly after receiving a dose to prevent a fungal infection in the mouth. Some devices use a powder or nonaerosolized spray for inhalation to avoid the compressed gas.

Proper administration of aerosolized medications is extremely important to ensure that medication reaches the lungs to control or relieve symptoms. The following technique is recommended:

1. Shake the canister well (otherwise only propellant may be administered).
2. "Prime" the canister by pressing down and activating a practice dose.
3. Prepare the MDI by inserting the canister into a mouthpiece or spacer to reduce the amount of drug deposited on the back of the throat. (This is especially helpful for young children or older adults who may have difficulty with eye-hand coordination.)
4. Breathe out and hold the spacer between the lips making a seal.
5. Activate the MDI and take a deep, slow inhalation at the same time.
6. Hold the breath briefly and slowly exhale through the nose.

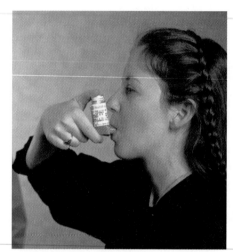

A metered-dose inhaler (MDI) is a common device used to administer a drug through inhalation into the lungs.

Another route of inhaled medication administration includes a nebulizer that creates a mist when a stream of air flows over a liquid. This route is commonly utilized for young children or elderly patients with asthma or lung disease.

Vaginal Medications Vaginal dose applications are generally indicated for bacterial or fungal infection or for hormone replacement therapy. The patient is instructed to use the medication for the prescribed period to ensure effective treatment. Many vaginal creams or ointments are delivered to the site with the use of an applicator tube.

If the medication is to be applied with an applicator, then the application should follow a specific technique:

1. Begin with an empty bladder and washed hands.
2. Open the container and place the dose in the applicator.
3. Lubricate the applicator with a water-soluble lubricant if it is not prelubricated.

4. Lie down, spread the legs, open the labia with one hand, and insert the applicator about 2 inches into the vagina with the other hand. (An alternative application is to insert the applicator and medication by standing with one foot on the edge of a bathtub.)
5. Release the labia; the free hand is used to push the applicator plunger, releasing the medication.
6. Withdraw the applicator and wash the hands.

Rectal Medications The patient or caregiver should be instructed to be sure the suppository is removed from its package. The suppository should then be inserted, small tapered end first, into the rectum with the index finger for the full length of the finger. The suppository may need to be lubricated with a water-soluble gel to ease insertion.

Safety Note
Refrigeration may make insertion of rectal medications easier in warm climates.

Another rectal dose form is the enema. An enema is a rectal injection of a solution used most commonly to evacuate the bowels for diagnostic procedures involving the lower GI tract.

PARENTERAL ROUTES OF ADMINISTRATION

Parenteral forms deserve special attention because of complexity, widespread use, and potential for therapeutic benefit and danger. The term *parenteral* comes from the Greek words *para,* meaning *outside,* and *enteron,* meaning *the intestine.* The derivation of the word refers to the fact that this route of administration bypasses the alimentary canal. Parenteral administration is injection or infusion by means of a needle or catheter inserted into the body. An IV injection or infusion goes directly into the bloodstream.

Parenteral Dose Forms

Parenteral preparations must be sterile (i.e., free of microorganisms). These medications are best prepared using aseptic techniques, special clothing (e.g., gowns, masks, hair net, gloves), and *laminar flow hoods* placed in special rooms to ensure sterility. Germ theory and aseptic technique are covered in more detail in Chapter 10, *Infection Control and Safe Handling of Hazardous Agents.*

Injections may be made into almost any part of the body. The most common sort of injection or infusion is one done by the IV route, directly into a vein. In the hospital and many home health-care pharmacies, antibiotics, chemotherapy, nutrition, and critical care medications are administered via this route. Other common forms of parenteral administration are intramuscular (IM) injections made into a muscle, subcutaneous injections made under the skin, and intradermal (ID) injections made into the skin.

Disposable syringes and needles are used to administer drugs by injection. Different sizes are available depending on the type of medication and injection needed.

Advantages and Disadvantages of the Parenteral Route

The IV route is the fastest of all methods for delivering systemic drugs, so it is the preferred administration in an emergency situation. It can also provide needed fluids, electrolytes, and nutrition to patients preoperatively or postoperatively who cannot take food or who have serious GI tract problems. The IV route provides a higher concentration of drug to the bloodstream or tissues, which is advantageous in the case of a serious bacterial infection. An IV infusion provides a continuous amount of needed medication without the fluctuation in blood levels experienced with other routes of administration; the infusion rate can be adjusted to provide more or less medication as the situation dictates.

The IV route does have associated dangers, including traumatic injury from the insertion of the needle or catheter into the body and the potential for introducing toxic agents, microbes, or pyrogens (i.e., fever-producing byproducts of microbial metabolism). If medication is injected directly into the body, then it is impossible to retrieve the drug if an adverse reaction occurs.

The intramuscular (IM) and subcutaneous routes of administration offer a convenient way to deliver medications. Although the onset of response of the medication is slower than the IV route, the duration of action is much longer, making it more practical for use outside the hospital. These routes are often used for drugs like insulin or heparin, which are not active if taken orally. The injection site needs to be "prepped" by use of an alcohol wipe and the correct syringe, needle, and technique must be used. With long-term use, the rotation of injection sites is important to prevent scarring and other skin changes that can influence drug absorption.

The major use of the intradermal (ID) route of administration is for diagnostic and allergy skin testing. If the patient is allergic or has been exposed to an allergen similar to tuberculosis (TB), then the patient may experience a severe local reaction.

Safety Note

Do not use SQ or SC abbreviations. Instead, write out *subcutaneous* to minimize potential medication errors.

Dispensing and Administering Parenteral Medications

The body is primarily an aqueous, or water-containing, vehicle; therefore, most parenteral preparations introduced into the body are made up of ingredients placed in a sterile-water medium. Parenteral preparations are either solutions (in which ingredients are dissolved with water or normal saline) or, much less commonly, suspensions (in which ingredients are suspended). IV injections and infusions must be free of air bubbles and particulate matter. The introduction of air or particles might cause an embolism, or blockage, in a vessel or a severe painful reaction at the injection site.

Intravenous Injections or Infusions IV drug administration, by injection or by infusion, is an extremely fast-acting route because the drug goes directly into the bloodstream. Because of the rapid delivery, IV injection and infusion are often used in the emergency department and in critical care areas. Not only is the IV route used for drug administration, but also it is commonly used for fluid and electrolyte replacement, as well as to provide necessary nutrition to the patient who is critically ill. Although other sites are also used, injections and infusions are usually administered into the superficial veins of the arm on the side opposite the elbow. Figure 4.3 shows an IV injection.

Intramuscular Injections IM injections are slower in delivery but longer in duration than IV injections. Care must be taken with deep IM injections to avoid hitting a vein, artery, or nerve. In adults, IM injections are generally given into the upper,

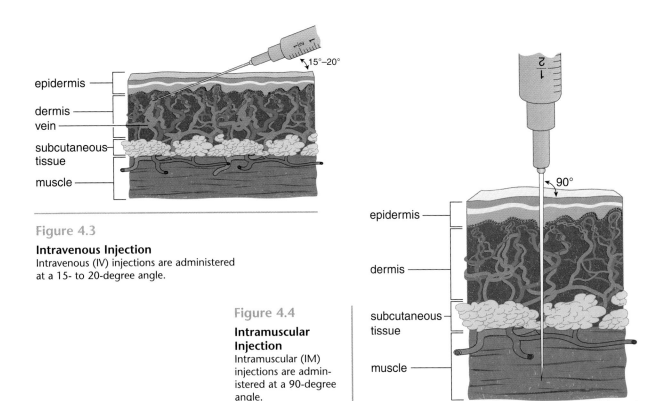

epidermis
dermis
vein
subcutaneous tissue
muscle

15°–20°

Figure 4.3

Intravenous Injection
Intravenous (IV) injections are administered at a 15- to 20-degree angle.

Figure 4.4

Intramuscular Injection
Intramuscular (IM) injections are administered at a 90-degree angle.

epidermis
dermis
subcutaneous tissue
muscle

90°

outer portion of the gluteus maximus, the large muscle on either side of the buttocks. Another common site, especially for children, is the deltoid muscles of the shoulders. The typical needle used for IM injections is a 22- to 25-gauge, ½ - to 1- inch needle.

The volume of injection is limited to less than 3 mL. The IM route is used to administer antibiotics, vitamins, iron, and several vaccines. The absorption of the drug by the IM route is often unpredictable in a patient who is unconscious or in a shocklike state; thus it is not recommended for these patients. Figure 4.4 shows the needle angle and injection depth for an IM injection.

Intradermal Injections ID injections, given into the more capillary-rich layer just below the epidermis (Figure 4.5), are given for local anesthesia and for various diagnostic tests and immunizations. Common examples of ID injections include a skin test for tuberculosis (TB) or fungal infections; the typical site is the upper forearm, below the area where IV injections are given. Another example of ID injections is allergy skin testing in which small amounts of various allergens are administered (usually on the back) to detect allergies before beginning desensitization "allergy shots."

Safety Note

To minimize medication errors, do not use SC or SQ as an abbreviation for subcutaneous.

Subcutaneous Injections Subcutaneous injections administer parenteral medications below the skin into the subcutaneous fat. Depending on the medication, a subcutaneous injection will often have a longer onset of action and a longer duration of action compared with an IM or IV injection. Subcutaneous injections are given just beneath the skin with the syringe held at a 45-degree angle (Figure 4.6), usually on the outside of the upper arm, the top of the thigh, or the lower portion of each side of the abdomen. In lean older patients with less tissue and obese patients with more tissue, the syringe should be held at more of a 90-degree angle. The needle used is normally a 25- or 26-gauge needle of ⅜ to ⅝ inch in length. The correct

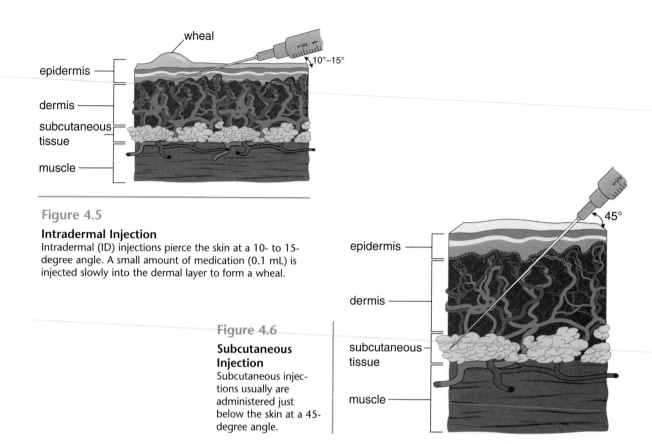

Figure 4.5

Intradermal Injection
Intradermal (ID) injections pierce the skin at a 10- to 15-degree angle. A small amount of medication (0.1 mL) is injected slowly into the dermal layer to form a wheal.

Figure 4.6

Subcutaneous Injection
Subcutaneous injections usually are administered just below the skin at a 45-degree angle.

length of the needle is determined by a skin pinch in the injection area. The proper needle length will be one half the thickness of the pinch. Subcutaneous injections should not be made into grossly adipose, hardened, inflamed, or swollen tissue. To avoid pressure on sensory nerves causing pain and discomfort, no more than 1.5 mL should be injected into the site.

Insulin, the most common type of subcutaneous injection, is given using 28- to 30-gauge short needles in a special syringe that measures the drug in units. The patient should carefully administer the insulin following a plan for site rotation. The site of insulin administration must be rotated to avoid or minimize local skin reactions. The absorption of insulin may vary depending on the site of administration and the activity level of the patient.

Patients should be instructed to keep insulin refrigerated and to check expiration dates frequently. Opened vials should generally be discarded after 1 month, because the insulin can lose its potency even if stored in ideal conditions. A vial of insulin is agitated and warmed by rolling between the hands and should never be shaken. The rubber stopper should be wiped with an alcohol wipe. The approximate amount of air should be injected into the vial equal to the amount of insulin to be withdrawn. To remove air bubbles from the syringe, the patient should hold the syringe needle up and tap it lightly. The air is gently pushed from the syringe with the plunger. The patient should be cautioned about planning meals, exercise, and insulin administration to gain the best advantage of the medication and avoid the chances of creating hypoglycemia.

Other common medications administered by this route include epinephrine (or adrenaline) for emergency asthmatic attacks or allergic reactions, heparin or low-molecular–weight heparins like Lovenox to prevent blood clots, sumatriptan or Imitrex for migraines, and many vaccines.

Safety Note
Do not shake insulin.

Chapter Terms

buccal administration oral administration in which a drug is placed between the gums and the inner lining of the cheek

drug tolerance occurs when the body requires higher doses of a drug to produce the same therapeutic effect

duration of action length of time a drug gives the desired response or is at the therapeutic level

first-pass effect extent to which a drug is metabolized by the liver before reaching systemic circulation

intrarespiratory route administration of a drug by inhalation into the lungs

local use site-specific application of a drug

metered-dose inhaler (MDI) device used to administer a drug in the form of compressed gas through inhalation into the lungs

oral administration medication administration (through swallowing) for absorption along the GI tract into systemic circulation; can also refer to topical administration such as for local treatment on the lips or mouth

route of administration way of getting a drug onto or into the body

sublingual administration oral administration where a drug is placed under the tongue and is rapidly absorbed into the bloodstream

systemic use application of a drug by means of absorption into the bloodstream

therapeutic effect desired pharmacological action of a drug on the body

topical administration administration of a drug to the skin or any mucous membrane such as eye, nose, ears, lungs, vagina, urethra, and colon; usually administration of a drug directly to the surface of the skin

toxicology study of the toxic effects of drugs or other substances in the body

urethral route administration of a drug by insertion into the urethra

vaginal route administration of a drug by application of a cream or insertion of a tablet into the vagina

Chapter Summary

- Factors influencing the decision on route of administration include the following: ease of administration, site, onset and duration of action, the quantity to be administered, drug metabolism by the liver or excretion by the kidney, and the toxicity of the drug.
- Major routes of medication administration are oral, topical, and parenteral.
- Tablets, capsules, liquids, solutions, suspensions, syrups, and elixirs are common dose forms for oral administration of drugs.
- Oral administration also includes specially formulated sublingual or buccal tablets and lozenges.
- Topical administration includes not only medication applied to the skin but also ophthalmic, nasal, otic, inhaled, vaginal, urethral, and rectal formulations.
- Topical agents often require additional counseling in technique for proper administration.
- Parenteral administration commonly includes IV, IM, subcutaneous, and ID injections, as well as IV infusions.
- Infusions are given for a variety of purposes, including the delivery of fluids and electrolytes, nutrients, and drugs.
- IV injections and infusions are injected directly into the bloodstream and special precautions must be taken in their preparation and administration to maintain sterility and to prevent air embolism.

Chapter Review

Choose the best answer from those provided.

1. The route of administration with the fastest onset of action is
   a. sublingual.
   b. subcutaneous.
   c. intramuscular (IM).
   d. intravenous (IV).

2. Nausea and vomiting might preclude the use of a(n)
   a. parenteral route of administration.
   b. topical route of administration.
   c. oral route of administration.
   d. urethral route of administration.

3. In the first-pass effect, some drugs taken orally are rapidly metabolized, or broken down, by the
   a. small intestine.
   b. stomach.
   c. liver.
   d. kidneys.

4. The study of toxic effects of drugs or other substances on the body is
   a. pharmacology.
   b. physiology.
   c. pharmacokinetics.
   d. toxicology.

5. The most common route of administration of drugs is
   a. parenteral.
   b. topical.
   c. oral.
   d. intravenous (IV).

6. Administration of gum placed between the gums and the inner lining of the cheek is called
   a. topical.
   b. sublingual.
   c. intradermal (ID).
   d. buccal.

7. A transdermal formulation makes use of which organ of the body for its site of absorption?
   a. skin
   b. eyes
   c. ears
   d. lungs

8. Suppositories are *usually* used for
   a. rectal administration.
   b. oral administration.
   c. buccal administration.
   d. parenteral administration.

9. The word *parenteral* means, literally, *outside the*
   a. *stomach.*
   b. *intestine.*
   c. *mouth.*
   d. *liver.*

10. Insulin needles for subcutaneous administration are usually
    a. 28 gauge.
    b. 22 gauge.
    c. 18 gauge.
    d. 15 gauge.

Pharmacy in Practice

1. Nitroglycerin is an example of a drug that comes in a wide variety of dose forms appropriate for a wide variety of routes of administration. Research the different routes of administration used for nitroglycerin. Refer to Internet sites or reference works, as well as to healthcare professionals. Pose the following questions: What are the dose forms of nitroglycerin? What routes of administration are used? Why do people choose one route of administration over another? For what purposes are the various routes of administration used?

2. In a small group, discuss the advantages and disadvantages of the various routes of administration. Which is the most convenient? Safest? Fastest onset? Longest duration? Poses the most compliance problems? Present your group's opinions to the class.

3. Create a chart with a schematic diagram of the human body illustrating the various routes of administration described in this lesson. To visualize administration techniques, get an orange and use IM, suctaneous, and ID techniques to inject it with water or normal saline.

4. Check the *Physician's Desk Reference (PDR)* for the following information on reconstituted antibiotic suspensions for the following drugs: amoxicillin, Biaxin and Omnicef. How should each of these medications be stored, and what expiration date is recommended after reconstitution? What auxiliary labels are needed for each?

Improving Communication Skills

1. A patient has come in to pick up some prescriptions for fertility drugs. Some of the medications are given subcutaneous and others IM. The pharmacist has selected the appropriate syringes for them.
   a. Which of the following syringes is for the IM injection, and which is for the subcutaneous injection?

22G1½ Needle Do not reshield used needles. Discard after single use. STERILE.	**27G ½** Needle Do not reshield used needles. Discard after single use. STERILE.

   b. Prepare a brief statement for the patient explaining which syringe is used for each type of injection, as well as the technique and location used for each injection.

2. Antiviral medications are available in a variety of dose forms and use a variety of routes for administration. Often the drug, dose form, and route of administration are selected because of a specific viral infection in a specific location. Research three antiviral medications that have different dose forms and routes of administration using a source such as *Drug Facts and Comparisons*. Make a list of the three drugs you have found, and prepare a brief paragraph on the drugs and their indications. Use lay terms to describe the medical terms that you find.

Internet Research

1. Visit a drug information site, such as www.drugs.com or www.Rxlist.com and research the following drugs. For each drug identify the dose forms and the route by which each dose form is administered. Each drug is available in at least two dose forms.
   a. Imitrex
   b. Compazine
   c. Valium
   d. morphine
   e. triamcinolone
   f. Proventil

2. Go to www.baxter.com, research five specialized products for administering medications manufactured by this company, and state how each is used.

3. Visit the following site and provide information on the proper use of the Duragesic transdermal patch:
   www.fda.gov/cder/drug/infopage/fentanyl/DuragesicPPI.pd

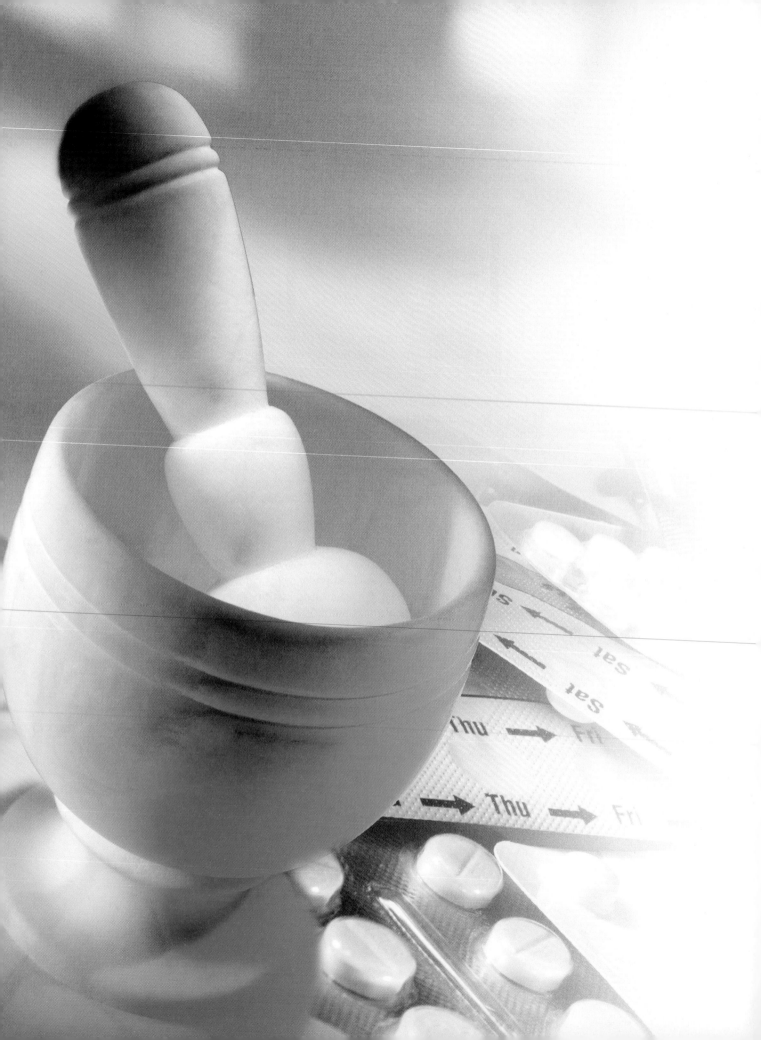

Basic Pharmaceutical Measurements and Calculations

Chapter **5**

Learning Objectives

- Describe four systems of measurement commonly used in pharmacy, and be able to convert units from one system to another.
- Explain the meanings of the prefixes most commonly used in metric measurement.
- Convert from one metric unit to another (e.g., grams to milligrams).
- Convert Roman numerals to Arabic numerals.
- Distinguish between proper, improper, and compound fractions.
- Perform basic operations with fractions, including finding the least common denominator; converting fractions to decimals; and adding, subtracting, multiplying, and dividing fractions.
- Perform basic operations with proportions, including identifying equivalent ratios and finding an unknown quantity in a proportion.
- Convert percents to and from fractions and ratios, and convert percents to decimals.
- Perform elementary dose calculations and conversions.
- Solve problems involving powder solutions and dilutions.
- Use the alligation method.

The daily activities of pharmacists and pharmacy technicians require making precise measurements. Because they measure liquids or reconstitute solutions (mixing water to a powder to make a solution) for pediatric patients, compound drugs, and prepare parenteral infusions, the amounts or quantities and calculations must always be precise. A mistake in calculation can have severe consequences such as drug toxicity. Therefore it is essential for the practicing pharmacy technician to grasp the basic measurement systems and mathematical techniques used in the field as discussed in this chapter.

SYSTEMS OF PHARMACEUTICAL MEASUREMENT

Systems of measurement are widely accepted standards used to determine such quantities as area, distance (or length), temperature, time, volume, and weight. Of these, temperature, distance, volume, and weight are the most important for the pharmacy profession.

- Quantities of temperature and weight are the simplest and most familiar.
- Distance is a measurement of extension in space in one dimension.
- Volume, the least intuitive of these quantities, is a measurement of extension in space in three dimensions (i.e., cubic volume).

Metric System

The **metric system** is the measurement system most commonly used today for pharmaceutical measurement and calculation. Developed in France in the 1700s, the metric system became the legal standard of measure in the United States in 1893. The metric system is the one to which other measurements are compared for legal purposes.

The metric system has several distinct advantages over other measurement systems:

- The metric system is based on decimal notation, in which units are described as multiples of ten (0.001, 0.01, 0.1, 1, 10, 100, 1000), and this decimal notation makes calculation simple.
- The metric system contains clear correlations among the units of measurement of length, volume, and weight, again simplifying calculation. For example, the standard metric unit for volume, the liter, is almost exactly equivalent to 1000 cubic centimeters. (A centimeter is a metric unit of length.)
- With slight variations in notation, the metric system is used worldwide, especially in scientific measurement, and so, like music, is a "universal language."

The modern metric system makes use of the standardized units of the Système International (SI), adopted by agreement among governments worldwide in 1960. Three basic units in this system are the (1) meter, (2) liter, and (3) gram. The **meter** is the unit for measuring distance, length, and area, and has limited use in pharmacy. Figure 5.1 shows an application of the metric system in measuring distance, area, and volume. Table 5.1 lists the prefixes in the SI language.

The major metric units used most commonly in pharmacy are the gram and the liter. The **gram**, the unit for measuring weight, is used for measuring the amount of medication in solid form and for indicating the amount of solid medication in a solution. The gram is the weight of 1 cubic centimeter of water at 4° C. The **liter** is the unit for measuring the volume of liquid medications and also liquids for solutions.

The metric units most commonly used in pharmacy practice, along with their abbreviations, are given in Table 5.2. Note that the same abbreviations are used for both singular and plural (e.g., 1 g, 3 g).

Figure 5.1

Measurements in the Metric System
(a) Distance or length. (b) Area. (c) Volume.

Prefixes—syllables placed at the beginnings of words—can be added to these basic metric units to specify a particular measure. Because SI is a decimal system, the prefixes denote powers of 10, as shown in Table 5.1.

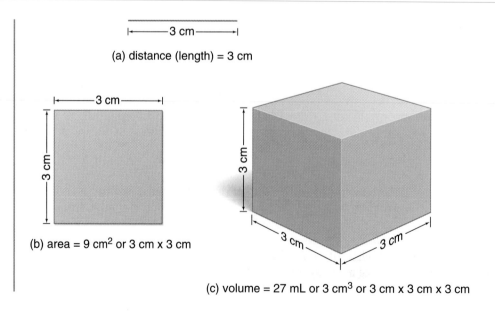

(a) distance (length) = 3 cm

(b) area = 9 cm^2 or 3 cm x 3 cm

(c) volume = 27 mL or 3 cm^3 or 3 cm x 3 cm x 3 cm

Table 5.1 Système International Prefixes

Prefix	Symbol	Meaning
micro-	mc	one millionth (basic unit $\times$ 10^{-6}, or unit $\times$ 0.000,001)
milli-	m	one thousandth (basic unit $\times$ 10^{-3}, or unit $\times$ 0.001)
centi-	c	one hundredth (basic unit $\times$ 10^{-2}, or unit $\times$ 0.01)
deci-	d	one tenth (basic unit $\times$ 10^{-1}, or unit $\times$ 0.1)
hecto-	h	one hundred times (basic unit $\times$ 10^{2}, or unit $\times$ 100)
kilo-	k	one thousand times (basic unit $\times$ 10^{3}, or unit $\times$ 1000)

Table 5.2 Common Metric Units

Measurement Unit	Equivalent
Weight: Gram	
1 gram (g)	1000 milligrams (mg)
1 milligram (mg)	1000 micrograms (mcg), one thousandth of a gram (g)
1 kilogram (kg)	1000 grams (g)
Length: Meter	
1 meter (m)	100 centimeters (cm)
1 centimeter (cm)	0.01 m; 10 millimeters (mm)
1 millimeter (mm)	0.001 m; 1000 micrometers, or microns (mcm)
Volume: Liter	
1 liter (L)	1000 milliliters (mL)
1 milliliter (mL)	0.001 L, 1000 microliters (mcL)

In prescriptions using the metric system, numbers are expressed as decimals rather than fractions. Weights are generally given in grams and volumes in milliliters.

For numbers less than 1, a zero is placed before the decimal point to prevent misreading, as in the following:

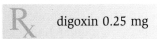 digoxin 0.25 mg

Note that an error of a single decimal place is an error by a factor of 10. It is therefore extremely important that decimals be written properly.

To convert from one metric unit to another, simply move the decimal point to the left (to convert to larger units) and to the right (to convert to smaller units). The most common metric calculations in pharmacy involve conversions to and from milliliters and liters, and to and from grams, milligrams, and kilograms. Table 5.3 shows how to do these conversions.

Common Measures

Like languages, measurement systems tend to evolve by folk processes. Thus a foot was, originally, a length approximately equal to that of the average person's foot. By its nature, common measure is approximate, and thus the metric system is the legal standard of measure in the United States. However, because many households still

Table 5.3 Common Metric Conversions

Conversion	Instruction	Example
kilograms (kg) to grams (g)	multiply by 1000 (move decimal point three places to the right)	6.25 kg = 6250 g
grams (g) to milligrams (mg)	multiply by 1000 (move decimal point three places to the right)	3.56 g = 3560 mg
milligrams (mg) to grams (g)	multiply by 0.001 (move decimal point three places to the left)	120 mg = 0.120 g
liters (L) to milliliters (mL)	multiply by 1000 (move decimal point three places to the right)	2.5 L = 2500 mL
milliliters (mL) to liters (L)	multiply by 0.001 (move decimal point three places to the left)	238 mL = 0.238 L

commonly use these common systems of measure, some U.S. pharmacies still use the common measure systems when dispensing medications.

Safety Note

For safety reasons, the use of the apothecary system is discouraged. Use the metric system.

Three types of common measures encountered in pharmacy are (1) apothecary, (2) avoirdupois, and (3) household. Table 5.4 provides a key to the symbols used in the apothecary system. Tables 5.5, 5.6, and 5.7 provide conversion equivalents for common units in these systems and compare them to the metric system.

When converting from fluid ounces to milliliters in pharmacy calculations, it is common practice to round up, for example, 29.57 mL up to 30 mL. In this chapter, use 30 mL when converting from apothecary, avoirdupois, or household measure fluid ounces. When the household system was formed, 1 f𝟥 became synonymous with 1 tsp or 5 mL, thus changing the equivalent to 6 f𝟥 = 1 f𝟪. Therefore, Table 5.5 states that there are 6 f𝟥 per 1 f𝟪 and 1 f𝟥 = 5 mL. For the purpose of this chapter, you will need to use these conversions.

Another calculation performed on a frequent basis is a conversion from ounces to grams. An apothecary ounce is 31.1 g and the avoirdupois ounce is 28.35 g. In both cases it is common practice to round to 30 g. Many physicians are accustomed to writing prescription orders in ounces of medication, in both liquid and solid forms; however, the metric system is considered more accurate and is becoming the system of choice in the United States. In addition, many pharmacy computer systems are programmed to accept only amounts with metric units.

As stated earlier, it is common practice to round a household fluid ounce (29.57 mL) up to 30 mL. When measuring this amount, it is often appropriate to make this estimation because the volume differs by such a small amount. However,

Table 5.4 Apothecary Symbols

Volume		Weight	
Unit of Measure	Symbol	Unit of Measure	Symbol
minim	♍	grain	gr
fluidram	f𝟥	scruple	Э
fluidounce	f𝟪	dram	𝟥
pint	pt	ounce	𝟪
quart	qt	pound	℔ or #
gallon	gal		

Table 5.5   Apothecary System

Measurement Unit	Equivalent within System	Metric Equivalent
Volume		
1 ℥ (℥)		0.06 mL
16.23 ℥		1 mL
1 f ℨ	60 ℥	5 mL (3.75 mL)*
1 f ℥	6 f ℨ	30 mL (29.57 mL)†
1 pt	16 f ℥	480 mL
1 qt	2 pt or 32 f ℥	960 mL
1 gal	4 qt or 8 pt	3840 mL
Weight		
1 gr		65 mg
15.432 gr		1 g
1 ℈	20 gr	1.3 g
1 ℨ	3 ℈ or 60 gr	3.9 g
1 ℥	8 ℨ or 480 gr	30 g (31.1 g)
1 #	12 ℥ or 5760 gr	373.2 g

*In reality, 1 f ℨ contains 3.75 mL; however, that number is usually rounded up to 5 mL or 1 tsp.
†In reality, 1 f ℥ contains 29.57 mL; however, that number is usually rounded up to 30 mL.

Table 5.6   Avoirdupois System

Measurement Unit	Equivalent within System	Metric Equivalent
1 gr (grain)		65 mg
1 oz (ounce)	437.5 gr	30 g (28.35 g)*
1 lb (pound)	16 oz or 7000 gr	454 g

*An avoirdupois ounce actually contains 28.34952 g; however, we often round up to 30 g. It is common practice to use 454 g as the equivalent for a pound (28.35 g × 16 oz/lb = 453.6 g/lb, rounded to 454 g/lb).

the discrepancy becomes far more apparent when measuring multiple fluid ounces that have been rounded up to the 30 mL equivalent. For example, if asked to measure a household pint (16 fl oz), one would measure roughly 480 mL. This becomes problematic as 29.57 mL multiplied by 16 is equal to only 473.12 mL, not 480 mL. Products in most stock bottles will be labeled 473 mL, yet pharmacies will bill according to the estimation of 480 mL and measure out fluid ounces in 30 mL increments. For the purposes of this chapter, use the rounded 30 mL and 480 mL.

Note that the only equivalent unit in both the apothecary and avoirdupois systems is the unit of dry measure known as the *grain*. This is the most commonly encountered nonmetric unit in pharmacy practice. Pharmacists sometimes make use of apothecaries' weights for extemporaneous compoundings that come in 5-grain, 4-grain, 3-grain, 2-grain, 1-grain, and ½-grain units. In Table 5.5, the grain is equal to 65 mg, but many other references use 60 mg instead. Most pharmacists use the 65-mg conversion.

Table 5.7 Household Measure

Measurement Unit	Equivalent within System	Metric Equivalent
Volume		
1 tsp (teaspoonful)		5 mL
1 tbsp (tablespoonful)	3 tsp	15 mL
1 fl oz (fluid ounce)	2 tbsp	30 mL (29.57 mL)*
1 cup	8 fl oz	240 mL
1 pt (pint)	2 cups	480 mL†
1 qt (quart)	2 pt	960 mL
1 gal (gallon)	4 qt	3840 mL
Weight		
1 oz (ounce)		30 g
1 lb (pound)		454 g
2.2 lb		1 kg

*In reality, 1 fl oz (household measure) contains less than 30 mL; however, 30 mL is usually used.
†When packaging a pint, companies will typically present 473 mL, rather than the full 480 mL, thus saving money over time.

Numeral Systems

Two types of numbers are used in pharmaceutical calculations: (1) Roman and (2) Arabic. The Arabic system uses numbers, fractions (such as ⅗), and decimals. In the Roman system, the numerals are expressed in either lowercase letters or as capital letters. The most frequently used numerals are the upper case I, V, and X, which represent the Arabic numbers 1, 5, and 10, respectively. A prescription using an apothecary measure is commonly written in lowercase Roman numerals that follow rather than precede the unit of measurement. Thus "aspirin gr vi" means "six grains of aspirin." Roman numerals are also sometimes used to express other quantities, as in tablets (C = 100 tablets) or volume (tbsp iii = 3 tablespoonsful). The lowercase Roman numerals i, ii, and iii are often written with a line above to prevent errors in interpretation (for example: ī, īī, īīī). Table 5.8 summarizes the Roman numeral system and gives equivalents in Arabic numerals.

Safety Note

New safety guidelines are discouraging use of Roman numerals.

  Roman numerals are equal or smaller when reading left to right; the total value equals the sum of their individual values. Thus iii = 3, and xi = 10 + 1 = 11. Otherwise, first subtract the value of each smaller numeral from the value of the larger numeral that it precedes, and then add the individual values. Thus iv = 5 − 1 = 4, and xxiv = 10 + 10 + (5 − 1) = 10 + 10 + 4 = 24.

Table 5.8 Comparison of Roman and Arabic Numerals

Roman	Arabic	Roman	Arabic
ss	0.5 or ½	L or l	50
I or i or ī	1	C or c	100
V or v	5	D or d	500
X or x	10	M or m	1000

BASIC MATHEMATICS USED IN PHARMACY PRACTICE

Many tasks in pharmacy—determining doses, compounding medications, and preparing solutions—use calculations involving the units of measure given in the preceding section. If you are fairly confident about your basic mathematical skills, you may wish to skip this section. However, it never hurts to review fundamental principles before undertaking mathematical work. Pharmacy work often requires performing fundamental operations involving fractions, decimals, ratios and proportions, and percentages.

Fractions

When something is divided into parts, each part is considered a **fraction** of the whole. For example, a pie might be divided into eight slices, each one of which is a fraction, or $\frac{1}{8}$, of the whole pie. In this example, 1 is a piece of the pie and 8 is the number of slices in the whole pie. A simple fraction consists of two numbers: a **numerator** (the number on the top) and a **denominator** (the number on the bottom).

$$\frac{1}{2} \quad \begin{matrix} \leftarrow & \text{numerator} \\ \leftarrow & \text{denominator} \end{matrix}$$

A fraction is simply a convenient way of representing an operation, the division of the numerator by the denominator. Thus the fraction $\frac{6}{3}$ equals 6 divided by 3, which equals 2. The fraction $\frac{7}{8}$ is 7 divided by 8, which equals 0.875. The number obtained upon dividing the numerator by the denominator is the value of the fraction.

Fractions with the same value are said to be equivalent fractions. The following are equivalent fractions:

$$\frac{1}{2} = 1 \div 2 = 0.5 \qquad\qquad \frac{3}{16} = 3 \div 16 = 0.1875$$

$$\frac{2}{4} = 2 \div 4 = 0.5 \qquad\qquad \frac{12}{64} = 12 \div 64 = 0.1875$$

$$\frac{4}{8} = 4 \div 8 = 0.5$$

A fraction with a value of less than 1 (the numerator smaller than the denominator) is called a **proper fraction**.

$$\frac{1}{4} \quad \frac{2}{3} \quad \frac{7}{8} \quad \frac{9}{10}$$

A fraction with a value greater than 1 (the numerator greater than the denominator) is called an **improper fraction**.

$$\frac{6}{5} \quad \frac{7}{5} \quad \frac{11}{6} \quad \frac{15}{8}$$

A **mixed number**, also called a *compound fraction*, is a whole number and a fraction.

$$5\frac{1}{2}, \qquad 13\frac{7}{8}, \qquad 99\frac{23}{24}, \qquad 111\frac{99}{100}$$

Safety Note

Be careful when reading compound fractions.

In pharmaceutical work, it is especially important not to misread a compound fraction as a simple one. For example, do not confuse the following fractions. They are not equal.

$$3\frac{3}{8} \neq \frac{33}{8}$$

Adding and Subtracting Fractions   To add or subtract fractions, first convert any compound fractions to improper fractions containing no whole numbers. To do this, multiply the whole number part of the compound fraction by the denominator and add the result to the numerator.

$$\text{compound fraction} = \frac{(\text{whole number} \times \text{denominator}) + \text{numerator}}{\text{denominator}}$$

$$3\frac{3}{8} = \frac{(3 \times 8) + 3}{8} = \frac{27}{8}$$

$$4\frac{1}{3} = \frac{(4 \times 3) + 1}{3} = \frac{13}{3}$$

The next step in adding or subtracting fractions is to check if the denominators are equal. If all of the fractions have the same denominator, addition or subtraction can proceed. If not, it is necessary to convert each fraction to an equivalent fraction such that all the fractions have the same denominator, or a **common denominator**. The **least common denominator** of a group of fractions is the smallest number that is evenly divisible by all of the denominators. To find the least common denominator, follow the steps shown in the following example.

Example 1

Find the least common denominator of the following fractions:

$$\frac{9}{28} \qquad \frac{1}{6}$$

Step 1. Find the prime factors (numbers divisible only by 1 and themselves) of each denominator. Make a list of all the different prime factors that you find. Include in the list each different factor as many times as the factor occurs for any one of the denominators of the given fractions.

The prime factors of 28 are 2, 2, and 7 (because 2 3 2 3 7 5 28).
The prime factors of 6 are 2 and 3 (because 2 3 3 5 6).

The number 2 occurs twice in one of the denominators, so it must occur twice in the list. The list will also include the unique factors 3 and 7; so the final list is 2, 2, 3, and 7.

Step 2. Multiply all the prime factors on your list. The result of this multiplication is the least common denominator.

$$2 \times 2 \times 3 \times 7 = 84$$

Step 3. To convert a fraction to an equivalent fraction with the common denominator, first divide the least common denominator by the denominator of the fraction, then multiply both the numerator and denominator by the result (the quotient).

The least common denominator of $\frac{9}{28}$ and $\frac{1}{6}$ is 84. In the first fraction, 84 divided by 28 is 3, so multiply both the numerator and the denominator by 3.

$$\frac{9}{28} = \frac{9 \times 3}{28 \times 3} = \frac{27}{84}$$

In the second fraction, 84 divided by 6 is 14, so multiply both the numerator and the denominator by 14.

$$\frac{1}{6} = \frac{1 \times 14}{6 \times 14} = \frac{14}{84}$$

The following are two equivalent fractions:

$$\frac{27}{84} \text{ and } \frac{14}{84}$$

Step 4. Once the fractions are converted to contain equal denominators, adding or subtracting them is straightforward. Simply add or subtract the numerators.

$$\frac{9}{28} + \frac{1}{6} = \frac{27}{84} + \frac{14}{84} = \frac{41}{84}$$

$$\frac{9}{28} - \frac{1}{6} = \frac{27}{84} - \frac{14}{84} = \frac{13}{84}$$

Multiplying and Dividing Fractions To multiply fractions, multiply numerators by numerators and denominators by denominators. Table 5.9 shows some guidelines for multiplying fractions.

$$\frac{1}{8} \times \frac{1}{2} = \frac{1 \times 1}{8 \times 2} = \frac{1}{16} \qquad \frac{3}{4} \times \frac{12}{17} = \frac{3 \times 12}{4 \times 17} = \frac{36}{68} = \frac{9}{17}$$

$$\frac{1}{8} \times \frac{1}{2} \times \frac{2}{3} = \frac{1 \times 1 \times 2}{8 \times 2 \times 3} = \frac{2}{48} = \frac{1}{24}$$

Table 5.9 Guidelines for Multiplying Fractions

1. Multiplying the numerator by a number increases the value of a fraction.

$$\frac{1}{4} \times \frac{2}{1} = \frac{1 \times 2}{4 \times 1} = \frac{2}{4} = \frac{1}{2}$$

2. Multiplying the denominator by a number decreases the value of a fraction.

$$\frac{1}{4} \times \frac{1}{2} = \frac{1 \times 1}{4 \times 2} = \frac{1}{8}$$

3. The value of a fraction is not altered by multiplying or dividing both numerator and denominator by the same number.

$$\frac{1}{4} \times \frac{4}{4} = \frac{1 \times 4}{4 \times 4} = \frac{4}{16} = \frac{1}{4}$$

4. Dividing the denominator by a number is the same as multiplying the numerator by that number.

$$\frac{3}{\frac{20}{5}} = \frac{3}{4} \qquad \frac{3 \times 5}{20} = \frac{15}{20} = \frac{3}{4}$$

5. Dividing the numerator by a number is the same as multiplying the denominator by that number.

$$\frac{\frac{6}{3}}{4} = \frac{2}{4} = \frac{1}{2} \qquad \frac{6}{4 \times 3} = \frac{6}{12} = \frac{1}{2}$$

To divide by a fraction, invert the fraction and multiply. The inverted fraction is known as the reciprocal of the original fraction. Note that if the numerator of the original fraction is 1, the reciprocal will be a whole number.

$$\frac{3}{4} \div \frac{1}{3} = \frac{3}{4} \times \frac{3}{1} = \frac{3 \times 3}{4 \times 1} = \frac{9}{4} = 2\frac{1}{4}$$

$$\frac{10}{\frac{1}{4}} = 10 \div \frac{1}{4} = \frac{10}{1} \times \frac{4}{1} = \frac{40}{1} = 40$$

Decimals

An understanding of decimals is crucial to dose calculations because most medication orders are written using decimals. A **decimal** is any number that can be written in decimal notation, using the integers 0, 1, 2, 3, 4, 5, 6, 7, 8, and 9 and a point (.) to divide the "ones" place from the "tenths" place. Figure 5.2 illustrates the relative value of each decimal unit and provides the names of the place values. Numbers to the left of the decimal point are whole numbers; numbers to the right of the decimal point are decimal fractions (parts of the whole).

0.131313   2.09   43.09

Safety Note

Use a leading zero to avoid misreading of decimals.

Notice that in the decimal expansion of a fraction, a zero (0) is placed before the decimal point if the number is less than 1. This zero is called a **leading zero**, and using this zero helps to prevent potential medication errors in reading decimals.

A fraction can be expressed as a decimal by dividing the numerator by the denominator.

$$\frac{1}{2} = 1 \div 2 = 0.5$$

$$\frac{1}{3} = 1 \div 3 = 0.33333$$

$$\frac{438}{64} = 438 \div 64 = 6.84375$$

Converting Fractions to Decimal Equivalents One way to add, subtract, multiply, or divide fractions is to first convert each fraction to a decimal equivalent and then perform the operation, as is shown in Example 2.

Example 2   **Multiply the two given fractions.**

$$\frac{24}{3} \times \frac{22}{4}$$

$$\frac{24}{3} = 24 \div 3 = 8 \qquad\qquad \frac{22}{4} = 22 \div 4 = 5.5$$

$$8 \times 5.5 = 44$$

Converting Decimals to Fractions The metric system generally uses numbers in decimal form. Any decimal number can be expressed as a decimal fraction that has a power of 10 as its denominator. The decimal-fraction equivalents shown in Table 5.10 correspond to the decimal place names previously presented in Figure 5.2.

To express a decimal number as a fraction, remove the decimal point and use the resulting number as the numerator. To obtain the denominator, count the number of places to the right of the decimal point. Use Table 5.10 to find the corresponding power of ten to put in the denominator.

$$2.33 = \frac{233}{100} \qquad 0.1234 = \frac{1234}{10,000} \qquad 0.00367 = \frac{367}{100,000}$$

Figure 5.2

Decimal Units and Values

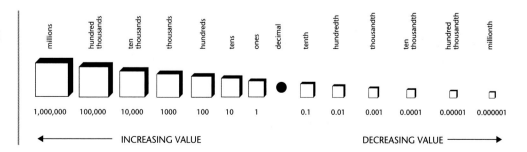

millions	hundred thousands	ten thousands	thousands	hundreds	tens	ones	decimal	tenth	hundredth	thousandth	ten thousandth	hundred thousandth	millionth
1,000,000	100,000	10,000	1000	100	10	1		0.1	0.01	0.001	0.0001	0.00001	0.000001

◄———— INCREASING VALUE   DECREASING VALUE ————►

Table 5.10   Decimals and Equivalent Decimal Fractions

$$1 = \frac{1}{1} \qquad\qquad 0.01 = \frac{1}{100} \qquad\qquad 0.0001 = \frac{1}{10,000}$$

$$0.1 = \frac{1}{10} \qquad\qquad 0.001 = \frac{1}{1000} \qquad\qquad 0.00001 = \frac{1}{100,000}$$

Once a decimal number is expressed as a fraction, the fraction can be simplified by dividing it by a fraction equivalent to 1.

$$0.84 = \frac{84}{100} = \frac{84}{100} \div \frac{4}{4} = \frac{21}{25}$$

$$0.1234 = \frac{1234}{10,000} = \frac{1234}{10,000} \div \frac{2}{2} = \frac{617}{5,000}$$

Adding and Subtracting Decimals   When adding or subtracting decimals, place the numbers in columns so that the decimal points are aligned directly under each other. Add or subtract from the far-right column to the left column.

$$
\begin{array}{r}
20.4 \\
+21.8 \\
\hline
42.2
\end{array}
\qquad
\begin{array}{r}
11.2 \\
13.6 \\
+16.0 \\
\hline
40.8
\end{array}
\qquad
\begin{array}{r}
15.36 \\
-3.80 \\
\hline
11.56
\end{array}
$$

Multiplying Decimals   Multiply the two decimals as whole numbers. Add the total number of decimal places that are in the two numbers being multiplied (count from right to left), count that number of places from right to left in the answer, and insert a decimal point.

$$
\begin{array}{r}
1.23 \\
\times\ \ 2.3 \\
\hline
369 \\
+\ 2460 \\
\hline
2.829
\end{array}
$$

(A zero is added to align the columns. Note that no value is added to the number.)

Dividing Decimals   To divide decimal numbers, change both the divisor (the number doing the dividing; the denominator) and the dividend (the number being divided; the numerator) to whole numbers by moving their decimal points the same number of places to the right. If the divisor and the dividend have a different number of digits after the decimal point, choose the one that has more digits and move its decimal point a sufficient number of places to make it a whole number. Then move the decimal point in the other number the same number of places, adding a zero at the end if necessary. In the first example, the divisor has more digits after the decimal point, so move its decimal point three places to the right to make it a whole number. Then move the decimal point in the dividend the same number of places, adding a zero at the end. In the second example, the dividend has more digits after the decimal point, so move its decimal point three places to the right to make it a whole number. Then move the decimal point in the divisor three places to the right also.

$$1.45 \div 3.625 = 0.4 \qquad\qquad 1.617 \div 2.31 = 0.7$$

$$\frac{1.45}{3.625} = \frac{1450}{3625} = 0.4 \qquad\qquad \frac{1.617}{2.31} = \frac{1617}{2310} = 0.7$$

Rounding Decimals To round off an answer to the nearest tenth, carry the division out two places, to the hundredth place. If the number in the hundredth place is 5 or greater, add 1 to the tenth place number. If the number in the hundredth place is less than 5, round the number down by omitting the digit in the hundredth place.

$$5.65 \text{ becomes } 5.7 \qquad 4.24 \text{ becomes } 4.2$$

The same procedure may be used when rounding to the nearest hundredth place or thousandth place.

$$3.8421 = 3.84 \text{ (hundredth)}$$
$$41.2674 = 41.27 \text{ (hundredth)}$$
$$0.3928 = 0.393 \text{ (thousandth)}$$
$$4.1111 = 4.111 \text{ (thousandth)}$$

When rounding numbers used in pharmacy calculations, it is common to round off to the nearest tenth. However, sometimes a dose is very small, and rounding to the nearest hundredth or thousandth may be more appropriate.

The exact dose calculated is 0.08752 g
Rounded to nearest tenth: 0.1 g
Rounded to nearest hundredth: 0.09 g
Rounded to nearest thousandth: 0.088 g

Ratios and Proportions

A **ratio** is a comparison of two like quantities and can be expressed in a fraction or in ratio notation, using a colon. For example, if a beaker contains two parts water and three parts alcohol, then the ratio of water to alcohol in the beaker can be expressed as the fraction ⅔ or as the ratio 2:3. The ratio is read not as a value (2 divided by 3) but as the expression "a ratio of 2 to 3."

One common use of ratios is as follows: The numerator is the number of parts of one substance contained in a known number of parts of another substance, which is the denominator. For example, suppose that 60 mL of sterile solution contains 3 mL of tetrahydrozoline hydrochloride. This can be expressed as the ratio ³⁄₆₀ or ¹⁄₂₀. In other words, the ratio of the active ingredient to the sterile solution is 1 to 20, or 1 part in 20 parts.

Two ratios that have the same value, such as ½ and ²⁄₄, are said to be equivalent ratios. This is similar to the concept of equivalent fractions discussed earlier. When ratios are equivalent, the product of the numerator of the first ratio and the denominator of the second ratio is equal to the product of the numerator of the second ratio and denominator of the first ratio.

Therefore if $\quad 2{:}3 = 6{:}9;\quad$ then $\quad \dfrac{2}{3} = \dfrac{6}{9};\quad$ thus $\quad 2 \times 9 = 3 \times 6 = 18$

The same thing is true of the reciprocals.

Therefore if $3:2 = 9:6$;   then $\dfrac{3}{6} = \dfrac{9}{2}$;   thus $3 \times 6 = 2 \times 9 = 18$

Two equivalent ratios are said to be in the same proportion. Equivalent, or proportional, ratios can be expressed in three different ways.

$$\frac{a}{b} = \frac{c}{d} \qquad \text{example: } \frac{1}{2} = \frac{2}{4}$$

$$a{:}b = c{:}d \qquad \text{example: } 1{:}2 = 2{:}4$$

$$a{:}b :: c{:}d \qquad \text{example: } 1{:}2 :: 2{:}4$$

Pairs of equivalent ratios are called a **proportion**. The first and fourth, or outside, numbers are called the extremes, and the second and third, or inside, numbers are called the means.

$$3{:}4 \quad = \quad 15{:}20$$

means

extremes

A very useful fact about proportions was illustrated in the previous examples: the product of the extremes equals the product of the means. If the proportion is expressed as a relationship between fractions, the numerator of the first fraction times the denominator of the second is equal to the denominator of the first fraction times the numerator of the second. This can be stated as a rule:

$$\text{If } \frac{a}{b} = \frac{c}{d}, \quad \text{then} \quad a \times d = b \times c$$

This equation proves extremely valuable because it can be used to calculate an unknown quantity in a proportion when the other three variables are known. In mathematics, it is common to express unknown quantities using letters from the lower end of the alphabet, especially x, y, and z.

When setting up ratios in the proportion, it is important that the numbers remain in the correct ratio and that the numbers have the correct units of measurement in both the numerator and denominator. Table 5.11 lists the rules for solving proportions. Table 5.12 lists the steps for solving for an unknown quantity, which we usually label x, using the ratio-proportion method.

Table 5.11   Rules for Solving Proportions

- Three of the four amounts must be known.
- The numerators must have the same unit of measurement.
- The denominators must have the same unit of measurement.

Table 5.12   Steps for Solving for an Unknown "x" Using the Ratio-Proportion Method

Step 1. Create the proportion by placing the ratios in fraction form so that the x is in the upper-left corner.

Step 2. Check that the unit of measurement in the numerators is the same and the unit of measurement in the denominators is the same.

Step 3. Solve for x by multiplying both sides of the proportion by the denominator of the ratio containing the unknown, and cancel.

Step 4. Check your answer by seeing if the product of the means equals the product of the extremes.

Example 3   Solve for x.

$$\frac{x}{35} = \frac{2}{7}$$

By the proportion rule,

$$7x = 70$$

Then, dividing both sides by 7,

$$\frac{7x}{7} = \frac{70}{7}$$

$$x = 10$$

Percents

The word *percent* comes from the Latin words *per centum*, meaning "in one hundred." A **percent** is a given part or amount in a hundred. Percents can be expressed in many ways, and all of the following expressions are equivalent.

- as an actual percent (example: 3% [or 3 percent])
- as a fraction with 100 as the denominator (example: $\frac{3}{100}$)
- as a decimal (example: 0.03)
- as a ratio (example 3:100)

Converting a Ratio to a Percent   To express a ratio as a percent, designate the first number of the ratio as the numerator and the second number as the denominator. Multiply the fraction by 100% (which does not change the value), and simplify as needed.

$$5:1 = \frac{5}{1} \times 100\% = 5 \times 100\% = 500\%$$

$$1:5 = \frac{1}{5} \times 100\% = \frac{100\%}{5} = 20\%$$

$$1:2 = \frac{1}{2} \times 100\% = \frac{100\%}{2} = 50\%$$

Converting a Percent to a Ratio   To convert a percent to a ratio, first change it to a fraction by dividing it by 100 and then reducing the fraction to its lowest terms. Express this as a ratio by making the numerator the first number of the ratio and the denominator the second number.

$$2\% \ = 2 \div 100 = \frac{2}{100} = \frac{1}{50} = 1{:}50$$

$$10\% \ = 10 \div 100 = \frac{10}{100} = \frac{1}{10} = 1{:}10$$

$$75\% \ = 75 \div 100 = \frac{75}{100} = \frac{3}{4} = 3{:}4$$

$$\frac{1}{2}\% \ = \frac{1}{2} \div 100 = \frac{\frac{1}{2}}{100} = \frac{1}{2} \times \frac{1}{100} = \frac{1}{200} = 1{:}200$$

Converting a Percent to a Decimal To convert a percent to a decimal, divide by 100% or insert a decimal point two places to the left of the last number, inserting zeros if necessary, and drop the percent symbol. To change a decimal to a percent, multiply by 100% or move the decimal point two places to the right and write in the percent symbol. (Just as multiplying or dividing a number by 1 does not change the value of the number, multiplying or dividing a number by 100% does not change the value of a number.)

Percent to Decimal

4% = 0.04	4 ÷ 100% = 0.04
15% = 0.15	15 ÷ 100% = 0.15
200% = 2.0	200 ÷ 100% = 2.0

Decimal to Percent

0.25 = 25%	0.25 × 100% = 25%
1.35 = 135%	1.35 × 100% = 135%
0.015 = 1.5%	0.015 × 100% = 1.5%

COMMON CALCULATIONS IN THE PHARMACY

Math skills typically used by the pharmacy technician involve converting units and calculating doses. For nearly all types of mathematics in the pharmacy, decimals and the metric system are preferred over Roman numerals, fractions, and the apothecary, avoirdupois, or household systems.

Converting Quantities between the Metric and Common Measure Systems

Many situations in pharmacy practice call for conversion of quantities within one measurement system or between different measurement systems. When possible, convert to the metric system, because it is the preferred system. To convert between metric measurements and apothecary units, it is necessary to know the equivalent measures shown in Table 5.5. The following examples will demonstrate some common pharmacy conversions.

Example 4   **How many milliliters are there in 1 gal, 12 fl oz?**

According to the values in Table 5.7, 3840 mL are found in 1 gal. In addition, because 1 fl oz contains 30 mL, you can use the ratio-proportion method to calculate the amount of milliliters in 12 fl oz as follows:

$$\frac{x \text{ mL}}{12 \text{ fl oz}} = \frac{30 \text{ mL}}{1 \text{ fl oz}}$$

$$\frac{(12 \text{ fl oz}) \, x \text{ mL}}{12 \text{ fl oz}} = \frac{(12 \text{ fl oz}) \, 30 \text{ mL}}{1 \text{ fl oz}}$$

$$x \text{ mL} = 360 \text{ mL}$$

Add the two values:

$$3840 \text{ mL} + 360 \text{ mL} = 4200 \text{ mL}$$

Example 5   **A solution is to be used to fill hypodermic syringes, each containing 60 mL, and 3 L of the solution is available. How many hypodermic syringes can be filled with the 3 L of solution?**

From Table 5.2, 1 L is 1000 mL. The available supply of solution is therefore

$$3 \times 1000 \text{ mL} = 3000 \text{ mL}$$

Determine the number of syringes by using the ratio-proportion method:

$$\frac{x \text{ syringes}}{3000 \text{ mL}} = \frac{1 \text{ syringe}}{60 \text{ mL}}$$

$$\frac{(3000 \text{ mL}) \, x \text{ syringes}}{3000 \text{ mL}} = \frac{(3000 \text{ mL}) \, 1 \text{ syringe}}{60 \text{ mL}}$$

$$x \text{ syringes} = 50 \text{ syringes}$$

Therefore 50 hypodermic syringes can be filled.

Example 6   **You are to dispense 300 mL of a liquid preparation. If the dose is 2 tsp, how many doses will there be in the final preparation?**

Begin solving this problem by converting to a common unit of measure using conversion values in Table 5.7.

$$1 \text{ dose} = 2 \text{ tsp} = 2 \times 5 \text{ mL} = 10 \text{ mL}$$

Using these converted measurements, the solution can be determined one of two ways.

Solution 1: Using the ratio-proportion method and the metric system,

$$\frac{x \text{ doses}}{300 \text{ mL}} = \frac{1 \text{ dose}}{10 \text{ mL}}$$

$$\frac{(300 \text{ mL}) \ x \text{ doses}}{300 \text{ mL}} = \frac{(300 \text{ mL}) \ 1 \text{ dose}}{10 \text{ mL}}$$

$$x \text{ doses} = 30 \text{ doses}$$

Solution 2: Using the dimensional analysis method,

$$300 \text{ mL} \times \frac{1 \text{ dose}}{10 \text{ mL}} = 30 \text{ doses}$$

Example 7

A prescription calls for acetaminophen 400 mg. How many grains of acetaminophen should be used in the prescription?

Solve this problem by using the ratio-proportion method. The unknown number of grains and the requested number of milligrams go on the left side, and the ratio of 1 gr = 65 mg goes on the right side, per Table 5.5.

$$\frac{x \text{ gr}}{400 \text{ mg}} = \frac{1 \text{ gr}}{65 \text{ mg}}$$

$$\frac{(400 \text{ mg}) \ x \text{ gr}}{400 \text{ mg}} = \frac{(400 \text{ mg}) \ 1 \text{ gr}}{65 \text{ mg}}$$

$$x \text{ gr} = 6.1538 \text{ gr, rounded to } 6 \text{ gr}$$

Rounding down, 6 gr should be used in the prescription.

Example 8

A physician wants a patient to be given 0.8 mg of nitroglycerin. On hand are tablets containing nitroglycerin 1/150 gr. How many tablets should the patient be given?

Begin solving this problem by determining the number of grains in a dose by setting up a proportion and solving for the unknown. The unknown number of grains and the requested number of milligrams go on the left side, and the ratio of 1 gr = 65 mg goes on the right side, per Table 5.5.

$$\frac{x \text{ gr}}{0.8 \text{ mg}} = \frac{1 \text{ gr}}{65 \text{ mg}}$$

$$\frac{(0.8 \text{ mg}) \ x \text{ gr}}{0.8 \text{ mg}} = \frac{(0.8 \text{ mg}) \ 1 \text{ gr}}{65 \text{ mg}}$$

$$x \text{ gr} = 0.0123076, \text{ rounded to } 0.012 \text{ gr}$$

Determine the number of tablets that the patient should receive by first converting the fraction value to a decimal value:

$$1/150 \text{ gr} = 0.00666 \text{ gr, rounded to } 0.0067 \text{ gr}$$

Then, set up another proportion and solve for the unknown:

$$\frac{x \text{ tablets}}{0.012 \text{ gr}} = \frac{1 \text{ tablet}}{0.0067 \text{ gr}}$$

$$\frac{(0.012 \text{ gr}) \ x \text{ tablets}}{0.012 \text{ gr}} = \frac{(0.012 \text{ gr}) \ 1 \text{ tablet}}{0.0067 \text{ gr}}$$

$$x \text{ gr} = 1.79 \text{ tablets, rounded to 2 tablets}$$

Calculation of Doses

One of the most common calculations in pharmacy practice is that of doses. The available supply is usually labeled as a ratio of an active ingredient to a solution.

$$\frac{\text{active ingredient (available)}}{\text{solution (available)}}$$

The prescription received in the pharmacy gives the amount of the active ingredient to be administered. The unknown quantity to be calculated is the amount of solution needed to achieve the desired dose of the active ingredient. This yields another ratio.

$$\frac{\text{active ingredient (to be administered)}}{\text{solution (needed)}}$$

The amount of solution needed can be determined by setting the two ratios into a proportion.

$$\frac{\text{active ingredient (to be administered)}}{\text{solution (needed)}} = \frac{\text{active ingredient (available)}}{\text{solution (available)}}$$

Safety Note

Always double-check the units in a proportion and double-check your calculations.

When solving medication-dosing problems, use ratios to describe the amount of drug in a dose form (tablet, capsule, or volume of solution). It is important to remember that the numerators and denominators of both fractions (ratios) must be in the same units. For example, in oral medications, the active ingredient is usually expressed in milligrams and the solution is expressed in milliliters. Similarly, the pharmacy stock will most likely be a milligram per milliliter solution. Because it is so easy to confuse units, setting up proportions with the units clearly shown is the safer way to solve these types of calculations.

Example 9

You have a stock solution that contains 10 mg of active ingredient per 5 mL of solution. The physician orders a dose of 4 mg. How many milliliters of the stock solution will have to be administered?

Using the information provided, set up a proportion, but flip the ratios so that the unknown variable is in the upper-left corner of the proportion.

$$\frac{\text{solution (needed)}}{\text{active ingredient (to be administered)}} = \frac{\text{solution (available)}}{\text{active ingredient (available)}}$$

$$\frac{x \text{ mL}}{4 \text{ mg}} = \frac{5 \text{ mL}}{10 \text{ mg}}$$

$$\frac{(4 \text{ mg}) \ x \text{ mL}}{4 \text{ mg}} = \frac{(4 \text{ mg}) \ 5 \text{ mL}}{10 \text{ mg}}$$

$$x \text{ mL} = 2 \text{ mL}$$

Thus 2 mL of solution are needed to provide the 4 mg dose.

Example 10

An order calls for Demerol 75 mg IM q4h prn pain. The supply available is in Demerol 100 mg/mL syringes. How many milliliters will the nurse give for one injection?

Using the abbreviations list in Appendix A, this order is calling for an intra-muscular (IM) injection of 75 mg every 4 hours as needed for pain. Determine the number of milliliters in an injection by setting up a proportion:

$$\frac{\text{solution (needed)}}{\text{active ingredient (to be administered)}} = \frac{\text{solution (available)}}{\text{active ingredient (available)}}$$

$$\frac{x \text{ mL}}{75 \text{ mg}} = \frac{1 \text{ mL}}{100 \text{ mg}}$$

$$\frac{(75 \text{ mg}) \, x \text{ mL}}{75 \text{ mg}} = \frac{(75 \text{ mg}) \, 1 \text{ mL}}{100 \text{ mg}}$$

$$x \text{ mL} = 0.75 \text{ mL}$$

Notice that 0.75 mL is three quarters of a syringe.

Proportions can be used to solve other types of dose calculations, such as converting an adult dose based on body surface area (BSA) to an appropriate child's dose. Many medications have a wide dose range, and the patient's response and adverse reactions can vary widely, even in adults. For this reason, many physicians prefer to prescribe to children only those medications that have a known pediatric-suggested dose. As you will see in Example 11, the calculated pediatric dose is rounded down, rather than up, for safety reasons.

Example 11

An average adult has a BSA of 1.72 m² and requires an adult dose of 12 mg of a given medication. The same medication is to be given to a child in a pediatric dose. If the child has a BSA of 0.60 m², and if the proper dose for pediatric and adult patients is a linear function of the BSA (in other words, think of the child as a small adult), what is the proper pediatric dose? Round off the final answer.

The assumptions regarding the calculation of pediatric doses make it possible to use a proportion to answer this question.

$$\frac{\text{child's dose}}{\text{child's BSA}} = \frac{\text{adult dose}}{\text{adult BSA}}$$

$$\frac{x \text{ mg}}{0.6 \text{ m}^2} = \frac{12 \text{ mg}}{1.72 \text{ m}^2}$$

$$\frac{(0.6 \text{ m}^2) \, x \text{ mg}}{0.6 \text{ m}^2} = \frac{(0.6 \text{ m}^2) 12 \text{ mg}}{1.72 \text{ m}^2}$$

$$x \text{ mg} = 4.186 \text{ mg, rounded to } 4 \text{ mg}$$

Because this dose is for a child, it is customary to round down to 4 mg rather than rounding up to 4.2 mg.

Preparation of Solutions

The pharmacy technician will need to calculate the amount of ingredients required to create prescribed solutions. For example, parenteral products are often reconstituted by adding a diluent to a lyophilized or freeze-dried powder to prepare a solution for intravenous administration. The product is commercially manufactured in powder form due to the instability of the drug in solution over a long period of time. In addition, the pharmacy technician may be asked to create solutions of a specific concentration by combining measured amounts of solutions of more and less concentrated ingredients. This section will present these types of calculations.

Preparing Solutions Using Powders In preparing solutions, although the active ingredient is discussed in terms of weight, it also occupies a certain amount of space. With dry pharmaceuticals, this space is referred to as **powder volume (pv)**. It is equal to the difference between the final volume (fv) and the volume of the diluting ingredient, or the diluent volume (dv), as expressed in the following equation:

$$\text{powder volume} = \text{final volume} - \text{diluent volume}$$
$$or \quad \text{pv} = \text{fv} - \text{dv}$$

Example 12

A dry powder antibiotic must be reconstituted for use. The label states that the dry powder occupies 0.5 mL. Using the formula for solving for powder volume, determine the diluent volume (the amount of solvent added). You are given the final volume for three different examples with the same powder volume.

Final Volume	Powder Volume
(1) 2 mL	0.5 mL
(2) 5 mL	0.5 mL
(3) 10 mL	0.5 mL

$$\text{dv} = \text{fv} - \text{pv}$$
(1) dv = 2 mL − 0.5 mL = 1.5 mL
(2) dv = 5 mL − 0.5 mL = 4.5 mL
(3) dv = 10 mL − 0.5 mL = 9.5 mL

Example 13

You are to reconstitute 1 g of dry powder. The label states that you are to add 9.3 mL of diluent to make a final solution of 100 mg/mL. What is the powder volume?

Step 1. Calculate the final volume. The strength of the final solution will be 100 mg/mL. Since you start with 1 g = 1000 mg of powder, for a final volume x of the solution, it will have strength 1000 mg/x mL.

Solution 1: Using the ratio-proportion method,

$$\frac{x \text{ mL}}{1000 \text{ mg}} = \frac{1 \text{ mL}}{100 \text{ mg}}$$

$$x \text{ mL} = \frac{(1000 \text{ mg}) \times 1 \text{ mL}}{100 \text{ mg}} = 10 \text{ mL}$$

Solution 2: Using the dimensional analysis method,

$$1000 \text{ mg} \times \frac{1 \text{ mL}}{100 \text{ mg}} = 10 \text{ mL}$$

Step 2. Using the calculated final volume and the given diluent volume, calculate the powder volume.

$$\text{pv} = \text{fv} - \text{dv}$$
$$\text{pv} = 10 \text{ mL} - 9.3 \text{ mL} = 0.7 \text{ mL}$$

Working with Dilutions Medications may be diluted for several reasons. They are sometimes diluted prior to administration to children, infants, and the elderly to meet the dosing requirements of those patients. Medications may also be diluted so that they can be measured more accurately and easily. For example, volumes less than 0.1 mL are usually considered too small to measure accurately. Therefore they must be diluted further. Many pharmacies have a policy as to how much an injection can be diluted. A rule of thumb is for the required dose to have a volume greater than 0.1 mL and less than 1 mL.

The following example will demonstrate the method for solving typical dilution problems. The first step is to use the ratio-proportion method to solve for the volume of the final product by using a ratio of diluted solution to desired concentration. The second step is to determine the amount of diluent simply by subtracting the concentrate from the total volume. Both of these volumes are approximate because they depend on the calibration and accuracy of the measuring devices used.

Although the second step is used to determine the amount of diluent added, the amount will actually be determined by adding "up to" the desired total quantity. The abbreviation QS for "sufficient quantity" is used to describe the process of adding enough of the last ingredient in a compound to reach the desired volume. It is helpful to calculate the necessary amount beforehand so that an adequate supply of medication is available.

Example 14

Dexamethasone is available as a 4 mg/mL preparation; an infant is to receive 0.35 mg. Prepare a dilution so that the final concentration is 1 mg/mL. How much diluent will you need if the original product is in a 1 mL vial and you dilute the entire vial?

Step 1. Determine the volume (in milliliters) of the final product. Since the strength of the dexamethasone is 4 mg/mL, a 1 mL vial will contain 4 mg of the active ingredient. Then, for a final volume x of solution, you will have a concentration of $(4/x)$ mg/mL.

Diluted solution	Desired concentration

$$\frac{x \text{ mL}}{4 \text{ mg}} = \frac{1 \text{ mL}}{1 \text{ mg}}$$

$$x \text{ mL} = \frac{(4 \text{ mg} \times 1 \text{ mL})}{1 \text{ mg}} = 4 \text{ mL final product}$$

Step 2. Subtract the volume of the concentrate from the total volume to determine the volume of diluent needed.

4 mL total volume − 1 mL concentrate = 3 mL diluent needed

Therefore an additional 3 mL of diluent are needed to dilute the original 1 mL of preparation to arrive at a final concentration of 1 mg/mL.

Using Alligation to Prepare Solutions Physicians prescribe concentrations of medications that are not commercially available, and these prescriptions must be compounded ("added" together) at the pharmacy. When an ordered concentration is not commercially available, it may be necessary to combine two different solutions with the same active ingredient in differing strengths. The resulting concentration will be greater than the weaker strength, but less than the stronger strength. For example, 1% and 5% hydrocortisone ointments may be combined to provide a 3% ointment. This is called an **alligation**. This method is used when the two quantities needed to prepare the desired concentration are both relatively large.

The amount of each stock product to be added together is calculated by using the alligation alternate method. This is the calculation used to determine the proportions of given percentages needed to prepare the desired concentration. The alligation alternate method requires changing the percentages to parts of a proportion and then using the proportion to obtain the amounts of the two ingredients. The answer can then be checked using the following formula.

milliliters × percent (expressed as a decimal) = grams

It is important to note that this formula works for any strength solution.

The following examples will demonstrate the application of the alligation alternate method.

Example 15

Prepare 250 mL of dextrose 7.5% weight in volume (w/v) using dextrose 5% (D_5W) w/v and dextrose 50% ($D_{50}W$) w/v. How many milliliters of each will be needed?

Step 1. Set up a box arrangement and at the upper-left corner, write the percent of the highest concentration (50%) as a whole number. At the lower-left corner, write the percent of the lowest concentration (5%) as a whole number, and in the center, write the desired concentration.

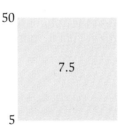

Step 2. Subtract the center number from the upper-left number (i.e., the smaller from the larger) and put it at the lower-right corner. Now subtract the lower-left number from the center number (i.e., the smaller from the larger), and put it at the upper-right corner.

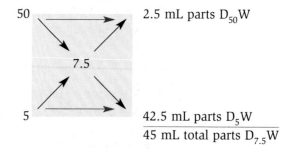

50   2.5 mL parts $D_{50}W$

7.5

5       $\dfrac{42.5 \text{ mL parts } D_5W}{45 \text{ mL total parts } D_{7.5}W}$

The number 2.5 mL represents the number of parts of the 50% solution that will be needed to make the final 7.5% solution, and the number 42.5 mL represents the number of parts of the 5% solution that will be needed. The sum of these two numbers, 2.5 mL + 42.5 mL = 45 mL, is the total number of parts of the 7.5% solution. In terms of ratios, the ratio of the 5% solution to the 7.5% solution is 42.5:45, and the ratio of the 50% solution to the 7.5% solution is 2.5:45. Much less of the 50% solution is needed to make the 7.5% solution.

Step 3. Calculate the volume needed of each dextrose solution.

50% Dextrose

$$\frac{x \text{ mL of } 50\%}{250 \text{ mL}} = \frac{2.5 \text{ mL parts } D_{50}W}{45 \text{ mL total parts } D_{7.5}W}$$

$$x \text{ mL} = \frac{(250 \text{ mL}) \times 2.5 \text{ mL parts}}{45 \text{ mL total parts}}$$

$$x \text{ mL} = 13.8888 \text{ mL } D_{50}W, \text{ rounded to } 13.89 \text{ mL}$$

5% Dextrose

$$\frac{x \text{ mL of } 5\%}{250 \text{ mL}} = \frac{42.5 \text{ mL parts } D_5W}{45 \text{ mL total parts } D_{7.5}W}$$

$$x \text{ mL} = \frac{(250 \text{ mL}) \times 42.5 \text{ mL parts}}{45 \text{ mL total parts}}$$

$$x \text{ mL} = 236.11 \text{ mL } D_5W$$

Step 4. Add the volumes of the two solutions together. The sum should equal the required volume of dextrose 7.5%.

$$
\begin{array}{r}
236.11 \text{ mL} \\
+13.89 \text{ mL} \\
\hline
250.00 \text{ mL}
\end{array}
$$

Step 5. Check your answer by calculating the amount of solute (dextrose) in all three solutions. The number of grams of solute should equal the sum of the grams of solutes from the 50% solution and the 5% solution, using the following formula.

$$\text{mL} \times \% \text{ (as a decimal)} = g$$

$$250 \text{ mL} \times 0.075 = 18.75 \text{ g}$$
$$13.89 \text{ mL D}_{50}\text{W} \times 0.5 = 6.945 \text{ g}$$
$$236.11 \text{ mL D}_5\text{W} \times 0.05 = 11.805 \text{ g}$$

$$
\begin{array}{r}
11.805 \text{ g} \\
+\ 6.945 \text{ g} \\
\hline
18.750 \text{ g}
\end{array}
$$

The amounts measured to prepare this prescription will be rounded to the nearest milliliter, 14 mL D$_{50}$W and 236 mL D$_5$W.

Example 16   **You are instructed to make 454 g of 3% zinc oxide cream. You have in stock 10% and 1% zinc oxide cream. How much of each percent will you use?**

Step 1.

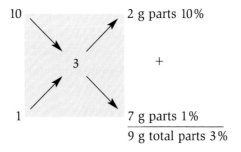

Step 2.

10% zinc oxide cream

$$\frac{x \text{ g of } 10\%}{454 \text{ g}} = \frac{2 \text{ g parts } 10\%}{9 \text{ g total parts } 3\%}$$

$$x \text{ g of } 10\% = 101 \text{ g of } 10\% \text{ zinc oxide cream}$$

1% zinc oxide cream

$$\frac{x \text{ g of } 1\%}{454 \text{ g}} = \frac{7 \text{ g parts } 1\%}{9 \text{ g total parts } 3\%}$$

$$x \text{ g of } 1\% = 353 \text{ g of } 1\% \text{ zinc oxide cream}$$

Step 3. Check your work.

$$353 \text{ g} + 101 \text{ g} = 454 \text{ g}$$

Math skills do not come easy for everyone; however, knowledge of the basic fundamentals of math, especially in the metric system, is critical to minimizing medication errors involving dose, flow rates, or concentrations. The end-of-chapter exercises, in addition to the Workbook, should assist you in gaining both confidence and competence in mathematical skills. Additional math skills are covered in Chapter 7, *The Business of Community Pharmacy* as well in Chapter 11, *Preparing Sterile Intravenous Products*.

Chapter Terms

alligation compounding of two or more products to obtain a desired concentration

common denominator a number into which each of the unlike denominators of two or more fractions can be divided evenly

decimal any number that can be written in decimal notation using the integers 0 through 9 and a point (.) to divide the "ones" place from the "tenths" place (e.g., 10.25 is equal to 10¼)

denominator the number on the bottom part of the fraction

fraction a portion of a whole that is represented as a ratio

gram the metric system's base unit for measuring weight

improper fraction a fraction with a value greater than 1 (the numerator's value is larger than the denominator's value)

leading zero a zero that is placed in the one's place in a number that is less than zero and is being represented by a decimal value

least common denominator the smallest number that is evenly divisible by all of the denominators in a group of fractions

liter the metric system's base unit for measuring volume

meter the metric system's base unit for measuring length

metric system measurement system based on subdivisions and multiples of 10; made up of three basic units: meter, gram, and liter

mixed number a whole number and a fraction

numerator the numeral on the upper part of the fraction

percent the number or ratio per 100

powder volume (pv) the amount of space occupied by a freeze-dried medication in a sterile vile, used for reconstitution; equal to the difference between the final volume and the volume of the diluting ingredient or the diluent volume

proper fraction a fraction with a value of less than 1 (the numerator's value is smaller than the denominator's value)

proportion a comparison of equal ratios

ratio a comparison of numeric values

Chapter Summary

- The metric system of measurement makes use of decimal units, including the basic units of the gram (for weight) and the liter (for volume). Pharmacy professionals should be able to convert between different systems such as metric, avoirdupois, apothecary, and household measures.
- The most widely used units of measure in pharmacy include milligrams, grams, kilograms, milliliters, and liters, as well as the grain.
- Pharmacists and pharmacy technicians should be familiar with the standard prefixes for abbreviating metric quantities and the basic mathematical principles used to calculate and convert doses and prepare reconstituted solutions from powdered drug products.
- Those working in the profession of pharmacy should be able to find an unknown quantity in a proportion when three elements of the proportion are known; they should also be able to use the alligation method to compound a solution from products with different concentrations.

Chapter Review

Knowledge Inventory

Choose the best answer from those provided.

1. The modern metric system makes use of the standardized units of the
   a. avoirdupois system.
   b. Système International (SI).
   c. Système Quebeçois.
   d. apothecaries' system.

2. The metric prefix meaning one millionth is
   a. nano-.
   b. micro-.
   c. milli-.
   d. deci-.

3. A gram is equal to
   a. 1000 micrograms.
   b. 1000 milligrams.
   c. 1000 centigrams.
   d. 1000 nanograms.

4. The liter is a standard measurement of
   a. distance.
   b. area.
   c. volume.
   d. weight.

5. Given ½, the fraction ²⁄₁ is its
   a. equivalent fraction.
   b. value.
   c. reciprocal.
   d. least common denominator.

6. A decimal fraction has as its denominator a power of
   a. 2.
   b. 5.
   c. 10.
   d. 25.

7. 58% means 58 out of one
   a. hundred.
   b. thousand.
   c. million.
   d. billion.

8. To find out if two fractions are equivalent,
    a. cross-multiply them and check to see if the products of the multiplication are equal.
    b. multiply their denominators and check to see if the product is equal.
    c. multiply their numerators and check to see if the product is equal.
    d. invert them, then cross-multiply them and check to see if the products of the multiplication are equal.

9. The only unit of measure that is the same in the apothecary and avoirdupois system is the
    a. grain.
    b. gram.
    c. liter.
    d. ounce.

10. The proper pediatric dose of a medication depends upon the child's
    a. body mass.
    b. weight.
    c. body surface area (BSA).
    d. None of the above

Pharmacy in Practice

1. Convert the following:
    a. 34.6 g = _____ mg
    b. 735 mg = _____ g
    c. 3400 mL = _____ L
    d. 1.2 L = _____ mL
    e. 7.48 kg = _____ g
    f. 4.27 mL = _____ L

2. Convert the following:
    a. 24 fl oz = _____ pt
    b. 40 gr (apothecary) = _____ Э (apothecary)
    c. 6 ℥ (apothecary) = _____ ℔ (apothecary)
    d. 6.25 tbsp = _____ tsp
    e. 8 qt = _____ gal
    f. viii = _____ (Arabic numeral)
    g. C = _____ (Arabic numeral)

3. Solve the following conversion problems:
    a. You have 2 L of solution in stock. The solution is to be used to fill vials that hold 40 mL each. How many vials can you fill with the 2 L of solution?
    b. The patient has received a bottle containing 400 mL of a liquid medication. The patient is to take 3 tsp of the medication per day. How many days will the bottle last?
    c. A prescription calls for codeine sulfate 40 mg. How many grains of codeine sulfate should be used in the prescription?
    d. A patient takes two 1/150-gr nitroglycerin tablets per day. How many mg of nitroglycerin does the patient receive each day?

4. Solve the following dose problems:
   a. In stock you have a solution that contains 8 mg of active ingredient per 10 mL of solution. A customer has a prescription calling for 4 doses of 6 mg each of the active ingredient. How many milliliters of the solution should the customer be given?
   b. A medication order calls for phenobarbital 60 mg. The supply available is phenobarbital 100 mg/mL of solution. How many milliliters of the solution will the patient be given?
   c. If the adult dose of a medication is 30 mg and the average adult body surface area (BSA) is 1.72 m^2, what would be the appropriate pediatric dose for a child with a BSA of 0.50 m^2?

5. Solve the following solution preparation problems:
   a. You have been asked to prepare a solution containing a powder with a volume of 0.7 mL. The total volume of the solution that you are to prepare should be 30 mL. How much diluent will you use in the solution, and what will be the percentage, by volume, of the powder in the solution?
   b. You are instructed to make 240 mL of a 0.45% w/v solution. You have a 3% concentrate in stock. How much of the full-strength solution will you use and how much diluent will be needed?
   c. You must prepare 300 mL of a solution containing 42.5% dextrose. In stock you have solutions containing 5% dextrose (Solution 1) and 50% dextrose (Solution 2). How many milliliters of each stock solution must you use in the solution that you prepare?

Improving Communication Skills

1. Interview a hospital and community pharmacy technician or pharmacist regarding their experience with calculations in their practice setting. Discuss your findings with the class.

2. Interview a lawyer about past litigation involving calculation errors in healthcare that may have led to serious disability or death. Report your findings to the class.

Internet Research

1. Visit www.malpracticeweb.com, and look under Miscellaneous to find legal summaries of the following cases. Describe the decision and explain how this decision affects pharmacy technicians.
   a. *J.C. vs. Osco Drug*
   b. *P.H. vs. Osco Drug*

Unit 2

Community Pharmacy

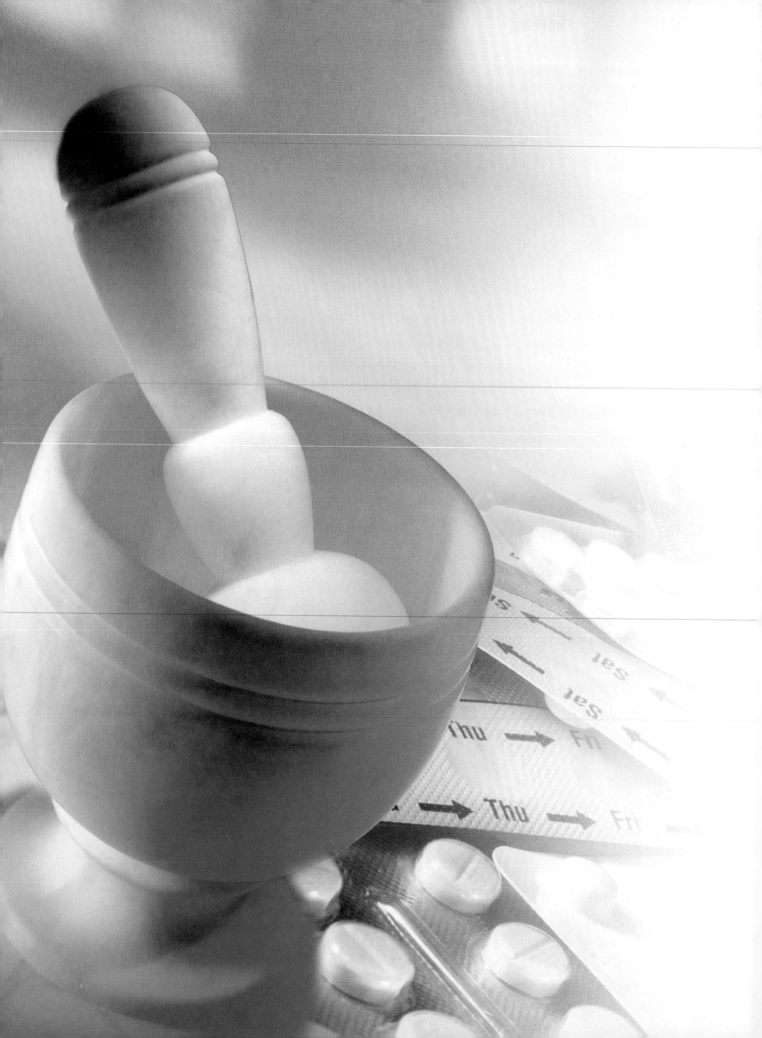

Dispensing Medications in the Community Pharmacy

Chapter 6

Learning Objectives

- Enumerate typical duties of pharmacy technicians with regard to dispensing of over-the-counter and prescription drugs.
- Explain the typical procedures for receiving and reviewing prescriptions.
- Describe the parts of a prescription and of a typical prescription label.
- Describe the parts of a patient profile, and detail the steps required to prepare, check, or update a profile.

The primary role of the pharmacist is to dispense medications safely, accurately, and in accordance with the law requiring receipt of a written order from a physician. The pharmacy technician provides necessary assistance in this process; thus reviewing the different parts of a prescription order is important. In this chapter you will learn some of what is involved in the dispensing of prescription and OTC medications, including the receipt and labeling of scheduled and nonscheduled medications. Of most importance is clarifying the legal responsibility of the pharmacy technician versus the pharmacist in the dispensing process, which may vary from state to state.

COMMUNITY PHARMACY OPERATIONS

A community pharmacy sells over-the-counter (OTC) and legend (Rx only or prescription) drugs, as well as vitamins, minerals, herbal medications, and other products that are sometimes classified as diet supplements. OTC drugs and diet supplements can be legally sold without a prescription, whereas legend drugs are required to bear on their labeling the legend "Rx only." Community pharmacies are generally organized into a "front area," where OTC drugs, toiletries, cosmetics, greeting cards, and other merchandise are sold, and a Rx area, where prescription merchandise and related items are sold. For obvious reasons, the Rx area is off-limits to customers and may be entered only by authorized employees.

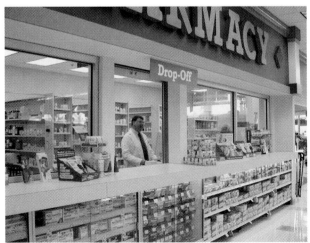

Only authorized employees can enter the Rx area of the pharmacy to limit access to legend drugs.

Technician Duties Related to Dispensing Over-the-Counter Drugs and Diet Supplements

Increasingly, customers are turning to products that they can purchase at will for self-administration to treat common everyday symptoms of illness or to maintain health. Self-administration of OTC drugs and diet supplements requires an accurate "self-diagnosis" by the patient in order to treat the symptoms. Inappropriate self-care may be harmful if diagnosis and necessary drug treatment are delayed. Customers often seek the counsel of the pharmacist to verify the assessment of their symptoms.

The increase in the use of OTC drugs and diet supplements is related to a number of factors, including the increased cost and inconvenience (e.g., taking time off work) of physician visits and the rising cost of prescription medications. In addition, many drugs that once could be purchased only with a prescription are now available over the counter. Although OTC medications may be purchased without a prescription, the active ingredients in these medications are sometimes the same as those found in higher-strength prescription versions.

The Food and Drug Administration (FDA) approves an OTC preparation only when the approval process leaves no doubt that the dose strength is generally recognized as *safe and effective* when taken according to labeled directions. The manufacturer is liable to provide all patient labeling for OTC drugs if purchased in the original container. To be approved by the FDA, the manufacturer must include all information on the product label that is necessary for the safe and effective use of the product by the consumer in language that is both understandable and readable. Such information should include dose and frequency of administration for different age groups, as well as precautions, warnings, and expiration dates. The FDA does not approve diet supplements with the same level of scrutiny; however, supplements, including herbals, vitamins, and minerals, must be *safe and correctly labeled*.

Currently, pharmacists are increasingly devoting a greater percentage of their time to recommending OTC products and diet supplements to customers and to counseling customers about their proper use. OTC drugs and diet supplements are also becoming an increasingly important part of the technician's responsibilities. Technicians often carry out such functions as stocking, taking inventory, removing stock when its shelf life has expired, and helping customers to locate items on the shelves. However, technicians should not counsel customers with regard to use of OTC drugs and diet supplements unless directed to do so by the pharmacist. Questions about indications, dose and administration, expected therapeutic effect, side effects, contraindications, and interactions should always be referred to the pharmacist.

Safety Note

Pharmacy technicians should not counsel patients about OTC products without the approval of the pharmacist.

Technician Duties Related to Dispensing Prescription Drugs

With regard to legend, or prescription, drugs, the technician may carry out a number of different duties, including the following:
- greeting customers and receiving written prescriptions
- answering the telephone and referring call-in prescriptions to the pharmacist
- updating the patient's computerized profile
- entering refill prescription information into the computer
- entering billing information for third-party reimbursement
- retrieving products from storage in the ℞ area
- assisting the pharmacist with compounding (in some states)
- packaging and repackaging products
- preparing labels for prescriptions
- accepting cash payments

Technicians are often responsible for preparing prescription medications, packaging and labeling them, and preparing a patient bill. All materials pertaining to a prescription are kept together for the pharmacist to check before dispensing to the patient. The process that begins with checking the prescription for completeness and ends with dispensing to the patient will take about 5 to 10 minutes, and 100% accuracy is expected. If prescriptions filled in a given day were 99% correct, then that would mean that the average pharmacy filling 200 prescriptions daily would have filled two prescriptions incorrectly. That is not acceptable. The prescription and product selection should be checked several times for accuracy during the fill process and should be mentally checked again before the stock bottle is returned to the shelf. Medication safety is discussed in more detail in Chapter 12.

Safety Note

100% accuracy is expected with all prescriptions.

Table 6.1 explains the path a single prescription follows once it crosses the threshold of a pharmacy, and the following sections of this chapter discuss certain steps in greater detail. Although a patient may bring in multiple prescriptions, each prescription follows the same critical path.

GUIDELINES FOR RECEIVING AND REVIEWING PRESCRIPTIONS

Prescriptions come into a pharmacy in a variety of ways. Most often, of course, customers carry in written prescriptions or physicians order them by telephone. A technician may, by law, receive a written prescription from a customer. By law, only a licensed pharmacist can take new telephone prescriptions in most states; taking prescription refill information by telephone is, in many instances, considered to be an acceptable activity for a pharmacy technician.

When taking a written prescription from a customer, the technician should first review it to make sure that it looks legitimate. Almost always, the prescription will be on a preprinted prescription form bearing the name, address, telephone number and

Table 6.1   The Critical Path of a Prescription

1. The patient drops off the prescription.
2. The pharmacy technician checks the prescription to make certain it is complete and authentic; then he or she verifies that the patient is in the pharmacy database. If the patient is not in the pharmacy database, the technician obtains necessary demographic, insurance, and allergy information from the patient and enters the information into the computer.
3. The pharmacy technician enters the prescription into the computer, bills the insurance company or the patient, and generates the medication label.
4. The pharmacy technician asks the pharmacist to check the drug use review (DUR) or drug interaction warning screen when required.
5. The pharmacy technician selects the appropriate medication and verifies the National Drug Code (NDC) number on the computer-generated medication label.
6. The pharmacy technician prepares the medication(s) (e.g., the prescribed number of tablets is counted or the liquid measured).
7. The pharmacy technician packages the medication in the appropriate container.
8. The pharmacy technician labels the prescription container with the computer-generated medication label. In some states the law requires the pharmacist to affix the label to the container.
9. The pharmacy technician prepares the filled prescription for the pharmacist to check.
10. The pharmacist checks the prescription(s) and may initial it.
11. The pharmacy technician bags the approved prescription for patient sale and attaches an information sheet about the prescription, including indications, interactions, and possible side effects.
12. The pharmacy technician returns the bulk product container to the shelf.
13. The pharmacy technician delivers the packaged prescription to the cash register area for patient pickup and pharmacist counseling.

Safety Note

Steps 5, 6, 9, 10, 12, and 13 in Table 6.1 should include verification that the proper product has been selected.

DEA number of the prescribing physician. When receiving a prescription, the pharmacy technician should always check the elements illustrated in Figure 6.1. Table 6.2 details the parts of a prescription. If there are any doubts about the authenticity or completeness of a prescription, these should be called to the attention of the pharmacist. A telephone call from the pharmacist to the prescribing physician might be necessary.

A trend exists for more prescriptions to be received by a pharmacy from a physician via fax or electronic transmission. In fact, with the increased use of pocket digital assistants (PDAs) by physicians, the use of the written prescriptions will probably continue to diminish each year. The advantages of the electronic submission are speed, accuracy, and improved billing. However, concerns about standardization and patient confidentiality must be resolved before widespread implementation. Importantly, pharmacy technicians must be aware of state laws regarding prescription faxing and the transferring of prescriptions electronically or via a database.

In some drugstore chains, as well as in many large managed-care organizations, a prescription may be entered (or phoned in, in the case of refills) into a central database and be accessed at a store or warehouse other than the one where the prescription was originally received. This model is similar to the mail-order pharmacy, except that the centralized pharmacy is located in the same geographic area (as opposed to out of state), and the patient picks up the prescription at the receiving pharmacy rather than receiving it through the mail. The advantage of centralizing these "filling" functions in a large off-site warehouse is the increased ability to use automation to fill a greater number of prescriptions per hour with less dispensing errors and liability (e.g., by double-checking bar codes). It also allows the pharmacist at the *receiving* pharmacy to spend more time in patient counseling on the medication(s).

Figure 6.1

Parts of a Prescription

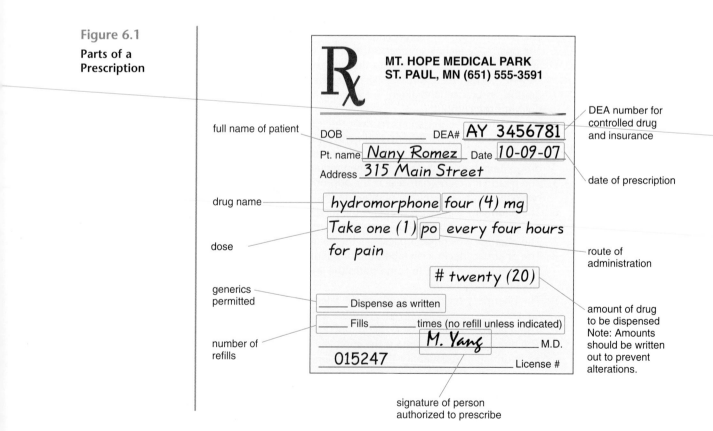

Table 6.2 Parts of a Prescription

Prescriber Information	Name, address, telephone number, and other information identifying the prescriber including state license number.
Date	Date on which the prescription was written.
Patient Information	Name, address, date of birth (needed to differentiate patients with same first/last names), and other pertinent information about the patient who receives the prescription. (If the patient is an infant, a toddler, an older adult, or someone with special needs, the prescription may include such information as weight and body surface area [BSA] of the patient—information needed by the pharmacist to calculate appropriate doses. If this information is missing, then the pharmacy technician may query the customer about it and add it to the prescription.)
℞	Symbol ℞, for the Latin word *recipe*, meaning *take*.
Inscription	Medication prescribed, including generic or brand name, strength, and amount. (States and most institutions have regulations and policies allowing pharmacists to substitute less expensive generic equivalents of brand name medications when appropriate.) A patient may request a brand name product, but his or her insurance may not cover the cost.
Subscription	Instructions to the pharmacist on dispensing the medication. (These instructions include such information as compounding or packaging instructions, labeling instructions, instructions on allowable refills, and instructions such as "No substitutions" or "No substitutions allowed" when a generic equivalent may not be substituted. The abbreviation *PBO* means *prescribe brand only*. The abbreviation *DAW* means *dispense as written*.)
Signa	Directions for the patient to follow (commonly called the *sig*).
Additional Instructions	Any additional instructions that the prescriber deems necessary.
Signature	The signature of the prescriber.
Drug Enforcement Administration (DEA) Number	Number that identifies the prescriber as someone authorized to prescribe controlled substances. (This number is required on all prescriptions for such substances, and is often required to file insurance claims.)

The following are some general guidelines when reviewing prescriptions:

- Patient name should be given in full, including at least the full first and last names. Initials alone are not acceptable. If necessary, rewrite the patient's name in full above the name on the prescription and verify the spelling of the patient's name when it is not legible.
- Patient address is needed for patient records. In most states, the address is required for all prescriptions.
- Preprinted prescriptions often contain a space for the patient's birth date. If this space is not filled in, then you should request this information. The patient birth date is helpful for third-party billing and for distinguishing among patients with the same name. Knowing the patient's age also helps the pharmacist evaluate the appropriateness of the drug, the quantity, and the dose form prescribed thus minimizing medication errors.
- The date the physician wrote the prescription should be provided. For pharmacy records, the date when the prescription is received should be written on the

prescription as well. If no date is written on the prescription, then the date the prescription is brought into the pharmacy should be recorded and noted as such. If the undated prescription is for an antibiotic, then the pharmacist may wish to verify that the patient is under the current care of a physician. The date on a prescription holds special importance for controlled substances (see *Receiving a Controlled-Drug Prescription* in next section).

- Drugs may be listed on a prescription using a brand or generic name. A given drug (i.e., one with a particular generic name) may be marketed under various brand names. For example, Prinivil and Zestril are two brand names under which the generic drug lisinopril is marketed. A generic drug is one that is marketed under the generic name rather than a brand name. Generic drugs are often less expensive than brand name drugs and are often substituted, under regulations now existing in every state, for brand name drugs. Such substitutions can be made, of course, only if the generic drug and the brand name drug are bioequivalent. (See *FDA Electronic Orange Book* in Chapter 3 under *Drug References*.) If the prescription for a brand name drug is filled with a generic equivalent, then the name, strength, and manufacturer of the generic substitution must be written on the medication container label.

- The **signa**, or directions for use, from the prescription must be placed on the label produced for the medication. The medication container label should read exactly as indicated on the prescription. In addition, any signa comments written on the prescription must be included on the label. Abbreviations used on prescriptions are included in Appendix A. You may wish to review this information or refer to it as you look at the sample prescriptions in this chapter.

- If the refill blank on the prescription is left blank, then there can be no refill for the prescription. The words *no refill* will appear on the medication label, and an indication of *no refill* will be entered into the patient's record. If the refill blank on the prescription indicates *as needed (prn)*, then this is not construed as indicating an unlimited duration. Most pharmacies and state laws require at least yearly updates on prn, or *as needed*, prescriptions.

- If refills are called for, then prescriptions should generally be refilled 1 or 2 days before the customer's supply will run out, although this is not a hard-and-fast rule. In some circumstances (e.g., when a customer is leaving on vacation) an early refill might be appropriate. Insurance companies often will not pay for these early refills, and the patient may need to pay for the prescription up front and send in the receipts for reimbursement.

- Regulations in a given state may require two signature lines at the bottom of the prescription: one reading *dispense as written* (DAW) and the other reading *substitution permitted*. If the DAW line is signed, then substitution of a generic equivalent is not permitted. Other states may require only one signature line, and if a prescriber wishes that only the brand name product be dispensed, *brand name medically necessary* must be noted on the prescription.

- Space for the DEA number on the prescription form is for the number issued to the physician authorizing him or her to prescribe controlled substances. (See next section for additional discussion.)

Checking for Patient Allergies

Importantly, the pharmacy technician must ask the patient about allergies to medications or food, as well as about past adverse drug reactions, when receiving each and every prescription. An **allergy** is a hypersensitivity to a specific substance that is manifested in a physiological disorder. Common allergic reactions include sweating, rashes, swelling, and difficulty in breathing. In extreme cases, allergic reactions can lead to shock, coma, or death. An **adverse drug reaction** is any negative consequence to any individual from taking a particular drug.

If the patient indicates that he or she does not have any allergies, the notation NKA, for *no known allergies*, should be made on the back of the prescription form and on the patient profile. If the patient indicates that he or she does have an allergy, then the allergy should be entered into the patient computerized profile.

Inquiring about allergies every time a patient comes to the pharmacy with a prescription for an antibiotic is a good practice. Antibiotics are the most common medication allergy, and allergies can begin at any age. A patient could have safely taken an antibiotic several times and become allergic to it on a subsequent occasion. Thus confirming and updating the patient's allergies in the profile is important. Some patients may think of stomach upset as an allergy. However, an upset stomach is a side effect, not an allergy. Therefore the patient should describe the allergy before entering the description into the computerized profile.

Receiving a Controlled-Drug Prescription

A prescription for a controlled drug requires additional care and scrutiny because of the potential for a patient to intentionally or nonintentionally abuse the drug. For example, federal law requires a physical address (not a post office box number) on prescriptions for controlled substances (substances with a high potential for abuse that are governed by the Controlled Substances Act [CSA], previously discussed in Chapter 2). The Joint Commission on Accreditation of Healthcare Organizations (JCAHO) has adopted additional standards to include full name and address of the patient, phone number of the pharmacy, amount of drug dispensed, and the name and initials of the dispensing pharmacist. Some states require veterinary labels to carry the name and address of the animal owner and species of the animal. In addition, refill information is often included on the medication label.

Medication labels for Schedule II, III, IV, and V drugs must contain the transfer warning "Caution: Federal law prohibits the transfer of this drug to any person other than the patient for whom it was prescribed." In addition, state regulations may dictate the length of time a controlled-substance prescription is valid (e.g., 6 months from the date of issue). State regulations may control the time period for filling a controlled-substance prescription. In some states a Schedule II prescription must be filled within 7 days of issue, and in other states it must be filled within 72 hours. Prescriptions for Schedule II controlled substances may be handwritten or typed. Some states do not allow a nurse practitioner or physician assistant to write the prescription, even if the physician signs it. Signatures on all Schedule II prescriptions must be handwritten, not stamped.

In an emergency situation, a person with the legal authority to issue prescriptions for Schedule II controlled substances may provide oral, rather than written, authorization for the prescription. However, the amount prescribed must not exceed the amount necessary for treatment during the emergency period, and the prescriber must provide a written prescription within 72 hours of the oral authorization.

The quantity of controlled substance dispensed may be limited in some states to 120 units or a 30-day supply, whichever is less. A prescription for a Schedule II drug cannot be altered in any way and cannot be refilled; such a medication requires a new prescription each time it is dispensed. This safeguard frequently causes an inconvenience to a parent whose child may be treated with a Schedule II drug like Ritalin for attention-deficit hyperactivity disorder (ADHD). A prescription for a Schedule III or IV drug may be refilled up to five times if allowed by the physician, but these refills must occur within a 6-month period, after which time a new prescription is required. A prescription for a Schedule V controlled substance (required in some states) may be refilled only if authorized by a prescribing physician.

Some physicians have their DEA number preprinted on their prescriptions, whereas others write it on the prescription when writing out the order for a Schedule II medication. Some states require all such prescriptions to be written on authorized "safety paper." Many insurance companies require a pharmacy to have a physician's DEA number on file to be reimbursed for prescriptions, even when the drug is for a nonscheduled medication. Pharmacy personnel can check for falsified DEA numbers by following this procedure:

1. Add the first, third, and fifth digits of the DEA number.
2. Add the second, fourth, and sixth digits of the number and multiply the sum by two.
3. Add the two results from steps 1 and 2. The last digit of this sum should be the same as the last digit of the DEA number.
4. The second letter of the DEA number is the same as the first letter of the doctor's last name.

PATIENT PROFILE

A **patient profile** is usually a computerized record that lists the patient's prescriptions and other relevant information. If the patient is a previous customer, then he or she may already have a profile on file that the technician can retrieve. If not, then a new profile will have to be created. Figure 6.2 is an example of a patient profile form. Figure 6.3 shows a computerized profile. The patient profile will generally contain the information listed in Table 6.3.

Different pharmacies follow different policies and procedures, generally explained in a *policy and procedure manual*. This manual reflects not only the requirements of the relevant state laws and regulations but also the guidelines for safe and effective operation established by the pharmacy itself. It is extremely important that confidentiality of patient medical information be maintained at all times (see Chapter 13, *Human Relations and Communications*). Part of the technician's job, as described in the policy and procedure manual, might be to enter data from a new prescription into the patient profile. Completing a patient profile might require asking questions related to each of the items indicated in Table 6.3. If a patient profile information sheet is not complete, then the technician may need to interview the patient to obtain necessary information. Any time the technician notices a patient having difficulty with filling out the form, assistance should be offered.

When the prescription is filled, the patient profile must be updated to reflect the prescription order. A technician who has received sufficient training may be given the task of recording the new prescription in the profile to provide such information as the prescription number, drug prescribed, dose form, quantity, number of refills authorized (if any), and the charge for the prescription. The pharmacy technician may need to update information in the patient profile by

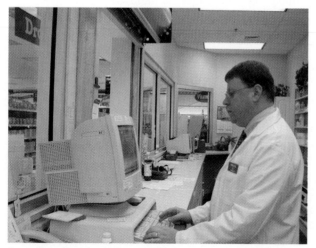

Records such as the patient profile must be kept up to date.

Figure 6.2

Patient Profile Form

PATIENT PROFILE

Patient Name

Last ______ First ______ Middle Initial ______

****

Street or PO Box ______

City ______ State ______ Zip ______

****

Phone ( ) ___ ___ Date of Birth ______ Month Day Year □ Male □ Female Social Security No. ___ ___ ____

□ Yes, I would like medication dispensed in a child-resistant container.
□ No, I do not want medication dispensed in a child-resistant container.

Medication Insurance □ Yes □ No

Card Holder Name ______
□ Card Holder □ Spouse □ Child □ Dependent Parent □ Disabled Dependent □ Full Time Student

MEDICAL HISTORY

HEALTH

□ Angina
□ Anemia
□ Arthritis
□ Asthma
□ Blood Clotting Disorders
□ High Blood Pressure
□ Breast Feeding
□ Cancer
□ Diabetes
□ Epilepsy
□ Glaucoma
□ Heart Condition
□ Kidney Disease
□ Liver Disease
□ Lung Disease
□ Parkinson's Disease
□ Pregnancy
□ Ulcers

Other Conditions ______

ALLERGIES AND DRUG REACTIONS

□ No known drug allergies or reactions
□ Aspirin
□ Cephalosporins
□ Codeine
□ Erythromycin
□ Penicillin
□ Sulfa Drugs
□ Tetracyclines
□ Xanthines

Other Allergies/Reactions ______

Prescription Medication Being Taken ______

OTC Medication Currently Being Taken ______

Would You Like Generic Medication Where Possible? □ Yes □ No

Comments ______

Health information changes periodically. Please notify the pharmacy of any new medications, allergies, drug reactions, or health conditions.

______ Signature ______ Date □ I do not wish to provide this information.

Figure 6.3

Computerized Patient Profile

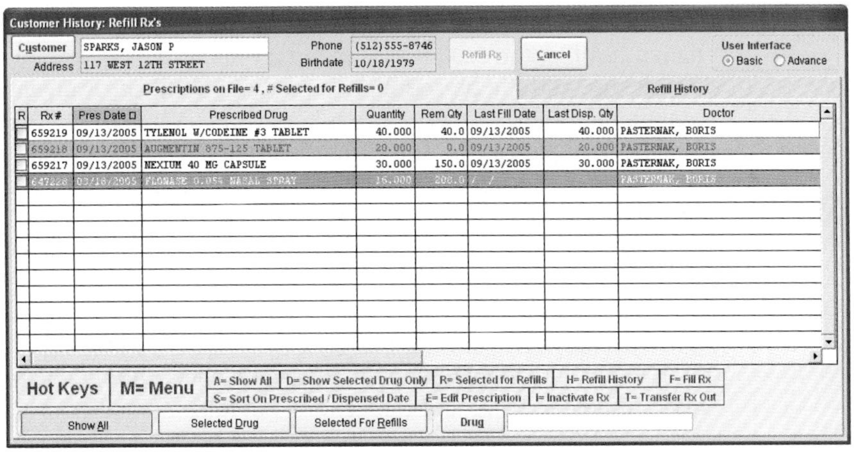

Customer History: Refill Rx's

Customer SPARKS, JASON P Phone (512)555-8746 Refill Rx Cancel User Interface ◉ Basic ○ Advance
Address 117 WEST 12TH STREET Birthdate 10/18/1979

Prescriptions on File= 4 , # Selected for Refills= 0 | Refill History

R	Rx#	Pres Date	Prescribed Drug	Quantity	Rem Qty	Last Fill Date	Last Disp. Qty	Doctor
□	659219	09/13/2005	TYLENOL W/CODEINE #3 TABLET	40.000	40.0	09/13/2005	40.000	PASTERNAK, BORIS
□	659218	09/13/2005	AUGMENTIN 875-125 TABLET	20.000	0.0	09/13/2005	20.000	PASTERNAK, BORIS
□	659217	09/13/2005	NEXIUM 40 MG CAPSULE	30.000	150.0	09/13/2005	30.000	PASTERNAK, BORIS
□	647228	03/18/2005	FLONASE 0.05% NASAL SPRAY	16.000	208.0	/ /		PASTERNAK, BORIS

Hot Keys | M= Menu | A= Show All | D= Show Selected Drug Only | R= Selected for Refills | H= Refill History | F= Fill Rx
S= Sort On Prescribed / Dispensed Date | E= Edit Prescription | I= Inactivate Rx | T= Transfer Rx Out

Show All | Selected Drug | Selected For Refills | Drug

Table 6.3 Parts of the Patient Profile

Identifying Information	Patient's full name with the middle initial, address, telephone number, birth date, and gender.
Insurance/Billing Information	Information necessary for billing. (If the patient has prescription insurance, then this should be indicated, along with information such as the name of the insurer, the group number, the patient's identification or card number, the effective date and expiration date of the insurance, the cardholder's name, the patient's relationship to the cardholder and the persons covered by the insurance, and other relevant information. Oftentimes the insurance card will have a BIN #, which assists in transmission for reimbursement.)
Medical History	Information concerning existing conditions (e.g., epilepsy, glaucoma) and known allergies and adverse drug reactions the patient has experienced. (The pharmacist reviews the medical history on the profile to make sure that the prescription is safe to fill for a given patient.)
Medication/ Prescription History	Any prescription and OTC medications currently being taken and a list of previous prescriptions filled for this patient, including information on refills. (The pharmacist reviews this information to make sure that the prescription will not cause adverse drug interactions [i.e., negative consequences] because of the combined effects of drugs and/or drugs and foods.)
Prescription Preferences	Patient preferences as they apply to his or her prescriptions (e.g., child-resistant or non-child-resistant containers or generic substitutions).
Refusal of Information	Statement of refusal by the patient to provide any or all of the previous information. (This statement is for the protection of the pharmacy.)

asking the patient for any changes in insurance coverage, medical conditions, or new medications including OTC drugs and diet supplements. The technician should confirm this new information with the pharmacist, because it may be essential to reviewing the computerized profile for dispensing the prescription and counseling the patient.

MEDICATION SELECTION AND PREPARATION

After the information for a new prescription or refill has been entered into the patient profile, the customer is given a time at which the prescription will be ready for pickup, and the prescription is ready to be filled. A given prescription may require either dispensing of drugs that come prepackaged in given dose forms (e.g., tablets, prefilled capsules, transdermal patches) or compounding before dispensing. Once the medication container label is available, the proper product should be selected from the stock area.

Figure 6.4 identifies the standard parts of a pharmacy stock drug label. When reading the stock drug label, the most important information to check before proceeding is the drug name and strength. Often in the pharmacy, drugs are arranged alphabetically, and drugs of a similar spelling and strength are nearby. The drug name and strength should always be checked immediately. The brand name is often in bolder print, and the generic name is in smaller print under or beside the

Figure 6.4

Parts of a Stock Drug Label
(a) Brand name,
(b) Generic name,
(c) Dose form,
(d) Strength per unit dose, (e) Package size,
(f) Manufacturer,
(g) National Drug Code (NDC),
(h) Special storage and handling requirements,
(i) Legend label,
(j) Expiration date and lot number.

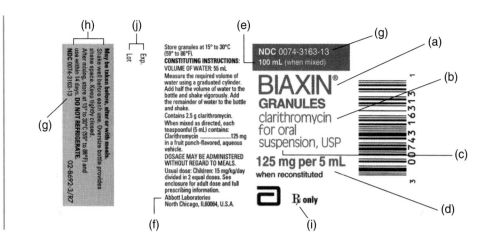

brand name. The dose form is also indicated in this area. The strength per unit or dose is prominently displayed near the drug name.

Other important features include the package size, expiration date, the manufacturer, and the National Drug Code (NDC). As described in Chapter 3, the NDC is a number assigned to every drug product. It consists of three parts, separated by dashes. The first part of the NDC represents the number assigned to the manufacturer of the drug product, the second represents the drug entity (generic name and strength), and the third indicates the package size of the drug. The NDC is used by many pharmacies to assist in identifying the exact drug and the package size it is using for the preparation of the prescription. The NDC is also used when managing inventory; when ordering drug supplies, it ensures the exact drug and package size is being ordered from the wholesaler. Some drugs may have special storage and handling requirements listed on their stock drug labels. The manufacturer's name and address also appear on this label. Some unit dose packaging and bulk-packaged products for larger institutions may have a stock drug label that contains only the drug name, dose, and manufacturer. The remainder of the information is on the reverse of a peel-off label, on a package insert inside the box, or attached to the drug container.

Pharmacy technicians handle and prepare medications more often than pharmacists do and are therefore in a better position to identify potential sources of error related to packaging and storage. A common error is the selection of the wrong pharmaceutical because two products look alike or have names that sound alike. Medication safety is more thoroughly discussed in Chapter 12, *Medication Safety*.

A good work habit is to read each stock drug label three times and to avoid basing product identification on size, color, package shape, or label design. The technician should develop the habit of making three checks to ensure the correct drug was selected: (1) when the product is initially being pulled from the inventory shelf, (2) at the time of preparation, and (3) when the product is returned to the shelf.

Safety Note

Review Appendix E for a listing of look-alike and sound-alike medications and recomendations by the ISMP.

Safety Note

Check each drug at least three times to confirm that the correct drug is dispensed.

Preparing Oral Dose Forms

Oral drug products are available in many different dose forms, and each dose form has its own dispensing requirements. The most commonly used dose form is the oral tablet or capsule. Often tablets and capsules must be counted out and placed in the appropriately sized vial. Liquid products commonly are poured directly into the dispensing bottle or are dispensed in their original packaging. Syrups and suspensions are frequently used for pediatric medications.

Figure 6.5 shows the equipment and procedure for counting tablets and capsules. A special counting tray is used. It has a trough on one side to hold counted tablets or capsules and a spout on the opposite side to pour unused medication back into the stock bottle. The technician should not touch the medication with his or her fingers, because germs and oils from the skin could contaminate the medication. Therefore the tablets and capsules should always be counted with a clean spatula and picked up with forceps if they are dropped on the counter. The spatula, tray, and forceps should be cleaned often throughout the workday with 70% isopropyl alcohol. Due to the frequency of severe patient allergies, this equipment should be cleaned after counting sulfa, penicillin, or aspirin products, as well as any product that leaves visible powder residue on the surfaces.

Dispensing Prepackaged Drugs

Filling a prescription often involves simply retrieving from stock a drug with the right name, manufacturer, and strength. Sometimes drugs come in prepackaged, unit-of-use form. A **unit of use** is a fixed number of dosage units in a drug stock container. Many drugs are prescribed as one dose daily, and many insurance companies reimburse for only a 1-month supply of medication. Unit-of-use packaging would consist of a month's supply or 30 tablets or capsules. Filling the prescription with medications in unit-of-use packaging thus amounts to little more than locating the correct drug, in the correct strength, in storage, and affixing a medication container label.

Sometimes filling a prescription involves retrieving a multiple-dose container of a premixed drug, measuring out the prescribed quantity, and placing it into a container with a label. This would be true, for example, of some powders and liquids. Again, the pharmacist must verify the quality of the technician's work that the proper drug, dose form, and amount were chosen and placed in the proper container, with a proper label prepared.

Dispensing Schedule V Over-the-Counter Drugs

Some Schedule V controlled substances may be dispensed without a prescription under specific conditions:

- The pharmacist must make the sale.

Figure 6.5

Counting Tablets
(a) Tablets should be counted by fives and moved to the trough with a spatula. (b) The unneeded tablets are returned to the stock container by pouring them from the spout. (c) The counted tablets are then poured into the appropriately sized medication vial.

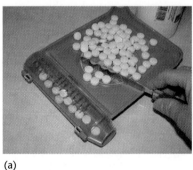
(a)

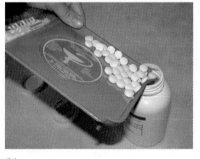
(b)

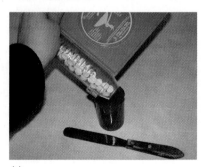
(c)

- Each state has different regulations on how much of an opium-containing controlled substance (like codeine cough medicines) can be sold to the same customer within a 48-hour period. Generally the amount is 120 to 480 mL or 4 to 8 oz of a Schedule V cough syrup.
- The purchaser must be 18 years of age and have proof of identity.

The pharmacy technician or the pharmacist must record all Schedule V controlled-substance sales in a record book. This record must include the name and address of the purchaser, date of birth, the date of purchase, the name and quantity of the Schedule V drug sold, and the name and initials of the pharmacist handling the sale.

Dispensing Drugs That Contain Ephedra

Many states have passed legislation restricting the access and sale of products containing ephedra and pseudoephedrine. These common ingredients of OTC cold medications are being used as raw products in the illegal manufacture of methamphetamine. These products must be stocked behind the counter and sold to the patient directly by the pharmacist in many states, and they may require a written record similar to the Schedule V drugs.

Choosing Containers

A wide variety of amber vial sizes are available and are named according to approximate *dram* size, even though the dram is a measure that is no longer used for writing prescriptions. (This unit of measure was discussed in Chapter 5.) Selecting the proper vial size is a skill that will be learned quickly. Most containers in the pharmacy are amber colored to prevent ultraviolet (UV) light exposure and subsequent degradation of the medication.

Other containers common to the retail pharmacy include amber liquid containers and solid-white ointment jars. Cardboard boxes may be available as well for products such as suppositories or tubes of cream. Many products such as metered-dose inhalers (MDIs) and oral contraceptives will not need a container, and the prescription label will be attached directly to the product. Some pharmacists prefer to apply prescription labels for topical products directly to the tube or jar, whereas others prefer to have the label placed on the box in which the product is packaged. A disadvantage to the latter method is that if the box is lost or discarded, the physician's directions to the patient will not be available.

Pediatric medications should always be dispensed in child-resistant containers, which are designed to be difficult for children to open. The Poison Prevention Packaging Act of 1970 requires (with some exceptions such as nitroglycerin sublingual tablets) that all prescription drugs be packaged in child-resistant containers but states that a non-child-resistant container may be used if the physician prescribing the drug or the patient receiving it makes a request for such a container. Many older patients, especially those with osteoarthritis, may have difficulty opening child-resistant containers.

The regulations of a given state may require the patient to make a special request for dispensing a prescription in a non-child-resistant container. Some pharmacies allow patients to complete a blanket request form for non-child-resistant containers. Others require patients to sign such a request for each prescription. Often pharmacies make use of a stamp on the back of the prescription for this purpose. Some OTC drugs such as

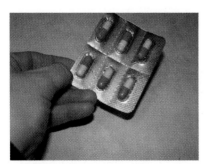

This medication is blister packed in unit dose form so that an individual dose may be prepared for the patient.

aspirin and iron that are potentially very toxic to children require the manufacturer to use child-resistant containers.

LABEL PREPARATION

From a legal point of view, a prescription drug label (i.e., medication container label) consists of all information provided on the prescription written by the physician and the **package insert** contains information on the appropriate use and common side effects of the product.

Manufacturers provide information to the pharmacist on the package inserts included with all prescription drug products. Legally, these package inserts are extensions of the labeling on the drug product, and the laws and regulations involving misbranding or mislabeling apply to them. These inserts are required by FDA regulation to contain the information listed in Table 6.4, in the order shown.

Physician's Desk Reference (PDR) is primarily a compilation of package inserts. It provides easy access to a great deal of information about prescription drugs, including a drug identification section. Pharmacy technicians can learn more about the drugs that they are helping the pharmacist to dispense by studying the *PDR* and package inserts.

A medication container label is usually generated by the computer data entry before the preparation of the prescription. This label may either be affixed directly to the container by the person generating the label, or it may be kept separate for review by the pharmacist before being affixed depending on policy and procedure of the pharmacy, as well as state laws and regulations. Figure 6.6 compares a prescription and a medication container label.

Most pharmacies of today generate medication labels on the computer. Less commonly, preprinted labels are used, requiring that information for a specific prescription be added, checked, or circled. Preprinted labels are generally discouraged because of the potential for labeling error (i.e., checking the wrong box on a preprinted label is too easy).

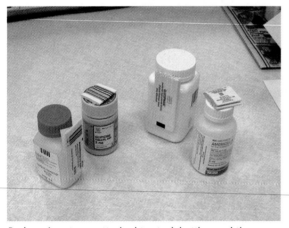

Package inserts are attached to stock bottles, and they provide detailed information about the drug. This information is regulated and is used to create patient information sheets.

Table 6.4   Organization of Package Insert Information

description
clinical pharmacology
indications and use
contraindications
warnings
precautions
adverse reactions
drug abuse and dependence
overdose
dose and administration
how supplied
date of the most recent revision of the labeling

Figure 6.6

Prescription and Label Comparison
(a) The original prescription contains the information that should be included on the label. (b) The medication container label translates the instructions for the patient.

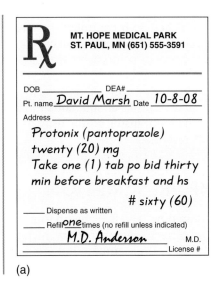

(a)

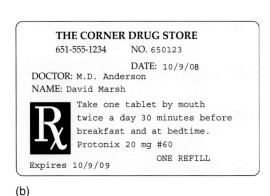

(b)

The information required on a label depends on the laws and regulations of a given state. As was indicated previously, manufacturers' labels for prescription medications must carry the legend "℞ only." Typical information required on a medication container label prepared by a pharmacy includes the information in Table 6.5.

Most computer software will print information for the patient to read and safely use the prescribed medication. In addition, auxiliary labels are the small, colorful labels that are added at the discretion of the pharmacist to supplement the labeled directions from the physician contained on the medication container (i.e., prescription label). The application of these auxiliary labels requires a thorough knowledge and understanding of the drug and is thus restricted to the professional judgment of the pharmacist. These labels could include such warnings as avoid exposure to sunlight, take with food, take on empty stomach, and avoid alcohol. For Schedule II, III, IV, and V controlled substances, the auxiliary label "Transfer Warning" is required.

Table 6.5   Label Information

Date when the prescription was filled

Serial number of the prescription

Name and address of the pharmacy

Name of the patient

Name of the prescribing physician

All directions for use given on the prescription

Any necessary auxiliary labels, containing patient precautions

Generic or brand name of the medication

Strength of the medication

Name of the drug manufacturer

Quantity of the drug

Expiration date of the drug or date after which the drug should not be used because of possible loss of potency or efficacy

Initials of the licensed pharmacist

Number of refills allowed or the phrase "No Refills"

Medication container labels for Schedule II controlled substances must contain the fill date; container labels for Schedule III, IV, and V drugs must show the date of initial filling. Labels for all prescriptions for controlled substances should include the pharmacy name and address, the serial number of the prescription, the name of the patient, the name of the physician, as well as directions for use and cautionary statements. Labels for Schedule II, III, and IV drugs should contain the cautionary statement "Caution: Federal law prohibits the transfer of this drug to any person other than the patient for whom it was prescribed."

FINAL CHECK OF THE PRESCRIPTION

It is extremely important, and required by law, that the pharmacist checks every prescription to make sure that it is correct. The pharmacist reviews the original prescription order, the computerized patient profile, the drug and quantity selected by the technician, the accuracy of the medication container label, and the price or insurance eligibility. After this review the pharmacist initials the medication container label. In doing so, the pharmacist assumes legal responsibility for the correctness of the prescription. However, the pharmacist does not necessarily assume, by this action, sole responsibility. Technicians have been held legally responsible for dispensing and labeling mistakes, especially in situations in which the dispensing error was the result of negligence on their part (e.g., improperly overriding a computerized adverse interaction warning).

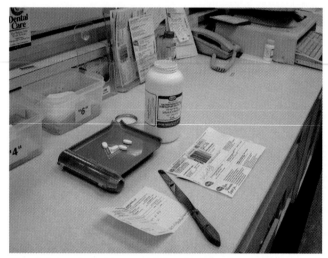

The pharmacy technician must have all prepared prescriptions checked by the supervising pharmacist.

Chapter Terms

adverse drug reaction a negative consequence to a patient from taking a particular drug

allergy a state of heightened sensitivity as a result of exposure to a particular substance

inscription the part of the prescription that lists the medication or medications prescribed, including the drug names, strengths, and amounts

package insert an information sheet required by the FDA and provided by a drug manufacturer that includes information on the product's indication and uses, dose, contraindications and warnings, as well as side effects and adverse reactions

patient profile a record kept by the pharmacy that lists a patient's identifying information, insurance information, medical history, prescription history, and prescription preferences

signa the part of the prescription that indicates the directions for the patient to follow

subscription the part of the prescription that lists instructions to the pharmacist about dispensing the medication, including information about compounding or packaging instructions, labeling instructions, refill information, and information about the appropriateness of dispensing drug equivalencies

unit of use a fixed number of dosage units in a drug stock container, usually consisting of a month's supply, or 30 tablets or capsules.

Chapter Summary

- In the community pharmacy, a pharmacy technician assumes a number of responsibilities related to both OTC and legend drugs, which depend on state laws and regulations.
- A technician can take written prescriptions from walk-in customers but cannot take new prescriptions by telephone and reduce them to writing.
- The parts of a prescription include prescriber information, the date, patient information, the symbol ℞, the inscription (i.e., the medication or medications prescribed and their amounts), the subscription (i.e., instructions to the pharmacist), the signa (i.e., directions to the patient), additional instructions, and the signature.
- The pharmacy technician is often responsible for entering the new prescription order and creating or updating the computerized patient profile including identifying information, insurance/billing information, medical history, medication/prescription history, and prescription preferences.
- The technician assists in the filling of the prescription, which commonly involves retrieving drugs, counting the prescribed quantity of medication, filling the appropriate container, and preparing labels.
- Prescriptions for controlled substances require special record-keeping procedures. Pharmacy technicins should be sure to follow any labeling requirements as determined under state and federal law.
- Medication container labels must contain a unique prescription number, the name of the patient, the date of the prescription, directions for use, the name and strength of the medication, the manufacturer of the medication, the quantity of the drug, the expiration date, the initials of the pharmacist, and the number of refills. Auxiliary labels may also be affixed to the container.
- The pharmacist is responsible for the final check of the original prescription, the patient profile, the drug and drug quantity used, and the accuracy of the medication label.

Chapter Review

Knowledge Inventory

Choose the best answer from those provided.

1. Technicians' duties with regard to over-the-counter (OTC) drugs typically include
   a. stocking them.
   b. taking inventory of them.
   c. removing expired drugs from the shelves.
   d. All of the above

2. In a prescription, the signa is the
   a. signature of the prescribing physician.
   b. initials of the pharmacist.
   c. directions for the patient to follow.
   d. instructions to the pharmacist on dispensing the medication.

3. The symbol ℞ stands for the Latin word *recipe* and means
   a. *give.*
   b. *take.*
   c. *prepare.*
   d. *mix.*

4. A signature on a prescription for a Schedule II controlled substance
   a. may be stamped.
   b. must be handwritten.
   c. must include the DEA number.
   d. may be that of the prescriber or his or her agent.

5. In most states, a generic drug may be substituted for a brand name or proprietary drug provided that the
   a. generic drug is cheaper.
   b. generic drug has undergone clinical trials.
   c. generic drug is bioequivalent to the brand name or proprietary drug.
   d. generic drug is nontoxic.

6. Pharmacy personnel can check to see if a DEA number has been falsified by
   a. looking up the number in the *FDA Electronic Orange Book.*
   b. performing a mathematic calculation.
   c. checking the number in *Drug Facts and Comparisons.*
   d. using a code to translate the number into an alphabetic form, which is the name of the prescriber.

7. An important purpose of the medication/prescription history on the patient profile is to
    a. identify potential adverse drug interactions.
    b. verify the authenticity of the current prescription.
    c. provide information on existing conditions, known allergies, and history of adverse drug interactions.
    d. provide the information used in the pharmacy's record of the controlled substances that it has dispensed.

8. A pharmacy technician can do all the following in most states *except*
    a. receive a new prescription from a patient.
    b. take a new prescription over the phone and immediately reduce it to writing.
    c. sell herbal medications.
    d. sell diet supplements.

9. A Schedule III prescription may be refilled how many times?
    a. once
    b. twice
    c. five times or within 6 months
    d. 12 times or within 1 year

10. A reference containing manufacturer patient package inserts is the
    a. *FDA Electronic Orange Book.*
    b. *United States Pharmacopeia.*
    c. *Physician's Desk Reference (PDR).*
    d. *National Formulary.*

Pharmacy in Practice

1. For each of the prescriptions on the next page, answer the following questions.
    a. Is any essential item missing from the prescription? If so, what is this item?
    b. What medication has been prescribed, in what strength, and in what amount?
    c. What special instructions, if any, are provided in the subscription?
    d. What directions are given for the patient to follow?

MT. HOPE MEDICAL PARK
MY TOWN, USA 555-3591

\# _127352_   DEA # _____

PT. NAME _Fred Figule_   DATE _____

ADDRESS _____ DOB _____

_____

Rx   Prednisone   5mg tabs
      Take AM   5 tabs day 1
                3   "   2
                2   "   3
                1 tab   "   4 and 5

REFILLS _____ TIMES (NO REFILL UNLESS INDICATED)

_____ M.D. _A Demomis_ _____ M.D.
DISPENSE AS WRITTEN   SUBSTITUTE PERMITTED

MT. HOPE MEDICAL PARK
MY TOWN, USA 555-3591

\# _42573_   DEA # _____

PT. NAME _H.R. Rubbins_   DATE _11-24-XX_

ADDRESS _____ DOB _____

_____

Rx   Tylenol/Codeine No.4
      Take 1 prn pain q4-6h

REFILLS _____ TIMES (NO REFILL UNLESS INDICATED)

_____ M.D. _J. Jutten_ _____ M.D.
DISPENSE AS WRITTEN   SUBSTITUTE PERMITTED

MT. HOPE MEDICAL PARK
MY TOWN, USA 555-3591

\#_____   DEA # _____

PT. NAME _Abby Gee_   DATE _9-10-XX_

ADDRESS _____ DOB _____

_____

Rx   Nexium 40 mg
      Take 1 cap before eating daily
                        #30

REFILLS _____ TIMES (NO REFILL UNLESS INDICATED)

C. Janew _____ M.D. _____ M.D.
DISPENSE AS WRITTEN   SUBSTITUTE PERMITTED

2. Prepare a medication container label for each of the prescriptions shown in the previous question.

a.

Paragon Pharmacy	AP 1111111
670 Main Street	220-555-3245
Anytown, USA	

Patient: _____ Prescriber: _____

Drug: _____

Date: _____ Refills: _____

b.

Paragon Pharmacy	AP 1111111
670 Main Street	220-555-3245
Anytown, USA	

Patient: _____ Prescriber: _____

Drug: _____

Date: _____ Refills: _____

c.

Paragon Pharmacy	AP 1111111
670 Main Street	220-555-3245
Anytown, USA	

Patient: _____ Prescriber: _____

Drug: _____

Date: _____ Refills: _____

3. Review the patient profile below; then answer the following questions:
   a. What essential information is missing from this profile? What questions should you ask of the customer to complete the profile?
   b. What allergies and drug reactions does the patient have?
   c. What known medical conditions does the patient have?
   d. What prescription and OTC medications is the patient currently taking?
   e. Should the customer's prescription be filled in a child-resistant container? Explain your answer.
   f. Does the customer have prescription insurance? If so, in whose name is this insurance held?

PATIENT PROFILE

Patient Name

Frames _____ Ted _____ R. _____
Last   First   Middle Initial

111 Black Road _____
Street or PO Box
Gaston _____ SC _____ 29052 _____
City   State   Zip

Phone (803) 555 7989   **Date of Birth** 07 28 38   ☒ Male ☐ Female   **Social Security No.** 249 00 0012
                            Month Day Year

☒ Yes, I would like medication dispensed in a child-resistant container.
☐ No, I do not want medication dispensed in a child-resistant container.
Medication Insurance   Card Holder Name __Ted Frames__
☒ Yes ☐ No   ☒ Card Holder   ☐ Child   ☐ Disabled Dependent
                   ☐ Spouse   ☐ Dependent Parent ☐ Full Time Student

---

MEDICAL HISTORY

HEALTH
☐ Angina
☐ Anemia
☒ Arthritis
☐ Asthma
☐ Blood Clotting Disorders
☐ High Blood Pressure
☐ Breast Feeding
☐ Cancer
☐ Diabetes
Other Conditions _____

☐ Epilepsy
☐ Glaucoma
☒ Heart Condition
☐ Kidney Disease
☐ Liver Disease
☐ Lung Disease
☐ Parkinson's Disease
☐ Pregnancy
☐ Ulcers

ALLERGIES AND DRUG REACTIONS
☐ No known drug allergies or reactions
☒ Aspirin
☐ Cephalosporins
☐ Codeine
☐ Erythromycin
☐ Penicillin
☒ Sulfa Drugs
☐ Tetracyclines
☐ Xanthines
Other Allergies/Reactions _____

Prescription Medication Being Taken
Feldene 20mg
Isoptin 80mg

OTC Medication Currently Being Taken
Nasalcrom

Would You Like Generic Medication Where Possible? ☒ Yes ☐ No

Comments

Health information changes periodically. Please notify the pharmacy of any new medications, allergies, drug reactions, or health conditions.
Ted Frames _____ Signature 9-9-XX Date ☐ I do not wish to provide this information.

4. Determine which of the following is a valid DEA number:
   AY 1234563
   AY 2749122

Improving Communication Skills

1. Sometimes customers have difficulty identifying the pharmacist and do not understand the different roles of the pharmacist and the pharmacy technician. This can be frustrating for a customer seeking assistance. What types of things could you do as a pharmacy technician to help the customers?

2. Discuss how you would handle a prescription for a controlled substance that you suspect is forged.

Internet Research

1. Visit the Web site of a local pharmacy chain drugstore.
   a. What types of services does the site provide?
   b. Does the site offer on-line counseling services?
   c. Does the site offer information regarding specific medications?

2. Visit www.dea.gov and research the effects of methamphetamine abuse. What is the Drug Endangered Children (DEC) Program?

The Business of Community Pharmacy

Chapter 7

Learning Objectives

- Explain the parts of a computer system.
- Explain the alternatives for third-party administration.
- Define and explain the terms *prescription benefits manager* and *tiered copay*.
- Discuss drug coverage for Medicaid and Medicare patients.
- Identify procedures for inventory management, including the purchasing, receiving, and storage of prescription and over-the-counter drugs.
- Identify procedures for the purchasing, receiving, storage, and inventory control of controlled-drug substances.
- Calculate inventory turnover, markup, and markup rate.
- Compute discounts.
- Apply average wholesale price to profit calculations.

In addition to assisting the pharmacist in the dispensing and preparing of medications in the community pharmacy environment, the pharmacy technician performs an important role in billing third-party insurance, as well as assisting in the purchasing, receiving, and inventorying of all pharmaceuticals including over-the-counter (OTC) drugs. The process of billing insurance companies on-line has greatly lessened the quantity of paperwork in the average retail pharmacy. This chapter discusses the Medicare Prescription Drug, Improvement, and Modernization Act (MMA) of 2003, which provides a drug insurance benefit to older adults. Pharmacy technicians also have the responsibility of monitoring and correcting insurance billing of prescription products. Inventory management is a duty assigned to the seasoned pharmacy technician who understands the movement of drug items on the shelf and how inventory levels are related to the cash flow in the pharmacy. The chapter provides an overview of the business functions that are critical to the success of the pharmacy operation. To aid in this success, the pharmacy technician must possess a basic understanding of both computer and mathematic skills.

MANAGING COMPUTER SYSTEMS

Computers are a critical tool needed for the safe and efficient dispensing of prescriptions in the community pharmacy. From their beginnings as simple order-input devices, contemporary pharmacy computer systems have evolved into complex systems offering a wide range of functions such as checking and updating patient profile information, checking for possible allergies and drug interactions, printing labels, calculating charges, and completing automated third-party billing. Most pharmacy computer systems contain automatic warnings about possible allergic or other adverse reactions. Systems vary from pharmacy to pharmacy. Some computer systems are capable of controlling automatic or robotic dispensing and compounding devices, tracking expenses and inventory reports, generating controlled-substances reports, performing special dosing calculations, or retrieving medical and pharmacy literature.

Because of the widespread use of computers in pharmacy, the aspiring technician should become familiar with computer systems and how they work. Becoming competent at basic keyboarding (i.e., typing) with a minimum competency of 30 words per minute is also essential. This section provides some elementary information about computer systems, but a thorough introduction to computers is beyond the scope of this book.

Parts of a Computer System

A **computer** is an electronic device for inputting, storing, processing, and/or outputting information. A digital computer represents information internally using binary numbers, which are constructed of strings of ones and zeros. Many types of digital computers exist today. In order of size and power, some types of computers available include supercomputers, mainframe computers, minicomputers, workstations, network computers, personal desktop or laptop computers, and handheld or palmtop computers. Some of the more important parts of a typical computer system include the following (Figure 7.1):

- one or more **input devices**, such as a keyboard, a mouse, or a touch screen, for getting information into the computer
- **central processing unit (CPU)** for processing (i.e., manipulating) data that are input before output or storage
- one or more **storage devices**, such as a floppy disk drive, hard drive, tape drive, compact disk (CD) drive, or removable disk drive (e.g., Zip, Jaz, SyQuest) for storing information that has been input into the computer
- **random-access memory (RAM)**, which is the temporary, nonpermanent memory of the computer in which information is held while it is being input and processed
- **read-only memory (ROM)**, which is permanent memory containing essential operating instructions for the computer
- **monitor**, or display screen, that provides a visual representation of data that have been input and/or processed
- **printer**, for creating hard copy, or paper output, such as patient profiles, medication labels, and receipts
- **scanner**, for inputting a photo version of the prescription into the computer system, used in some pharmacies to save the step of pulling out a hard copy of the prescription if a question about its original intent occurs
- **modem**, a device for connecting a computer to a remote computer via telephone lines
- **operating system**, a software program that performs essential functions such as maintaining a list of file names, issuing processing instructions, and controlling output
- **applications**, software programs that perform particular functions, such as word processing or spreadsheets

Figure 7.1

A Desktop Computer System

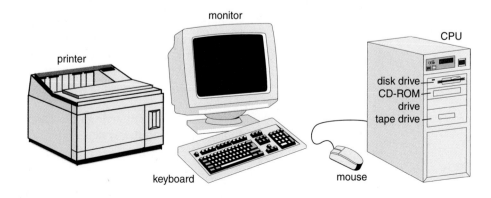

Figure 7.2

VisualScript Database Management System

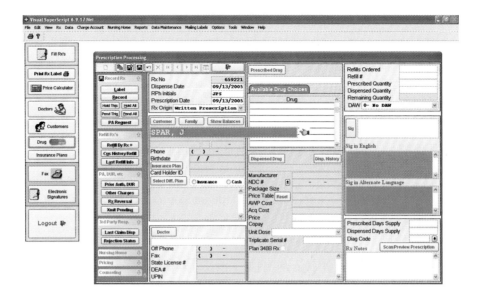

A software program application that allows one to enter, retrieve, and query records is known as a **database management system (DBMS).** A DBMS is the kind of application most commonly used in pharmacy. A DBMS contains many fields of information that can be sorted (or queried) and studied in various ways. The DBMS is usually specifically written and/or altered to meet the needs of that pharmacy or drug chain. Such a program, known as a *vertically integrated application*, meets a wide variety of needs from customer record keeping (i.e., mailing refill reminders to patients) to inventory control and billing. Often the pharmacy DBMS is menu driven, allowing the operator to choose functions from a menu of options on the screen by typing a single number, letter, or function key on the keyboard. A sample interface is shown in Figure 7.2.

How Pharmacy Computer Systems Work

In most small, independent pharmacies, the computer is a *smart terminal* or a computer device that contains its own storage and processing capabilities. In larger pharmacies, including most drug chains, the operator works at a *dumb terminal*, a computer device that contains a keyboard and a monitor but does not contain its own storage and processing capabilities. The terminal is connected to a *remote computer*—often a minicomputer or a mainframe—that stores and processes data.

Pharmacy computer systems differ dramatically from one another. In large retail chains, computers are commonly connected to a single large mainframe system at the company headquarters or home office. In such systems, customer records are stored remotely, backed up at the home office computer site, and accessed via telecommunications (i.e., connecting to the remote computer via telephone lines, digital subscriber line [DSL], cable, or wireless connections). Wireless communications involve the transmission of data or voice signals through the air and involve transmitters, receivers, and, often, satellites. Wireless communications are critical for determining patient eligibility and on-line processing of prescription claims (discussed later in this chapter).

Pharmacy computer systems often allow the operator to call up patient profiles onscreen and to enter new prescription information. A hard-copy patient profile might then be generated for backup filing. Drugs are generally identified on computer screens by product name, manufacturer, strength, and unique National Drug Code (NDC) number. The computer system may automatically print medication container labels that include information keyed into the profile for a given prescription. Many systems in use today contain automatic capabilities to compare the patient profile with new prescription information entered and warn of possible adverse drug interactions or potential problems with allergic reactions to a given prescription. Such systems typically prevent the filling of an order until a pharmacist intervenes. In no situation should a pharmacy technician override such a warning on his or her own initiative. In all cases the pharmacist should review the warning and make the professional decision as to whether the prescription should be filled.

Computers are fallible machines. They often break down and are susceptible to such problems as power failures and surges. Therefore copies, or backups, of all data should be made at regular intervals. Often pharmacy computer systems make use of tape backup devices. A tape backup device stores backup data on magnetic tape.

BILLING AND THIRD-PARTY ADMINISTRATION

Most patients have major medical coverage through either their employer or that of their spouse. In the past this coverage was limited to hospitalizations and emergency room coverage. A patient would have to pay cash for each physician visit and at the time of picking up a prescription. Today most patients have insurance coverage from a private insurance company through their employer or from the state (i.e., Medicaid) or federal government (i.e., Medicare). Unfortunately, the cost of health-care, including health insurance, is far outpacing the rate of inflation.

Private health insurance usually includes some combination of individual and family deductible, copays per visit or prescription, and limits on total or lifetime benefits. The first $1500 paid on a new General Motors automobile covers health benefits for General Motors' employees and retirees. An employer may or may not elect to provide drug benefit coverage; Medicaid and Medicare both offer drug benefit coverage with some limitations and restrictions. It is important to remember that as of 2006 there are 45 million adults and children in the United States who do not have any type of health insurance. For individuals who are either unemployed, work part-time, or are underinsured by their employers, the cost of private health insurance is prohibitive.

Many pharmacy customers have prescription drug insurance, which requires billing to be sent from the pharmacy to a third party. If the customer has such insurance, then he or she may carry a prescription card containing information such as the following: the name of the insured person, the insurance carrier, a group number, a cardholder identification number, information on coverage of dependents, an expiration date, and the amount of the charges paid for prescriptions or other medical care. The technician must request this information and either enter it into the computer system or, if the pharmacy uses a manual system for third-party billing, onto a form—generally a **universal claim form (UCF)**. A UCF is sometimes used to submit a reimbursement to a third-party insurer for unusual prescriptions. However, the use of these forms is decreasing.

Processing Prescription Drug Claims

When a new prescription is received, the pharmacy technician must obtain all necessary insurance information from the customer, including deductibles plus any copay or coinsurance percent amount. Most of this information is available on the patient's prescription card. The **deductible** is an amount that must be paid by the insured, (e.g., $250), usually at the beginning of the year, before the insurance company will consider paying its portion of the medical cost. A **copayment** (or copay) is the flat amount the patient is to pay for each prescription; copays vary by both drug and insurance company. **Coinsurance** is the term for a percentage-based plan whereby the patient must pay a certain percentage of the prescription price. The deductible, copay, or coinsurance are all methods by which an insurance company tries to control healthcare costs.

Billing policies and procedures differ from pharmacy to pharmacy and from customer to customer. In some cases the customer pays for the prescription at the time he or she receives it. The customer may or may not then be reimbursed by an insurer for "out-of-pocket" cost. In other cases billing involves **third-party administration (TPA)** or direct billing by the pharmacy to the customer's insurer. After the computer calculates the price of the prescription at the time of filling, the pharmacist verifies insurance coverage.

Billing of the third party may be handled in a variety of ways:
- transferring the bill to the third party electronically via modem
- placing the bill on a computer diskette that is then mailed to the insurer
- generating a bill that is mailed to the third party
- submitting a manually prepared bill, usually one on a UCF, to the insurer

Most insurance companies today will accept or reject a claim on-line while the pharmacy technician and pharmacist are processing the prescription. Many insurance companies elect to *outsource* (or contract outside the insurance company) for this administrative function. A **prescription benefits manager (PBM)** is a company that provides this service on-line by administering the prescription drug benefits from many different insurance companies. This process, called *on-line adjudication*, takes less than 1 minute during the prescription fill process and saves the pharmacy a great deal of paperwork when performed properly.

When the prescription is billed to a PBM (or individual insurance company), the pharmacy will be notified within a few minutes what amount it should charge the patient and what amount the pharmacy will be reimbursed. In some cases the PBM advises the pharmacy that a deductible needs to be met before benefits will be paid. The PBM may also inform the pharmacy of the appropriate copay or coinsurance that the patient is responsible for paying. In some cases a patient may have a dual copay—one copay for brand names and a lower one for generics (e.g., $25.00 for brand names; $10.00 for generics). Similarly, coinsurance coverage is the option in which a higher percentage (e.g., 30%) is in effect for brand name medications and usually a lower percentage is in effect for generic medications (e.g., 10%). Copays are for each drug and generally are paid for each 30- or 90-day supply of medication. Five or six copays may be available at the time of each refill for a patient with medications for high blood pressure, diabetes, and high cholesterol.

More common today is the use of a *tiered copay* by many PBMs and insurance companies. The tiered copay has an escalating cost for a generic, a *preferred* brand, and a *nonpreferred* brand. The PBM has a formulary of preferred medications for various medical conditions for which it will pay maximum benefits and a list of drugs that are either not fully covered or not covered at all. To complicate matters, each insurance company/PBM has a unique formulary that is constantly changing; on-line adjudication can greatly assist in this complex process.

Patients are often provided with these lists of preferred drugs and encouraged to share them with their physicians so that *appropriate and preferred medications* may be selected from the list whenever possible. Physicians cannot remember which drug is on which PBM formulary, so the patient, or the pharmacist acting as the patient advocate, may need to discuss therapy options with the physician, especially if drug affordability is an issue. For example, a PBM may elect to cover the generic drug lovastatin and the brand name drug Zocor for the treatment of high cholesterol. The

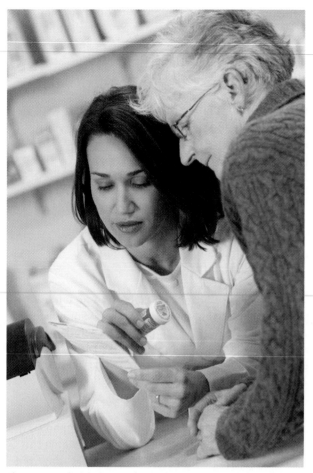

Pharmacy technicians may discuss insurance coverage with patients to help them understand their medication expenses.

copay for lovastatin may be $10, the copay for the Zocor may be $25, and the copay for Lipitor (the *nonpreferred* brand name drug) may be $50.

When the physician decides the patient must have a medication that is not on the insurance company's formulary, it may be necessary to obtain an override number (or *prior approval* or *prior authorization*) from the insurance company/PBM for the prescription to be properly covered. For example, in the previous patient example, if the patient's cholesterol could not be controlled with lovastatin and the patient suffered an adverse reaction to the Zocor, the PBM would, in most cases, approve drug coverage for Lipitor at the *preferred brand* copay amount ($25 as opposed to $50 in this example).

In some cases these *nonpreferred prescriptions* cannot be adjudicated on-line and must be hand-billed on a UCF to the appropriate insurance company/PBM. Many of these cases require weeks or even months to resolve, thus delaying reimbursement to the pharmacy. Cases exist in which the medication selected by the physician and needed by the patient is not covered by the insurance under any circumstance. This lack of coverage is true for newly marketed innovative drugs that are extremely expensive, as well as drugs that have less costly alternatives. If a question about coverage arises, then having a photocopy of the patient's insurance card on file with appropriate contact phone numbers is often helpful. The pharmacy technician often has to be empathetic to a patient who does not fully understand why his or her medications are so expensive and not fully covered by the insurance company.

Medicaid Prescription Billing

Each state has its own policies, procedures, and regulations on the reimbursement of prescription drugs for Medicaid patients. Medicaid subsidizes the cost of healthcare, including drugs, for indigent and disabled citizens of its state who meet age and income eligibility requirements. Eligibility is renewed monthly and must be verified by the pharmacy technician at the receipt of the prescription. If a patient does not present his or her Medicaid card and turns out to be ineligible for benefits during a specific month, then the pharmacy will receive no reimbursement. Today Medicaid eligibility can often be verified online.

Most community pharmacies sign a contract to agree to provide prescription benefits to this disadvantaged population according to the terms of that state. With few exceptions, OTC drugs are not covered. Some states may have a formulary of acceptable drugs they will cover. Other states will provide a maximum number of prescriptions (usually five) that can be covered in any 1 month. Most states have instituted a minimal copay (usually less than $5.00) per prescription to discourage misuse.

The state reimbursement rate to pharmacies is generally *usual and customary charges*. This means that the pharmacy cannot charge the state more for the same prescription dispensed to a private or commercial insurance patient. Thus the pharmacist must avoid agreeing to nonprofitable contracts with PBMs or insurance companies, because Medicaid patients would add more financial loss to the balance sheet. In fact, because of the rising nature of drug costs and shrinking state tax revenues, some states are *outsourcing* their drug coverage to PBMs and others. Some community pharmacies elect not to accept Medicaid coverage because of low reimbursement, delays or errors in receipt of payment, and challenges on legitimate drug claims from accounting audits. The pharmacy can receive stiff financial and civil penalties for intentional or unintentional errors in billing.

Medicare Prescription Drug, Improvement, and Modernization Act of 2003

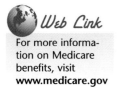

Web Link

For more information on Medicare benefits, visit
www.medicare.gov

Congress passed the original Medicare bill in 1965 to assist in the coverage of *major medical* healthcare costs (Medicare Part A and B) of citizens over the age of 65. Major medical coverage included costs for hospitalizations, emergency room and physician visits, laboratory tests and X-rays, and short-term nursing home admissions. However, coverage of prescription drugs outside the hospital (as well as long-term nursing home care) was not included at that time. For the past 40 years, older adult patients have had to pay out of pocket for medications or pay extra for supplemental insurance for drug coverage through their employers or commercial insurers. The cost of prescription drugs has outpaced inflation, and many patients on fixed income social security benefits have often had to choose between food and heat or drugs for their discretionary dollars. Some patients have resorted to the "illegal" importation of drugs from Canada. However, enforcement of the law to individuals purchasing small, personal quantities of prescription medications has been discouraged.

The **Medicare Prescription Drug, Improvement, and Modernization Act (MMA) of 2003**, also called Medicare Part D, offers eligible patients the option to add drug insurance to their health coverage. Starting in January 2006, patients who qualified for Medicare coverage were eligible to add drug benefit coverage for an additional monthly charge to their current premium. The initial enrollment started in November 2005 and proceeded through May 2006. Nearly 30 million Medicare patients were expected to take advantage of this insurance program. If eligible patients opted not to join initially, then the monthly cost may be higher if they decide to join in the future.

In this voluntary program a patient may elect to continue current drug coverage through his or her existing supplemental health insurance or employer. The plan has special provisions for low-income seniors who would likely benefit most from this program. This Medicare plan provides catastrophic coverage for all patients who develop serious medical conditions requiring expensive drug treatments.

This plan is complex with many choices for coverage, but each patient is expected to save an average of 25% to 30% from his or her current annual out-of-pocket cost of prescriptions. Older adults can choose from several insurance plans that are available in each region of the country. Each plan has its advantages and disadvantages, and each has a different list of lower-cost, *preferred* drugs. For example, a $250.00 deductible and a monthly premium must be paid before the patient is eligible for benefits. After the deductible is met, patients will pay an average of 25%

of the cost for their new and refilled prescriptions until they have spent a total of $2250.00. From $2250.00 to $5100.00 patients are responsible for 100% of the cost of their medications. Once $5100.00 in drug costs have been reached in the calendar year, the patient will only pay 5% of the cost of the medications. The premium, as well the annual drug costs, is adjusted annually with inflation.

Although far from perfect, the MMA of 2003 addresses the important issue of partial insurance coverage for prescription drugs. Patients will be frustrated and confused, and continue to have many questions about this insurance coverage. The pharmacy technician can provide a valuable service by educating patients on drug insurance coverage for their individual drug regimens. The MMA also provides for the reimbursement of pharmacists to review the medication profile of high-risk patients with high-cost drugs to ensure safe and cost-effective therapy. The cost for reimbursing pharmacists is expected to be offset by fewer unnecessary hospitalizations and emergency department visits.

INVENTORY MANAGEMENT

The primary purpose of inventory management is the timely purchase and receipt of pharmaceuticals and to establish and maintain appropriate levels of materials in stock. Purchasing, receiving, and inventory processes should be as uncomplicated as possible so as not to disrupt or to interfere with the other activities of the pharmacy. Community pharmacies must stock, or have ready access to, all drugs that may be written by the physicians in their practice area. In the community pharmacy most pharmaceutical products are purchased through a local wholesaler. To minimize the cost of doing business, inventory levels must be adequate but not excessive with a rapid turnover of drug stock on the shelf. The purchasing, receipt, and inventory of controlled-drug substances requires special procedures and record-keeping requirements.

Purchasing

Purchasing is defined as the ordering of products for use or sale by the pharmacy and is usually carried out by either an independent or group process. In independent purchasing, the pharmacist or technician deals directly with a drug wholesaler (or rarely the pharmaceutical manufacturer) regarding matters such as price and terms. In group purchasing, a number of pharmacies work together to negotiate a discount for high-volume purchases and more favorable contractual terms. The state pharmacy association may act as a facilitator for group purchasing contracting for its members as a benefit. Some independent purchasing exists in almost all pharmacy settings, because some drug products are not available through group purchasing.

Several purchasing methods or systems are used in pharmacies:

- **Direct purchasing** requires completion of a purchase order, generally a preprinted form with a unique number, on which the product name(s), amount(s), and price(s) are entered. If the pharmacy uses a purchasing agent, then a purchase requisition is sent to that agent. The order is then transmitted directly to the manufacturer. An advantage of direct purchasing is a lower cost and the lack of add-on fees. A disadvantage is the commitment of time and staff on the part of the pharmacy since there are multiple requisitions to be completed and mailed to multiple pharmaceutical companies.
- **Wholesaler purchasing** enables the pharmacy to use a single source to purchase numerous products from numerous manufacturers. Some pharmacies utilize more than one wholesaler. Most drug ordering is done on-line. Advantages

to wholesaler purchasing include reduced turnaround time for orders, lower inventory and lower associated costs, and reduced commitment of time and staff. Disadvantages include higher purchase cost, supply difficulties, loss of the control provided by in-house purchase orders, and unavailability of some pharmaceuticals.

- **Prime vendor purchasing** involves an agreement made by a pharmacy for a specified percentage or dollar volume of purchases. Such a system offers the advantages of lower acquisition costs, competitive service fees, electronic order entry, and emergency delivery services.
- **Just-in-time (JIT) purchasing** involves frequent purchasing in quantities that just meet supply needs until the next ordering time. JIT reduces the quantity of each product on the shelves and thus reduces the amount of money committed to inventory. However, such a system can be used only when supplies are readily available and pharmaceutical needs can be accurately predicted.

As expected, controlled-substance pharmaceuticals require special consideration. The Controlled Substances Act (CSA) defines procedures for purchasing and receiving and requirements for inventory and record keeping. Each pharmacy must register with the Drug Enforcement Administration (DEA) to purchase Schedule II drugs. The purchase of such controlled substances must be authorized by a pharmacist and executed on a DEA 222 form (Figure 7.3). This form provides the record of any Schedule II substances sold or delivered to another DEA-registered dispenser.

Receiving

Delivery of an order of products initiates a series of procedures known as **receiving**. Institutions and pharmacies should have a system of checks and balances for purchasing and receiving. In other words, full control should not reside with a single person, and the person ordering should not be the same as the person receiving. The pharmaceutical products received must be carefully checked against the purchase order or requisition. The shipment should be compared for name of product, quantity, product strength, and product package size. Products damaged in shipment or

Figure 7.3

DEA 222 Form
This form must be completed and signed by the pharmacist for the ordering of all Schedule II controlled substances.

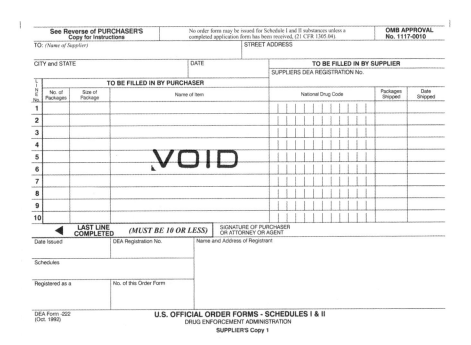

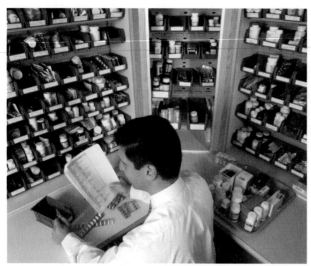
The pharmacy tech often cross-checks delivery of drugs with an order and updates pricing in the computer.

improperly shipped or stored must be reported to the pharmacist and vendor immediately. Stringent laws regulate the return of pharmaceuticals to manufacturers. In the case of a damaged or incorrect shipment, the manufacturer should be notified immediately and authorization should be secured for the return of the defective shipment.

Pharmaceuticals in a shipment should be carefully checked by the pharmacy technician for price updates and expiration dates. Each pharmacy has a policy for an acceptable range of product expiration dates. A typical requirement might be that products have expiration dates of at least 6 months from the date of receipt. After products are received and checked, they are placed in a proper storage location. The expiration dates of stored products on the shelf are periodically checked, and expired products are removed from stock. An accepted method for stocking pharmaceuticals is to position the units of product with the shortest expiration dates where they will be the first units selected for use.

Occasionally a pharmaceutical product will be temporarily or permanently unavailable from a supplier. It then becomes necessary to borrow or purchase a small quantity from another institution or pharmacy. A policy and procedure for control and accountability for loaned or borrowed products is necessary.

The DEA-registered pharmacy must maintain complete and accurate records of controlled substances. Receiving records include the DEA order form with the DEA number of the supplier, as well as receipts, sales, and dispensing. The record must contain substance name, dose form, strength or concentration per dose unit, and amount of dose units per commercial container. In the community pharmacy, the prescription is the written record of controlled substances dispensed. The DEA has a "paper trail" for each Schedule II drug from the drug manufacturer to the patient (if an audit is ever needed).

The pharmacist usually is responsible for the receipt and secure storage of Schedule II drugs. All commercial controlled-substance containers must be clearly marked with their *schedule* on the product label. This mark is an uppercase Roman numeral with or without a *C* symbol.

II or C-II
III or C-III
IV or C-IV
V or C-V

The symbol *C* and/or the Roman numeral must be at least twice the size of the largest letters printed on the label. When a bottle is too small to receive the symbol or numerals, then the box and package insert must contain them. Symbols and/or numerals are generally not required on the containers of dispensed medications.

Inventory Management Processes

The entire stock of products on hand for sale at a given time in a community pharmacy is known as **inventory**. **Inventory value** is defined as the total value of the drugs and merchandise in stock on a given day. In addition to prescription drugs,

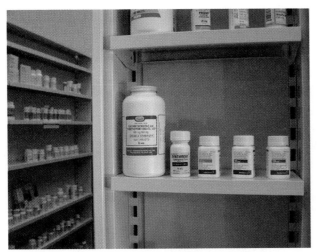
The pharmacy inventory must be carefully maintained.

inventory includes OTC drugs, diet supplements, supplies, and front-end merchandise. Pharmacies must maintain a record of drugs and other supplies and merchandise purchased and sold to know when to reorder and when to adjust inventory levels of each item. Unlike some businesses, however, a pharmacy may need to keep some very slow-moving drugs in stock as a service to a few customers.

Several important issues with regard to inventory management include how much inventory should be maintained, when inventory levels should be adjusted, and where inventory should be stored. Factors that bear on decisions regarding these issues include floor space allocation, design and arrangement of shelves, and demands on available refrigerator or freezer space.

Keeping medications on the shelf is a cost to a pharmacy, and an excessive inventory can hinder cash flow. Keeping excess inventory in stock has a number of associated costs, including the capital that is tied up in the inventory, waste because of product expiration, and increased likelihood of theft or contamination. Inventory management should be designed so that medications arrive shortly before they are dispensed and sold to minimize shelf space and maximize cash flow. The pharmacy technician is often in charge of restocking the OTC drug shelves. Proper shelf labeling, location of stock, setting inventory levels, rotating stock, and checking expiration dates are all important roles in the pharmacy. Checking for expired vitamins and herbs is especially important, because they can lose their labeled potency quickly.

Today a variety of methods may be used for inventory management. In some systems the pharmacist or pharmacy technician determines when a product needs to be reordered and enters it into an order book. Other systems make use of inventory records on which an ongoing usage report is kept. Some systems make use of predetermined minimum and maximum product levels based on historical or seasonal use. In still other systems, purchasing is based on calculation of the most economic order quantity or value.

Today many community pharmacies use a computerized inventory control system, which can automatically generate purchase orders under predetermined conditions. An important goal of computerized inventory control is to reduce the time and staff required for inventory management, as well as to maintain a balance of adequate stock with adequate turnover. Each time drugs are purchased from the wholesaler, the quantity and price are entered into the computer database. As a customer purchases the prescription product, the computer system automatically adjusts the inventory record. Pharmacies usually establish an inventory range for each item (i.e., a maximum and a minimum number of units to have on hand). When the inventory drops to the minimum level, the item is purchased to restock the supply. This predetermined order point and the order quantity is based on historical use of each drug. The following is an example of inventory management.

Example 1 **The maximum inventory level for ampicillin capsules is 1000. At the end of the day, the computer prints a list of items to be reordered; the list indicates an inventory level of 75 ampicillin capsules. How many capsules should be ordered to restock the inventory to the maximum? If the drug wholesaler supplies ampicillin in bottles of 25, 100, 250, and 500 capsules, how many**

of each bottle size will fill the order (assuming that you begin with one 500-capsule bottle)?

To replenish the ampicillin inventory to the maximum level (1000 capsules), first determine how much the present level differs.

$$1000 \text{ capsules} - 75 \text{ capsules} = 925 \text{ capsules}$$

According to this calculation, 925 capsules need to be purchased. The drug can be purchased in bottles of 500, 250, 100, and 25 capsules. It is good business practice to purchase the smallest possible number of bottles because large-quantity containers are usually a more economical purchase.

1 bottle of 500 capsules + 1 bottle of 250 capsules + 1 bottle of 100 capsules
+ 3 bottles of 25 capsules = 925 capsules

Although this example is important to illustrate the calculation, realistically, in this situation, a single package of 1000 would most likely be ordered.

Often today's pharmacies have $100,000 to $250,000 or more in inventory sitting on the shelves as drug products. If a large chain has 10 stores in a particular region, then the amount of money in goods sitting on the shelf adds up very quickly.

A physical inventory, or counting of items in stock, is taken when no perpetual inventory system is in place. Pharmacies may take an inventory as often as once a month or once a year. An inventory value is used to determine average inventory and turnover rate. The **average inventory** allows a pharmacy to determine the number of times that pharmaceuticals are repurchased in a specific period of time, usually annually. The following equation is used to calculate average inventory:

$$\text{average inventory} = \frac{\text{beginning inventory} + \text{ending inventory}}{2}$$

Turnover rate is the number of times the entire stock is used and replaced each year and calculated with the following formula:

$$\text{turnover rate} = \frac{\text{annual dollar purchases}}{\text{average inventory}}$$

Large companies often set goals for lowering the inventory to improve cash flow. One method used to set inventory goals for a pharmacy is called *days' supply*, which refers to making the value of the inventory approximately equal to the cost to the pharmacy of the products sold in a certain number of days. A common number is in the 25- to 35-day range. For example, if a pharmacy has a goal of *30 days' supply*, it means that the goal is to reduce the value of the inventory to equal the total cost to the pharmacy of the products sold every 30 days. Thus the average inventory would *turn over* each month or 12 times per year.

Sometimes a pharmacy does not know the best number of days to use as a goal in calculating costs for inventory turnover. What the pharmacy does know is the current inventory value, and average daily costs are easily calculated (weekly costs ÷ 7 days). With this information, it can be determined how many days it will take the average daily product costs to equal the value of the inventory, known as the *days' supply*. Then the pharmacy can revise the goal as necessary. The following equation is used to calculate the number of days' supply:

$$\text{number of days' supply} = \frac{\text{value of inventory}}{\text{average daily cost of products sold}}$$

The following is an example of how a community pharmacy can calculate its desired days' supply of inventory.

Example 2

Tom's Pharmacy has a total inventory value of $103,699.00. It had sales last week of $37,546.00, and the cost to the pharmacy of the products sold was $28,837.00. What should Tom's days' supply be to keep its inventory value stable?

Tom's average daily product costs were the following:

$$\$28{,}837.00 \div 7 \text{ days} = \$4120.00 \text{ (rounded)}$$

Now, according to the previous formula, dividing the value of the inventory by the average daily product costs approximately equals the number of days' supply.

$$\text{number of days' supply} = \frac{\$103{,}699.00}{\$4120.00} = 25$$

Thus, in 25 days, Tom's will have sold products approximately equal to the value of its inventory.

The pharmacy technician is often responsible for handling drug returns for credits to the wholesaler or manufacturer. These returns may be because of expired drugs, damaged drugs or supplies received, drug recalls by the drug manufacturer or FDA, reformulated drugs, drugs in new packaging, or drugs that are no longer manufactured. This process often involves a lot of paperwork and is time-consuming; however, it is an important part of inventory management and maintaining a profitable business. Importantly, prescription vials returned by the patient—even if unopened—cannot, by law, be returned to stock or for credit except in the case of a drug recall. Depending on the policy of the pharmacy, the cost of returned drugs may or may not allow a reimbursement to the patient.

Safety Note

Prescription vials returned by the patient cannot be returned to stock, even if they are unopened.

Inventory Management Requirements for Controlled Substances

The DEA requires that a complete inventory of all controlled substances must be taken every 2 years. Some states have more stringent requirements such as a yearly inventory. An exact count is required for Schedule II drugs. For Schedules III, IV, and V, an estimated count and/or measure is permitted unless a container holds more than 1000 capsules or tablets. If the container has been opened, then an exact count is required. The taking of an actual inventory should not vary more than 4 days from the biennial inventory date.

The complete inventory must include an inventory record and an extemporaneous compounding record. The inventory record must contain the following information for each controlled substance:

- name of the drug
- dose form and strength
- number of dose units or volume in each container
- number of containers

An extemporaneous compounding record must contain the following information:

- name of the drug
- total quantity in units or to the nearest metric unit weight
- the reason the drug is maintained in inventory (i.e., stocked for prescription compounding)

Schedule III, IV, and V controlled substances must be stored in a secured area or cabinet or otherwise distributed throughout all drug inventory. Most states require stricter management of stored Schedule II controlled substances, such as in a locked cabinet or vault. Many community pharmacies use a *perpetual* inventory to maintain close control of the Schedule II drug stock. A perpetual inventory is a method of maintaining ongoing accountability for Schedule II medications on a tablet-by-tablet (or other dose form) basis. Access to Schedule II substances is sometimes limited to the pharmacist.

All Schedule II records must be kept separate from other prescription records. All Schedule III, IV, and V records may be kept in a readily retrievable form. These records must be maintained for a minimum of 2 years. Some states require holding records for 5 years.

A pharmacy may file *schedule substance records* in one of the following ways:

- Schedule II alone; Schedules III, IV, and V together; and a file for all other prescriptions
- Schedule II alone and a file for all other prescriptions (A red *C* or symbol at least 1-inch tall is to be stamped in the lower-right corner of the Schedule III, IV, and V prescriptions.)
- All Schedule II prescriptions together with Schedule III, IV, and V stamped with a red *C* or symbol at least 1-inch tall in the lower-right corner of the prescription and a file for all other prescriptions

BUSINESS MATH USED IN PHARMACY PRACTICE

A community pharmacy operates under the same principles as any other business: it deals with expenses and receipts. In addition, like any other business, the pharmacy must make a **profit** (i.e., it must have more receipts than expenses to continue to provide customer services). One of the responsibilities of the pharmacy technician is to help ensure that the receipts are greater than the expenses.

The technician often takes care of pricing in the pharmacy by marking products up a certain percentage over the cost and by marking products down by a percentage discount at other times. Insurance companies most often use either a percentage-based payment for prescription products or a capitation fee. The successful pharmacy technician will need to master basic mathematic skills that are used in markup, discount, average wholesale price (AWP), capitation fee, and inventory management.

Markup

Like all businesses, pharmacies purchase their products (i.e., drugs) at one price and sell them at a higher price. This difference is called **gross profit** or **markup**. Prescription pricing is subject to governmental laws and regulations, as well as competition within the marketplace. Markup plays an important part in the pricing system. The markup is computed as follows:

$$\text{selling price} - \text{purchase price} = \text{markup or gross profit}$$

The markup rate is calculated as follows:

$$\frac{\text{markup}}{\text{cost}} \times 100\% = \text{markup rate}$$

Example 3

A 30-day supply of an antidiabetic agent sells for $45.00 and costs the pharmacy $30.00. What is the markup and markup rate?

The markup is computed as follows:

$$\$45.00 \text{ selling price} - \$30.00 \text{ purchase price} = \$15.00 = \text{markup or gross profit}$$

The markup rate is computed as follows:

$$\frac{\text{markup}}{\text{cost}} \times 100\% = \text{markup rate}$$

$$\frac{\$15.00 \text{ markup}}{\$30.00 \text{ purchase price}} \times 100\% = \text{markup rate}$$

$$50\% = \text{markup rate}$$

Discount

Sometimes a manufacturer or a supplier offers an item at a lower price to a pharmacy. This reduced price is a **discount**. Similarly, a pharmacy may offer a consumer a discount, or a deduction from what is normally charged, as an incentive to purchase an item. Discount and discounted price is calculated with the following formulas:

$$\text{purchase price} \times \text{discount rate} = \text{discount}$$

$$\text{purchase price} - \text{discount} = \text{discounted price}$$

Example 4

Assume the pharmacy purchases five cases of dermatologic cream at $100.00 per case. If the account is paid in full within 15 days, the supplier offers a 15% discount on the purchase. What is the total discounted purchase price?

First calculate the total purchase price.

$$\text{quantity of product} \times \text{cost per unit} = \text{total purchase price}$$
$$5 \text{ cases} \times \$100.00 \text{ per case} = \$500.00$$

Next calculate the discount for payment within 15 days.

$$\text{total purchase price} \times \text{discount rate} = \text{discount}$$
$$\$500.00 \times 0.15 = \$75.00$$

Finally, to obtain the discounted price, subtract the discount from the original price.

$$\text{total purchase price} - \text{discount} = \text{discounted purchase price}$$
$$\$500.00 \times \$75.00 = \$425.00$$

Average Wholesale Price Applications

A pharmacy may potentially receive payment for the drug product and its services from several different sources. Historically, patients have been responsible for paying for their own medications, but this responsibility is occurring much less often than in the past. More recently, health maintenance organizations (HMOs) and health insurance companies (or PBMs) have become major players in determining the cost of healthcare, including patient medications. The very survival of a pharmacy depends on its ability to contain drug costs. The **average wholesale price (AWP)** of a drug is an *average* price that wholesalers charge the pharmacy. Usually, third parties reimburse a pharmacy based on the AWP less an agreed on discount. Therefore the pharmacy has an incentive to purchase a drug as far below its AWP as possible. Drugs are sold below AWP in some situations (e.g., via group purchasing, volume discounts, contract situations, rebates from manufacturers). The AWP is used to calculate a prescription reimbursement with the following formula:

$$\text{prescription reimbursement} = \text{AWP} \pm \text{percentage} + \text{dispensing fee}$$

Example 5

A certain tablet comes in a quantity of 60 and has an AWP of $100.00. The pharmacy has an agreement with the supplier to purchase the drug at the AWP minus 15%. The insurer is willing to pay the AWP plus 5% plus a $2.00 dispensing fee. A patient on this insurer's plan purchases 30 tablets for $54.50. How much profit does the pharmacy make on this prescription?

First calculate the amount of the discount.

$$\$100.00 \times 0.15 = \$15.00$$

Then, calculate the purchase price of the drug.

$$\$100.00 - \$15.00 = \$85.00$$

Therefore, the pharmacy can purchase this drug at $85.00 per 60 tablets. The insurance company will pay the pharmacy AWP plus 5%.
(Note that 5% = 0.05.)

$$\$100.00 + (\$100.00 \times 0.05) = \$100.00 + \$5.00 = \$105.00$$

At that price, the amount the insurance company will pay to fill a prescription for 30 pills is:

$$(\$105.00 \div 2) + \$2 \text{ (dispensing fee)} = \$52.50 + \$2.00 = \$54.50$$

Compare this to the pharmacy's cost of 30 tablets.

$$\$85.00 \div 2 = \$42.50$$

Therefore, the pharmacy's profit on 30 tablets is:

$$\$54.50 - \$42.50 = \$12.00$$

Capitation Fee

Occasionally an insurer will provide a form of reimbursement to the pharmacy in the form of a monthly fee, called a **capitation fee,** to cover its members. The insurer pays the pharmacy the monthly fee whether or not the patient receives any prescriptions during that month. The pharmacy in turn must dispense all the patient's prescriptions, even if they cost more than the monthly fee. This reimbursement plan is infrequently used because it places all risk on the pharmacy without adequate controls in place to control prescribing.

Example 6

The Corner Drug Store receives a monthly capitation fee of $250.00 for John Jones. During April, John fills three prescriptions totaling $198.75. How much profit does the capitation fee provide?

In this case the monthly fee exceeds the sum of the prescription costs, yielding a profit for the pharmacy.

$$\$250.00 - \$198.75 = \$51.25$$

Understanding the terminology and mathematics used in community pharmacy is an important part of the pharmacy technician's job and can directly affect the profitability of the business.

Chapter Terms

applications computer software programs that perform particular functions such as word processing, spreadsheets, or databases

average inventory the beginning inventory plus the ending inventory divided by two

average wholesale price (AWP) average price that wholesalers charge the pharmacy for a drug

capitation fee monthly fee paid to the pharmacy by an insurer, whether or not the patient receives any prescriptions during that month

central processing unit (CPU) device used for manipulating computerized data input before output or storage

coinsurance percentage-based insurance plan whereby the patient must pay a certain percentage of the prescription price

computer an electronic device for inputting, storing, processing, and/or outputting information

copayment the amount the patient is to pay for each prescription, also called *copay*

database management system (DBMS) application that allows one to enter, retrieve, and query records

deductible amount that must be paid by the insured before the insurance company will consider paying its portion of a medical cost

direct purchasing ordering of drugs from a pharmaceutical manufacturer

discount reduced price

gross profit the difference between the purchase price and the selling price; also called *markup*

input devices devices used for getting information into the computer such as a keyboard, mouse, or touch screen

inventory the entire stock of products on hand for sale at a given time

inventory value the total value of the entire stock of products on hand for sale on a given day

markup *see* gross profit

Medicare Prescription Drug, Improvement, and Modernization Act (MMA) of 2003 voluntary insurance program started in January 2006 that provides partial coverage of prescriptions for patients eligible for Medicare

modem a device for connecting a computer to a remote computer via telephone lines

monitor a display screen that provides a visual representation of data that have been input and/or processed

operating system a software program that performs essential functions such as maintaining a list of file names, issuing processing instructions, and controlling output

prescription benefits manager (PBM) a company that administers drug benefits from many different insurance companies

prime vendor purchasing an agreement made by a pharmacy for a specified percentage or dollar volume of purchases

printer a device for creating hard copy or paper output

profit the amount of revenue received that exceeds the expense of the sold product

purchasing ordering of products for use or sale by the pharmacy

random-access memory (RAM) temporary, nonpermanent memory of the computer in which information is held while it is being input and processed

read-only memory (ROM) permanent memory containing essential operating instructions for the computer

receiving series of procedures for delivery of products

scanner a device for inputting images into the computer

storage devices devices used to store information that has been input into the computer such as floppy disk drive, hard drive, tape drive, CD drive, or removable disk drive

third-party administration (TPA) direct billing by the pharmacy to the customer's insurer

turnover rate the number of times the entire stock is used and replaced each year, calculated by the annual dollar purchases divided by the average inventory

universal claim form (UCF) a form used for requesting an insurance company to provide coverage for a prescription

wholesaler purchasing ordering of drugs and supplies from a local vendor who delivers the product to the pharmacy on a daily basis

Chapter Summary

- The pharmacy technician has an important role not only in assisting the pharmacist in the dispensing and preparing of pharmaceuticals but also in helping with the business operations of the pharmacy.
- The technician's responsibilities in billing, purchasing, receiving, and inventory management must be understood to run a profitable pharmacy.
- The technician needs to be knowledgeable in the billing for insurance companies, PBMs, Medicaid, and Medicare.
- Inventory management includes knowledge of the importance of turnover ratios.
- Purchasing, receiving, inventorying, and record keeping of controlled substances require specific legal procedures.
- Calculating the markup on the products and computing any discounts is often the responsibility of the technician.
- Understanding of average wholesale price is necessary for billing insurance companies.
- A basic knowledge of both computer and mathematic skills is necessary for the technician to successfully manage pharmacy business functions.

Chapter Review

Knowledge Inventory

Choose the best answer from those provided.

1. A computer term for typing is called
   a. keyboarding.
   b. networking.
   c. modem.
   d. optical scanning.

2. A digital computer uses what kind of numbers in processing information?
   a. decimals
   b. fractions
   c. whole numbers
   d. binary numbers

3. A computer application that can enter, retrieve, and query records is a(n)
   a. spreadsheet.
   b. word processing system.
   c. database management system (DBMS).
   d. Internet Web browser.

4. In a manual third-party administration (TPA) system, billing is typically done by means of a
   a. computer-generated form.
   b. purchase order.
   c. purchase requisition.
   d. universal claim form (UCF).

5. A PBM is best described as a(n)
   a. insurance company.
   b. company that contracts with several insurance companies.
   c. drug wholesaler.
   d. prime vendor.

6. If an insurance company has three different copays for each class of medications, its payment structure is best described as
   a. usual and customary.
   b. out of pocket.
   c. tiered copay.
   d. due copay.

7. In Medicare Part D which of the following apply?
   a. a monthly premium added to the current Medicare Part A/B premium
   b. a $250 deductible
   c. no coverage for medication costs between $2250 and $5100
   d. All of the above

8. Which type of purchasing arrangement will provide the lowest acquisition cost for most medications?
   a. direct from the manufacturer
   b. purchasing off the Internet
   c. purchasing from the wholesaler
   d. borrowing from the hospital pharmacy

9. A DEA 222 form must be used to order which of the following controlled substances?
   a. Schedule I
   b. Schedule II
   c. Schedule III
   d. Schedule IV
   e. Schedule V

10. The average price that wholesalers charge a pharmacy for a medication is better known as
    a. AWP.
    b. usual and customary.
    c. markup.
    d. capitation.

Pharmacy in Practice

1. Create a diagram of a typical computer system. Label the following parts: keyboard, mouse, central processing unit (CPU), floppy disk drive, monitor, printer, and modem.

2. Solve the following business math problems:
   a. Eyedrops with antihistamine are purchased in cases of 36 drop-dispenser bottles. The pharmacy desires a markup of $1.75 per bottle. The purchase price is $111.60 per case. What is the selling price per bottle?
   b. Identify the markup and the selling price of an oral antibiotic suspension that costs the pharmacy $15.60 per bottle if the markup rate is 25%.
   c. A month's supply of an asthma tablet costs the pharmacy $24.80, and the selling price is $30.75. Calculate the markup rate.
   d. John's Drug Shop purchases five cases of dermatologic cream at $100/case. The invoice specifies a 15% discount if the account is paid in full within 15 days. What is the discounted price?
   e. In question d, each case contains 24 tubes of cream. You are to mark each tube up by 20% based on the discounted cost. What will the selling price be per tube?
   f. A prescription is written for a tube of ointment. The AWP is $62.00. Smith's Pharmacy purchases the tube at AWP, and Jones' Pharmacy purchases the tube at AWP minus 10%. The insurer will reimburse at AWP plus 2% plus a $1.50 dispensing fee. How much profit does each pharmacy make?

g. Sinus tablets have an AWP of $37.50 per 50 tablets. The Corner Drug Store dispensed prescriptions for a total of 300 sinus tablets during May. They were purchased at AWP minus 15%. The insurer reimburses at AWP plus 1.5% plus a $2.00 dispensing fee. Fifteen prescriptions of 20 tablets each were filled that month. How much profit was made?

h. Mountain Health Maintenance pays a capitation fee of $310.00 per month. Six patients on this plan bring in prescriptions during July. They are as follows, with the cost reflected as the pharmacy cost for each:

   Patient #1: $15.75, $106.50, $27.80
   Patient #2: $210.00
   Patient #3: $47.50, $105.25, $160.00, $52.60
   Patient #4: $150.00, $210.00, $76.00
   Patient #5: $10.50, $28.00, $62.50
   Patient #6: $210.00, $210.00, $17.00
   (1) What is the total capitation?
   (2) What is the pharmacy cost?
   (3) Was the profit positive or negative?
   (4) What was the profit?

i. In the preceding question, if the drugs dispensed were allowed AWP (assuming all drugs were purchased at AWP) plus 3% and a $2.00 dispensing fee, would more profit have been made? How much total profit would be made? Is it more or less than on capitation? How much more or less?

j. Review the following inventory list and calculate the necessary purchases to reestablish maximum inventory. Write your answers in the *Purchased* column.

	A	B	C	D	E	F	G
1	JOHN'S DRUG SHOP						
2	Current Drug		Max.	Dispensed	Min.	Current	Purchased
3	Date		Level	Today	Level	Inventory	
4	Eucerin cream, jars		10	1	3	3	
5	Ampicillin caps		4500	500	4000	2400	
6	Eyedrops, bottles		24	4	4	4	
7	Nystatin oral solution		1000 mL	100 mL	200 mL	400 mL	
8	Sterile saline		600 mL	315 mL	100 mL	75 mL	
9							
10							
11							
12							
13							

k. Kathy's Pharmacy has an inventory of $184,520. Her cost of sales last week were $28,223, and she made a 26% profit. Her days' supply goal is 34 days.
   (1) What was the amount sold last week?
   (2) What is the days' supply?
   (3) How much is the value above or below inventory in dollars?

Improving Communication Skills

1. A pharmacy technician working in a retail environment should be familiar with various terms related to health insurance. Patients often have a difficult time understanding how their insurance works, and the technician can often act as an intermediary and advocate for the patient with regards to prescription drug benefits. Research the following insurance terms and define them in words that would be easily understood by a customer of the pharmacy.
    a. major medical insurance
    b. Medicare, Parts A, B, and D
    c. Medicaid
    d. deductible
    e. copay
    f. coinsurance
    g. preferred formulary
    h. prescription benefits manager (PBM)
    i. usual and customary
    j. dual and tiered copays

Internet Research

1. Visit the AmerisourceBergen Web site at www.amerisourcebergen.net
    a. What type of company is this? Check under About Us.
    b. What three inventory management services are available to independent community pharmacies?

2. Go to www.dea.gov. Check for contact phone numbers for your state and any local or regional news on drug enforcement. Check the most recent federal drug seizures in your state for cocaine, heroin, methamphetamine, marijuana, ecstasy, and meth labs. Find three "club" drugs.

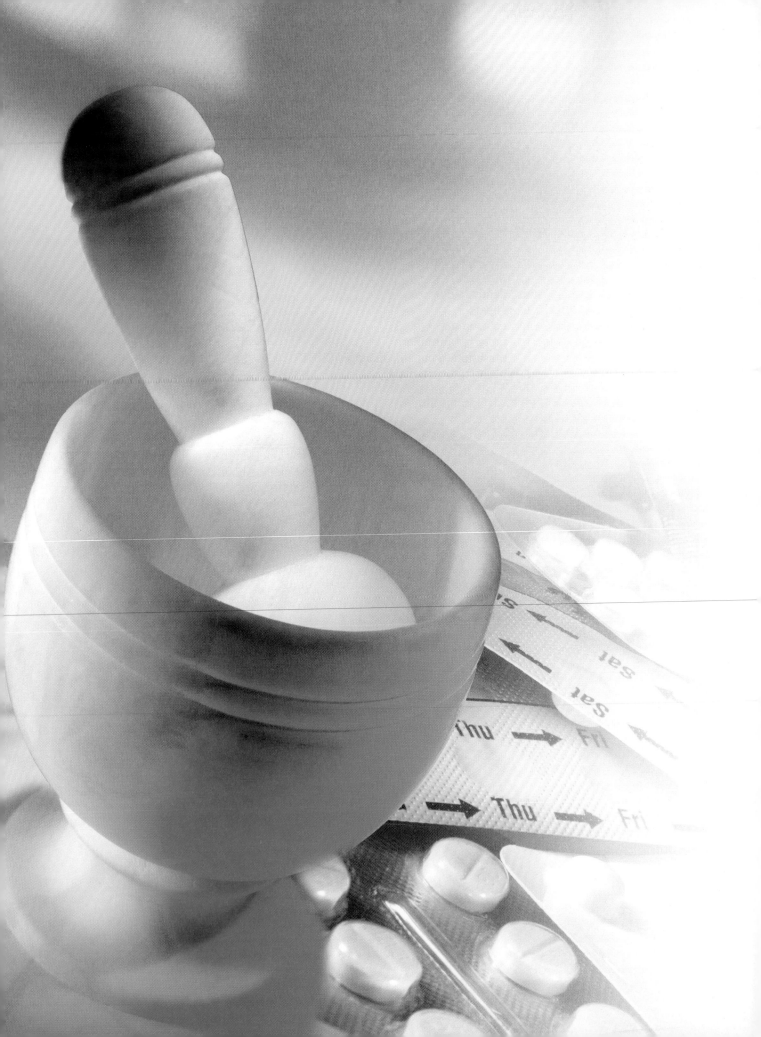

Extemporaneous Compounding

Chapter 8

Learning Objectives

- Define the term *extemporaneous compounding*, and describe common situations in which compounding is required.
- Identify and describe the equipment used for the weighing, measuring, and compounding of pharmaceuticals.
- Use the proper technique for weighing pharmaceutical ingredients.
- Use the proper technique for measuring liquid volumes.
- Define the term *percentage of error*.
- Explain the common methods used for comminution and blending of pharmaceutical ingredients.
- Explain the use of the geometric dilution method.
- Explain the processes by which solutions, suspensions, ointments, creams, powders, suppositories, and capsules are prepared.

Compounding remains an important part of pharmacy practice, and, in many states, pharmacy technicians assist in or carry out compounding tasks. The pharmacy technician may be required to retrieve from storage in the pharmacy area the necessary constituents of a compound (e.g., liquids, powders, capsules, containers), to prepare necessary equipment for the compounding process, to count or weigh materials, to compound the prescription, to return the products, and to clean up the compounding area and equipment after the procedure. In any case, compounding duties undertaken by the technician must be directly supervised and checked by the pharmacist. This chapter deals with the extemporaneous compounding of nonsterile products, ones compounded without using special aseptic techniques. Compounding of sterile products will be covered in Unit 3, *Institutional Pharmacy*.

NEED FOR EXTEMPORANEOUS COMPOUNDING

Extemporaneous compounding is the production of medication on demand in an appropriate quantity and dose form from pharmaceutical ingredients. Compounding might involve, for example, mixing a powdered active ingredient with a diluent powder and filling a given number of capsules with the combined materials. Until the emergence of modern, large-scale pharmaceutical manufacturing in the nineteenth century, pharmacists prepared (i.e., compounded) all medications from raw pharmaceutical ingredients. With these advancements, the need for extemporaneous compounding has decreased, but not to the vanishing point. In fact, on many occasions the pharmacist and his or her technician are called on to practice this ancient art.

For example, a national trend exists where a growing number of pharmacies practice only specialty compounding. Reimbursement is based more on the time and experience of the pharmacist rather than on the cost of the active ingredients. Many high-volume, chain pharmacies do not have the time for compounding and refer these prescriptions to independent community pharmacies that have the necessary equipment and expertise. However, many physicians, especially dermatologists and gynecologists, prefer to individualize their prescriptions for their patients.

Compounding is often required to meet these needs. In addition, pharmacists compound prescriptions from veterinarians for animals of all sizes and types. It is important to note, products formulated for "veterinary use only" cannot be used in humans, even if the medication and dose are identical.

The law addresses compounding and quality issues by defining and requiring **good manufacturing practice (GMP)**. Being able to compound by following GMP is a skill that is learned in pharmacy schools, as well as with experience during internship and on-the-job practice. The pharmacist's duty is to ensure that all compounded products are prepared using GMP. (For more information on using GMP, see Chapter 1075, entitled *Good Compounding Practices*, in the 2005 edition of the *United States Pharmacopeia*.)

One portion of the Food and Drug Administration (FDA) Modernization Act of 1997 addresses the issue of compounding medications by pharmacists. Essentially, Section 127 allows pharmacists to compound medications for an individual patient if they use quality approved bulk chemicals that meet the standard of the United States Pharmacopeia (USP) (contained in Chapter 795 of the 2005 edition of the *United States Pharmacopeia*). In most cases, compounds are prepared for an individual patient and not made until the prescription is received by the pharmacy. Pharmacies are allowed to advertise their compounding services but not the compounding of a specific drug product. Some examples of situations that require extemporaneous compounding include the following:

- The prescription calls for doses smaller than those that are commercially available, as is sometimes the case with pediatric medications. For example, a prescription might call for 15 mg per dose of a medication available only in unscored tablets containing 30 mg of the active ingredient. Therefore the pharmacist might have to pulverize, or triturate, the tablets, mix the resultant powder with a suitable diluent, and then use the diluted powder to fill 15 mg capsules.
- A medication normally available in a solid dose form might have to be prepared in another dose form, such as a liquid or a suppository, for administration to a patient who cannot or will not swallow the solid form.
- A medication with an unpleasant taste might have to be prepared in a more palatable masking syrup base to ensure compliance by a pediatric patient.
- A medication may be available only in commercial forms containing preservatives, colorings, or other materials to which a patient is allergic; therefore an alternative without the unwanted ingredients might need to be prepared.
- The strength or dose form called for in the prescription may not be in stock or readily available.
- A dose form other than those commercially available may be desired to customize the rate of delivery, rate of onset, site of action, or other pharmacokinetic properties of the drug.
- A noncommercially available medication must be prepared for a veterinary application.

The federal law affects those pharmacies specializing their business by making the prescription product in bulk in advance. If a community pharmacy is selling compounded drug products directly to health professionals (rather than to an individual patient), then it must apply to the FDA for a manufacturing license.

A need exists for extemporaneous compounding to prepare doses of therapeutic agents for individual patients. This activity is a true example of the art of pharmacy, but it requires special expertise and technique to prepare a quality product. The pharmacy technician often assists the pharmacist in this function.

EQUIPMENT FOR WEIGHING, MEASURING, AND COMPOUNDING

Proper compounding requires an intimate knowledge of pharmaceutical equipment and of the techniques for using that equipment properly to weigh, measure, reduce, and combine ingredients.

Balances

A **Class III prescription balance**, formerly known as a *Class A prescription balance*, is required equipment in every pharmacy. The Class III prescription balance is a two-pan balance that can be used for weighing small amounts of material (120 g or less) and that has a sensitivity requirement (SR) of 6 mg. This means that a 6 mg weight will move the indicator on the balance 1 degree.

A **counterbalance**, which also has two pans, is used for weighing larger amounts of material, up to about 5 kg. It has a sensitivity requirement of 100 mg. Because of its lesser sensitivity, a counterbalance is not used in prescription compounding but rather for tasks such as measuring bulk products (e.g., Epsom salts).

Balance measurements using a counterbalance are made using sets of standardized pharmaceutical weights. Typical weight sets contain both metric weights and apothecary weights. (For information about the metric and apothecary measurement systems, see Chapter 5.) Weights are generally made of polished brass and may be coated with a noncorrosive material such as nickel or chromium. Typical metric sets may contain gram weights of 1, 2, 5, 10, 20, 50, and 100 g, which are conically shaped, with a handle and flattened top. Fractional gram weights (e.g., 10, 20, 50, 100, 200, 500 mg) are also available. These are made of aluminum and are usually flat, with one raised edge to facilitate picking up the weight using forceps. Forceps are used to lift weights to prevent oil or body perspiration from causing a weighing error on small measurements such as for a pediatric patient. Avoirdupois weights (see Chapter 5) of $\frac{1}{32}$, $\frac{1}{16}$, $\frac{1}{8}$, $\frac{1}{4}$, $\frac{1}{2}$, 1, 2, 4, and 8 oz may also be used. Weights come in a container in which they should be stored when not in use. Care should be taken not to touch or drop a weight or otherwise expose it to damage or contamination.

An electronic balance uses a single pan. An electronic balance is easier to learn and use and is more accurate than other types of balances. However, electronic balances tend to be much more costly than other pharmacy balances. For this reason, they are typically only used in large-scale pharmacy

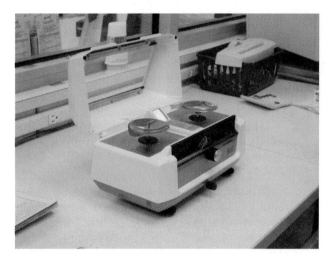

The Class III prescription balance accurately weighs small amounts of material.

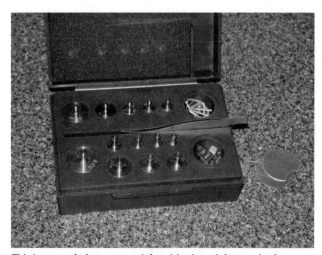

This is a set of pharmacy weights. Metric weights are in the front row and apothecary weights are in the back row.

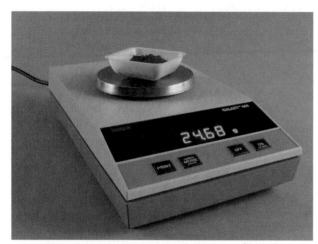

This Mettler Toledo balance is an example of an electronic balance used in a compounding pharmacy.

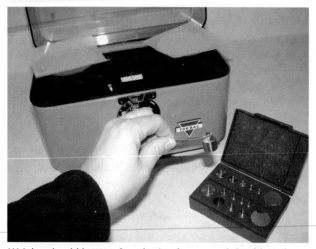

Weights should be transferred using forceps and should not be touched with bare skin. Moisture or oils will affect their accuracy.

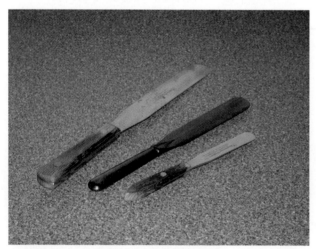

Spatulas are a common tool in the pharmacy.

compounding labs or hospitals. The procedure for measuring using an electronic balance can be outlined in a series of three steps: (1) locate the zero point, including the weight of the powder paper; (2) place the chemical or drug to be measured on powder paper; and (3) read the digital reading. Because the equipment is so sensitive and costly, the pharmacy technician must be fully trained on its proper use.

Forceps and Spatulas

Forceps are instruments for grasping small objects. They are provided with weight sets to use for picking up weights and transferring them to and from balances to avoid transferring moisture or oil to the weights, thereby changing their weight. Weights should not be transferred using the hands and fingers. The product and the weights should always be placed on weighing papers. Weighing papers are placed on balances to avoid contact between pharmaceutical ingredients and the balance tray. Typically, glassine paper is used. Glassine paper is a thin paper coated with a nonabsorbent paraffin wax.

    Spatulas are stainless steel, plastic, or hard rubber instruments used for transferring solid pharmaceutical ingredients to weighing pans and for various compounding tasks such as preparing ointments and creams or loosening material from the surfaces of a mortar and pestle. Hard rubber spatulas are used when corrosive materials such as iodine and mercuric salts are handled.

Compounding Slab

A **compounding slab**, also known as an *ointment slab,* is a plate made of ground glass that has a flat, hard, nonabsorbent surface ideal for mixing compounds. In lieu of a compounding or ointment slab, compounding may be performed on special disposable nonabsorbent parchment paper that is discarded after the compounding operation is completed.

Mortar and Pestle

A **mortar and pestle** are used for grinding and mixing pharmaceutical ingredients. These devices come in glass, porcelain, and Wedgwood varieties. Paradoxically, the coarser the surface of the mortar and pestle, the finer

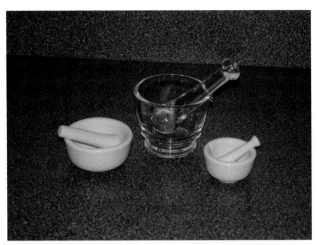

The mortar and pestle are used to mix or grind substances.

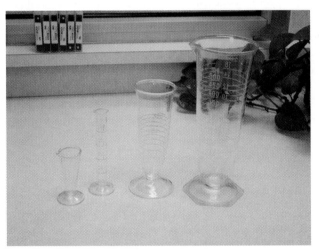

Graduates come in a variety of sizes and shapes. Cylindrical graduates are more accurate than conical graduates. The second graduate from the left is cylindrical.

the triturating, or grinding, that can be done. As a result, a coarse-grained porcelain or Wedgwood mortar and pestle set is used for triturating of crystals, granules, and powders, whereas a glass mortar and pestle, with its smooth surface, is preferred for mixing of liquids and semisolid dose forms. A glass mortar and pestle also has the advantages of being nonporous and nonstaining.

Graduates and Pipettes

Graduates are glass or polypropylene flasks used for measuring liquids. They come in two varieties: (1) conical and (2) cylindrical. Conical graduates have wide tops and wide bases and taper from the top to the bottom. These graduates are calibrated in both metric and apothecary units. Cylindrical graduates, which are more accurate, have the shape of a uniform column. Cylindrical graduates are generally calibrated in metric units (i.e., cubic centimeters). Both kinds of graduates are available in a wide variety of sizes, ranging from 5 mL to more than 1000 mL.

A **pipette** is a long, thin, calibrated hollow tube used for measurement of volumes of liquid less than 1.5 mL. A pipette filler is a device used instead of the mouth for drawing a dangerous solution, such as an acid, into the pipette.

Master Formula Sheet

Of course, in addition to the equipment described previously, the compounding of a medication requires the necessary ingredients. Figure 8.1 shows an example of a **master formula sheet**, also known as a *pharmacy compounding log*. The master formula sheet, prepared by the pharmacist, will indicate the amount of each ingredient needed, list the procedures to follow, and provide the labeling instructions. The example in Figure 8.1 lists the directions and ingredients for compounding a preparation called *Magic Mouthwash*. Some pharmacies keep this information on large index cards, similar to recipe cards. This formula has many variations in different regions of the country.

TECHNIQUE FOR WEIGHING PHARMACEUTICAL INGREDIENTS

Weighing of the product is one of the most essential parts of the compounding process. One must continually practice to feel confident and comfortable with weighing products on a prescription balance. The balance is accurate to within a very small quantity, and variations in technique could easily result in a slight but serious error. Weighing the exact amount prescribed is essential in compounds for several

Figure 8.1

Master Formula Sheet
This formula sheet is for Magic Mouthwash, a commonly made formula.

MASTER FORMULA SHEET

PRODUCT _____ MTC LOT NUMBER _____

_____

LABEL: Date MFG:
MAGIC MOUTHWASH

Take 1 teaspoonful 3 times
daily. Swish and swallow.

STRENGTH: _____

QUANTITY MFG: _____

	MANUFACTURER'S LOT NUMBER	INGREDIENTS	AMOUNT NEEDED	WEIGHED OR MEASURED BY	CHECKED BY
1		Decadron or hydrocortisone	4.5 mg 120 mg		
2		nystatin (Mycostatin)	2,000,000 units		
3		tetracycline	1 g		
4		diphenhydramine (Benadryl)	qs to 120 mL		
5					
6					
7					
8					

DIRECTIONS FOR MANUFACTURING

1. Draw up, by syringe, 4.5 mg Decadron or 120 mg of hydrocortisone or equivalent steroid.
2. Crush nystatin tablets and mix with 5 mL sterile water or measure 2,000,000 units of liquid.
3. Measure 1 g of liquid tetracycline or dissolve tablets or capsules in 5 mL sterile water.
4. Add each ingredient to liquid container and qs with diphenhydramine to 120 mL.
5. Attach label.

Manufactured by _____
Approved by _____
Date _____

_____

Auxiliary Labeling: SHAKE WELL

_____

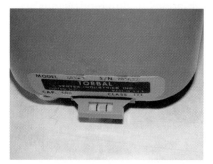

The balance is leveled front to back and side to side when the bubble is centered.

reasons: the product cannot be "checked" for content once mixed, the quantities weighed out are often very small, and a slight overage could mean a serious overdose for the patient.

Table 8.1 outlines the procedure for weighing pharmaceutical ingredients. A pharmacist or an experienced technician may need to check your weighing technique and results for a while after you begin training.

The balance should be placed on a secure, level surface, at waist height, where it cannot be easily jarred. It should be in the locked or "arrested" position when not in use and when moved. The area where the balance is placed should be well lighted and free from drafts, dust, corrosive vapors, or high humidity that

Table 8.1 Weighing Pharmaceutical Ingredients

1. Unlock the balance and confirm that it is leveled, front to back and side to side, using the leveling screws at its base. Once this is done, the balance is ready to use. Lock the balance once again, before transferring weight to it.
2. Place weighing papers on the two pans of the balance. These papers should be of exactly the same size and weight. The edges of the paper on the left-hand pan may be folded upward, to hold the substance to be weighed. Do not place any materials on the weighing pans without using weighing papers.
3. Unlock the balance to confirm that the balance is still leveled, and then lock it again.
4. Add the desired weight to the right-hand pan, using forceps to transfer the weight from the weight container.
5. Place an approximate amount of the material to be weighed onto the left-hand pan, using a spatula to transfer it.
6. Slowly release the beam using the unlocking device at the front of the balance, and check the balance.
7. If the amount of the substance being weighed is too great or too small, lock the balance again and use a spatula to add or remove material (Figure 8.2, a).
8. Slowly release the beam using the unlocking device and check for equilibrium.
9. Once a nearly precise amount of material has been transferred to the pan, a very small adjustment upward can be made by placing a small amount of material on the spatula, holding the spatula over the left pan, and lightly tapping the spatula with the forefinger to knock a bit of the substance onto the pan. This is done with the balance unlocked and the balance beam free to move.
10. Lock the balance, close the lid, and then unlock the balance to make a final measurement. (At this point, have the pharmacist check the measurement.) (Figure 8.2, b).
11. Lock the balance before removing the measured substance. Use transfer forceps to remove the weights and return them to their storage case.

might affect the ingredients or the measurements. Avoid spilling materials onto the balance. If any materials are spilled on the balance, then wipe them off immediately. Do not place materials onto the balance while it is released (i.e., unlocked), because doing so may force the pan down suddenly and cause damage to the instrument.

The balance must be perfectly level, both side to side and front to back. Leveling is often the most time-consuming process for beginners. Front-to-back leveling is done by adjusting the pegs on the front of the scale so that the leveling bubble is centered. The side-to-side leveling is adjusted in a similar way. The released, empty

Figure 8.2

A Prescription Balance
(a) Transferring a substance to the scale. (b) The final measurement is taken with the lid closed.

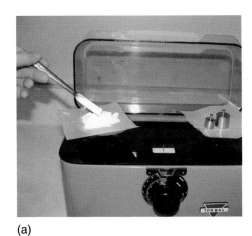

(a)

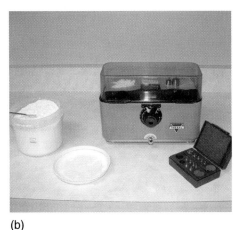

(b)

scales will register as equal when the scale is balanced. The levelness should be checked often throughout the day when the balance is heavily used. Remember that the scale must be in an arrested (i.e., locked) position whenever the balance is moved or the pegs are adjusted.

TECHNIQUE FOR MEASURING LIQUID VOLUMES

Liquid volumes are often much easier to measure than solid volumes that must be weighed, and a wide variety of containers are available to assist in volumetric measurement. A general rule of thumb is to always select the device that will give you the most accurate volume. Selecting a container that will be at least half full when measuring, or using the smallest device that will hold the required volume, is considered good practice.

Most commonly, the upper surface of the liquid will be a **meniscus**, or moon-shaped body (i.e., slightly concave or bowed inward toward the center) (Figure 8.3). In other words, the level of the liquid will be slightly higher at the edges. Therefore do not measure the level by looking down on the graduate. Instead measure by placing the eyes at the level of the liquid. Read the level of the liquid at the *bottom* of the meniscus. Table 8.2 outlines the procedure for measuring liquid volumes.

Safety Note

Use the smallest device that will hold the required volume when measuring a liquid.

Safety Note

Always measure liquids on a solid, level surface at eye level.

Table 8.2 **Measuring Liquid Volumes**

1. Choose a graduate with a capacity that equals or very slightly exceeds the total volume of the liquid to be measured. Doing so reduces the percentage of error in the measurement. In no case should the volume to be measured be less than 20% of the total capacity of the graduate. For example, 10 mL of liquid should not be measured in a graduate exceeding 50 mL in capacity. Again, the closer the total capacity of the graduate to the volume to be measured, the more accurate the measurement will be.
2. Bear in mind that the more narrow the column of liquid in the graduate, the less substantial any reading error will be. Thus for very small volume measurements, a pipette is preferable to a cylindrical graduate, and for larger measurements, a cylindrical graduate is preferable to a conical graduate.
3. Pour the liquid to be measured slowly into the graduate, watching the level of the liquid in the graduate as you do so. If the liquid is viscous, or thick, then you should attempt to pour it toward the center of the graduate to avoid having some of the liquid cling to the sides.
4. Wait for liquid clinging to the sides of the graduate to settle before taking a measurement.
5. Measure the level of the liquid at eye level and read the liquid at the bottom of the meniscus (see Figure 8.3).
6. When pouring the liquid out of the graduate, allow ample time for all of the liquid to drain. Bear in mind that depending on the viscosity of the liquid, more or less will cling to the sides of the graduate. For a particularly viscous liquid, some compensation or adjustment for this clinging may have to be made.

Figure 8.3

Meniscus
Liquid in a narrow column usually forms a concave meniscus. Measurements should be taken at the bottom of the concavity when read at eye level.

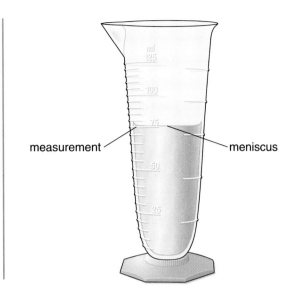

measurement — meniscus

PERCENTAGE OF ERROR

Percentages are used in a variety of ways when preparing medication doses. As discussed in Chapter 7, percentages are used when doing the business of the pharmacy (e.g., calculating percentage of sales, percentage of discount, percentage of markup). In the compounding pharmacy, percentages are used in determining the possible percentage of error and the least weighable quantity of a substance for safe preparation.

Error in measurement in pharmacy-prepared products is expected, and allowances are made for a certain percentage of error over or under the target measurement. This percent of error is considered to be a range both above and below the target measurement, and being over or under (i.e., positive or negative) within this range is not consequential.

Pharmacy scales are generally very accurate when compared with other small scales. However, knowing the margin of error that a particular scale has is important. When weighing any substance, the scale will appear to have measured correctly. However, a very small sample may have an unacceptable margin of error. Pharmacy scales are generally marked with their degree of accuracy. This degree of accurateness has been determined by comparing quantities weighed on the scale and then weighed on another scale of greater known accuracy. This function is performed in the factory and is not associated with a function normally practiced in the pharmacy.

If a substance was weighed or measured incorrectly, and we have something that will allow us to more accurately measure the amount in question, we may determine the **percentage of error**. This can be found by using the following formula:

$$\frac{\text{amount of error}}{\text{quantity desired}} \times 100\% = \text{percentage of error}$$

In this equation the amount of error is the difference between the measured amount and the actual amount, or

$$\text{actual amount} - \text{measured amount} = \text{amount of error}$$

For example, a new brand of vitamins claims to have a range of 9% bioavailability of a national brand of 1000 mg of vitamin C. The range of error is +/– 90 mg or 910 mg to 1090 mg. This is 9% less and 9% more than the labeled amount of 1000 mg. Some more potent compounded drugs require a lower range of error, usually less than or no greater than 5%.

COMMINUTION AND BLENDING OF DRUGS

Comminution is the act of reducing a substance to small, fine particles. **Blending** is the act of combining two substances. Techniques for comminution and blending include trituration, levigation, pulverization by intervention, spatulation, sifting, and tumbling. **Trituration** is the process of rubbing, grinding, or pulverizing a substance to create fine particles, generally by means of a mortar and pestle. A rapid motion with minimal pressure provides the best results.

Other forms of comminution include levigation and pulverization by intervention. **Levigation** is typically used when reducing the particle size of a solid during the preparation of an ointment. A paste is formed of a solid material and a tiny amount of a liquid levigating agent, such as castor oil or mineral oil, that is miscible, or mixable, with the solid but in which the solid is not soluble. The paste is then triturated to reduce the particle size and added to the ointment base. The levigating agent becomes part of the final product.

Pulverization by intervention is the process of reducing the size of particles in a solid with the aid of an additional material in which the substance is soluble—a volatile solvent such as camphor and alcohol or iodine and ether. The solvent is added, then the mixture is triturated. The solvent is permitted to evaporate and so does not become part of the final product.

Spatulation is the process of combining substances by means of a spatula, generally on an ointment tile. Sifting, like the sifting of flour in baking, can be used to blend or combine powders. Powders can also be combined by tumbling—placing the powders into a bag or container and shaking it.

Geometric Dilution Method

Often a mortar and pestle are used to combine more than one drug. To combine drugs in a mortar and pestle, you can use the **geometric dilution method**. Place the most potent ingredient, which will most likely be the ingredient that occurs in the smallest amount, into the mortar first. Then add an equal amount of the next most potent ingredient and mix well. Continue in this manner, adding, each time, an amount equal to the amount in the mortar, until successively larger amounts of all the ingredients are added. Then add any excess amount of any ingredient and mix well.

Examples of Compounding Preparations

In practice, a pharmacy technician will, if the laws of the state allow, assist in compounding only after instruction by a pharmacist in specific techniques for specific preparations, and compounding will be done in accordance with instructions in a master formula sheet. Any compounding tasks undertaken by the technician must, in any case, be supervised and checked by the pharmacist.

The following are some common examples of compounding in the community pharmacy: solutions, suspensions, ointments and creams, powders, suppositories, and capsules.

Solutions As defined in Chapter 3, a solution is a liquid dose form in which active ingredients are dissolved in a liquid vehicle. The vehicle that makes up the greater part of a solution is known as a *solvent*. An ingredient dissolved in a solution is known as a *solute*. Solutions may be aqueous (or water), alcoholic, or hydroalcoholic. Hydroalcoholic solutions contain both water and alcohol, which may be needed to dissolve some solutes. Solutions are prepared by dissolving the solute in the liquid solvent or by combining or diluting existing solutions. Careful measurement is important for solutions, as it is for all extemporaneous compounding. Colorings or flavoring agents may be added to solutions if needed. A simple syrup, known as *Syrup NF*, can be made by combining 85 g of sucrose with 100 mL of purified water.

When mixing solids and liquids, reducing the particle size of the solid through triturating or gently heating the liquid (if the liquid is stable or nonvolatile) will generally make the solid dissolve faster and more uniformly. In addition, there will be less precipitation or clinging together of the solute into particles of unacceptably large size. An example of a compounding formula for an otic solution to remove ear wax is contained in Table 8.3.

When mixing two liquids, a possible precipitation of solutes within the liquids can sometimes be avoided by making each portion as dilute as possible before mixing the liquids together. Before preparing a solution for compounding, the technician should gather the master formula sheet, ingredients, equipment, glassware, and packaging material. Providing adequate and uninterrupted time to the person who is compounding the prescription to prepare the product is also important.

Figure 8.4, *a*, shows an example of a master formula sheet for a prescription for a dog. To prepare this medication, the technician would follow the steps in Table 8.1 for weighing the product (potassium bromide) (Figure 8.4, *b*). Then, the product is placed in a mortar to be triturated and combined with the flavoring (Figure 8.4, *c*). Figure 8.4, *d*, shows the mixed ingredients, but at this stage, more trituration is needed to get the particles to a more even texture. The mixed and triturated ingredients are put into an amber bottle using a glass funnel. In Figure 8.4, *e*, a wall-mounted source of distilled water is added to mix the veterinary prescription. Then, the bottle is shaken well and labeled, and the preparation is checked by the pharmacist before the bottle is bagged for customer pickup (Figure 8.4, *f*).

A good example of the need for compounding is when a drug that is not available in a solution is prescribed for a pediatric patient less than 6 years of age. The heart drug captopril is available in 12.5 mg, 25 mg, 50 mg, and 100 mg tablets. The pediatric dose is approximately 0.2 mg/kg. For a 10-kg patient, the dose would be 2 mg. Tablets must be crushed and a suitable vehicle and flavoring agents must be

Table 8.3   Formula for Otic Solution Compound

Compound Title:

     urea and hydrogen peroxide otic solution

Compound Ingredients:

     carbamide peroxide 6.5 g

     glycerin qs, 100 mL

Compounding Procedure:

Dissolve the carbamide peroxide in sufficient glycerin to volume; then package and label. A beyond-use date of up to 6 months can be used for this preparation.

Source: Compounding for otic disorders. *Secundum Artem*, vol. 13, no. 1 (2005), www.paddock labs.com/secundum_artem.html (accessed September 25, 2005). Used with permission of Loyd V. Allen, Jr., PhD.

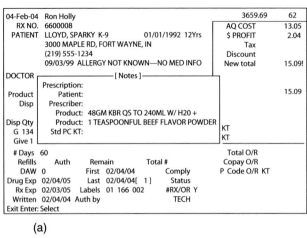

04-Feb-04	Ron Holly			3659.69	62
RX NO.	6600008			AQ COST	13.05
PATIENT	LLOYD, SPARKY K-9	01/01/1992 12Yrs		$ PROFIT	2.04
	3000 MAPLE RD, FORT WAYNE, IN			Tax	
	(219) 555-1234			Discount	
	09/03/99 ALLERGY NOT KNOWN—NO MED INFO			New total	15.09!

DOCTOR ———————[Notes]———————
Prescription:
Product   Patient:
Disp   Prescriber:
        Product: 48GM KBR QS TO 240ML W/ H20 +
Disp Qty   Product: 1 TEASPOONFUL BEEF FLAVOR POWDER   KT
G 134   Std PC KT: KT
Give 1

15.09

# Days	60				Total O/R	
Refills	Auth	Remain		Total #	Copay O/R	
DAW	0	First	02/04/04	Comply	P Code O/R KT	
Drug Exp	02/04/05	Last	02/04/04[1]	Status		
Rx Exp	02/03/05	Labels	01 166 002	#RX/OR Y		
Written	02/04/04	Auth by		TECH		
Exit Enter: Select						

(a)

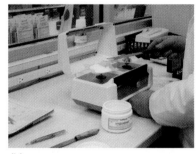

(b)

Figure 8.4

Preparing a Solution for Sparky the Dog
(a) Master formula sheet. (b) Weighing the potassium bromide. (c) Potassium bromide and beef flavoring. (d) Not yet fully triturated. (e) Adding distilled water. (f) Prepared prescription waiting for pharmacist approval.

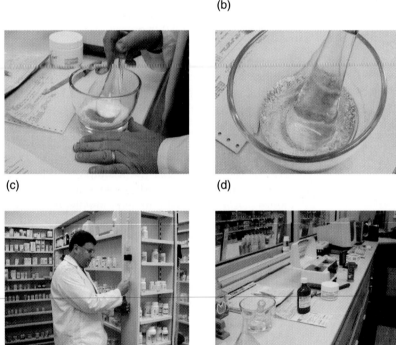

(c)

(d)

(e)

(f)

identified for stability and palatability. Flavoring agents may sometimes be incompatible with the active ingredient because of its pH or acid/base ratio. Many vendors provide flavoring vehicles that have been proven to be safe and effective in children.

Suspensions In a suspension, as opposed to a solution, the active ingredient is not dissolved in the liquid vehicle but rather is dispersed throughout it. Many commercially unavailable pediatric suspensions can be extemporaneously prepared in the pharmacy from adult tablets or capsules. An obvious problem with suspensions is the tendency of the active ingredient to settle. To avoid settling of the insoluble drug, a suspending agent is sometimes added. Such suspending agents include tragacanth, acacia, and carboxymethylcellulose (CMC). The point at which the suspending agent is added in the mixing procedure can be crucial. Therefore the technician must always remember to add the ingredients in the proper order, according to the master formula sheet.

Safety Note

Regardless of their apparent stability, all suspensions should be dispensed with an auxiliary label reading "Shake Well."

Ointments and Creams Ointments and creams are semisolid dose forms that are meant for topical application. Gynecologists in particular are requesting more compounded formulations to individualize hormone treatments for their patients. An ointment is usually a water-in-oil (w/o) emulsion that is occlusive, greasy, and not water washable. A cream is an oil-in-water (o/w) emulsion that is nonocclusive, not greasy, and water washable. A lotion is a liquid suspension or oil-in-water emulsion used topically in areas of the body where a lubricating effect is desirable.

Emulsions require the addition of an emulsifying agent(s) to help disperse the immiscible liquids. A common example for an oil-in-water (o/w) emulsion would use an agent with hydrophilic (i.e., water soluble) properties, whereas an example for a water-in-oil (w/o) emulsion would use one with more lipophilic (i.e., fat soluble) properties. A cream is best prepared with glass equipment, whereas an ointment is best prepared using water-repellant plastic equipment.

Water-soluble bases are commonly called *creams* even though they are officially defined as *ointments*. The properties of "ointment" bases such as lanolin, petrolatum, and Aquaphor vary in the degree of occlusiveness, emolliency, water washability, and water absorption. An occlusive base has the ability to hold moisture in the skin and is best used where additional hydration is needed. An emollient base has the ability to soften skin such as in bath oils. White petrolatum is an example of a lipophilic base with high occlusive and emollient properties. Water washability and absorption relate to cosmetic appearance such as vanishing creams. Polyethylene glycol ointment is an example of a water-soluble base. An example of a compounding formula for an emollient cream base is included in Table 8.4. Most ointment bases are commercially available from the wholesaler or pharmacy compounding vendor.

Dermatologic therapies may call for combining existing ointments or creams. Most ointments and creams are prepared via mechanical incorporation of materials, levigation, or mixing in a mortar and pestle. Levigation involves forming a paste containing a small amount of liquid, generally using a spatula and an ointment slab, before addition to the base of the ointment or cream.

Table 8.4 Formula for Emollient Cream Base Compound

Compound Title:

     emollient cream base, 120 g

Compound Ingredients:

anhydrous ointment base	40 g
polysorbate 80	2.4 g
purified water	78 mL

Compounding Procedure:

Melt ointment base at 70° C and add polysorbate 80. Heat water to 70° C and add to base. Stir with electric mixer without heat until cream thickens and is uniform.

Keep refrigerated after compounding.

Use either 0.02% sodium benzoate or 1/2000 methylparaben and 1/4000 propylaparaben as preservative.

Source: Ointment compounding: basic concepts. *Secundum Artem*, vol. 1, no. 1 (1993), www.paddocklabs.com/secundum_artem.html (accessed September 25, 2005). Used with permission of Loyd V. Allen, Jr., PhD.

Table 8.5 Formula for Topical Compound

Compound Title:

    ketoprofen 10% and ibuprofen 2.5% in pluronic lecithin organogel

Compound Ingredients:

ketoprofen	10 g
ibuprofen	2.5 g
lecithin:isopropyl palmitate 1:1 solution	22 mL
Pluronic F127 20% gel qs	100 mL

Compounding Procedure:

Mix the ketoprofen and ibuprofen powders with propylene glycol to form a smooth paste. Incorporate the lecithin:isopropyl palmitate solution and mix well. Add sufficient Pluronic F127 gel to volume and mix using high-shearing action until uniform. Package and label.

Source: Compounding for sports injuries. *Secundum Artem*, vol. 12, no. 4 (2004), www.paddock labs.com/secundum_artem.html (accessed September 25, 2005). Used with permission of Loyd V. Allen, Jr., PhD.

In some cases the dry ingredients of an ointment or cream may have to be triturated, or reduced to a fine powder, in a mortar and pestle before being added to the ointment or cream base. When placing a powder into an ointment, adding the powder in small amounts and constantly working the mixture with the spatula or pestle to reduce particle size and to obtain a smooth, nongritty product are important. If mixing three or more ingredients to the base, then adding them sequentially rather than mixing together is important; this allows for more drug stability and a more elegant end product. When an ointment slab and spatula are used, the edge of the spatula should press against the slab to provide a shearing force, which allows for a smoother end product.

A good example of the importance of compounding topical products is provided by the nonsteroidal anti-inflammatory drugs (NSAIDs). You may recognize some of their names, such as ibuprofen tablets, which are available in both prescription and over-the-counter (OTC) forms. Oral NSAIDs have very good analgesic and anti-inflammatory properties, but they can cause gastric ulcers if used in high doses, for long periods of time, or in some patients with a history of ulcer disease. Using a compounded topical formula (Table 8.5) can localize the beneficial properties of NSAIDs to the site of the sports injury and reduce the risk of adverse effects on the stomach.

Powders In the past it was common for the pharmacist/apothecary to prepare medicines in the form of powders. Often the pharmacist would dispense powders that were prepared, measured, mixed, divided into separate units, and placed on pieces of paper that were then folded and given to the patient. However, powders dispensed in bulk amounts had the disadvantage of leading to inaccuracy in the dose taken by the patient. Today dispensing of medicines in the divided powder dose form is rare; however, fresh herbs are commonly prepared in this manner in the Chinese culture.

To a layperson a **powder** is any finely ground substance. To a pharmacist a powder is a finely divided combination, or admixture, of drugs and/or chemicals ranging in size from extremely fine to very coarse. Official definitions of powder size include very coarse (No. 8 powder), coarse (No. 20 powder), moderately coarse (No. 40 powder), fine (No. 60 powder), or very fine (No. 80 powder), according to the amount of the powder that can pass through mechanical sieves made of wire cloth of various dimensions (e.g., No. 8 sieves, No. 20 sieves).

Safety Note

The *qs* abbreviation means to add "as much as necessary" to the specified amount. JCAHO recommends using text words rather than abbreviations to minimize a medication error.

Powders are combined and mixed by a variety of means, including spatulation, trituration, sifting, and tumbling in a container or blending machine. They may also be levigated (i.e., formed into a paste using a small amount of liquid) in preparation for being added to an ointment base. Spatulation, or blending with a spatula, is used for small amounts of powder having a uniform and desired particle size and density. Trituration is used when a potent drug is mixed with a diluent. At first equal amounts of the potent drug and the diluent are triturated with a mortar and pestle. When these are thoroughly mixed, more of the diluent is added, equal to the amount already in the mortar. This process is continued until all of the diluent is incorporated. Tumbling is used to combine powders that have little or no toxic potential. The powders to be combined are placed in a bag or in a wide-mouthed container and shaken well.

Suppositories Suppositories are solid dose forms that are inserted into bodily orifices, generally the rectum or the vagina or, less commonly, the urethra. They are composed of one or more active ingredients placed into one of a variety of bases, such as cocoa butter, hydrogenated vegetable oil, or glycerinated gelatin, which melts or dissolves when exposed to body heat and fluids. Suppositories are produced by molding and by compression. The preparation of suppositories involves melting the base material, adding the active ingredient(s), pouring the resultant liquid into a mold, and then chilling the mold immediately to solidify the suppository before the suspended ingredients have time to settle.

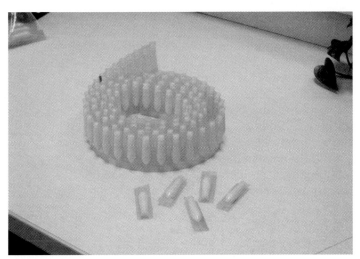

Disposable suppository molds are commonly used to dispense and shape suppositories.

Capsules A capsule is a solid dose form consisting of a gelatin shell that encloses the medicinal preparation, which may be a powder, granules, a liquid, or some combination thereof. Extemporaneous compounding of ingredients for capsules is often done to provide unusual dose forms, such as dose forms containing less of an active ingredient than is readily available in commercial tablets or capsules.

Hard gelatin shells are made of gelatin, sugar, and water and consist of two parts: (1) the body, which is the longer and narrower part, and (2) the cap, which is shorter and fits over the body. In some cases capsules have a snap-fit design, with grooves on the cap and the body that fit into one another to ensure proper closure (Figure 8.5).

Hard gelatin shells commonly contain powders or granules and are used for extemporaneous (i.e., to order) hand-filling operations. Hard-shell capsules come in standard sizes indicated by the numbers 000, 00, 0, 1, 2, 3, 4, 5 (from largest to smallest). The largest capsule, size 000, can contain about 1040 mg of aspirin; the smallest, size 5, about 97 mg (Figure 8.6).

Figure 8.5

Types of Hard-Shell Capsules
(a) Regular, (b) Snap Fit.

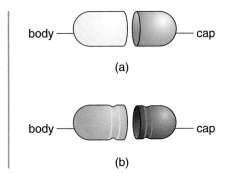

body — cap

(a)

body — cap

(b)

Figure 8.6

Hard-Shell Capsule Sizes
The sizes in which hard-shell capsules are available range from 5, the smallest, to 000, the largest.

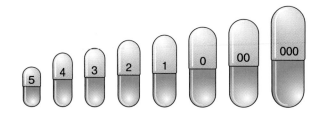

When hand-filling a capsule with powder, a pharmacist or technician generally uses the **punch method**. First, the number of capsules to be filled is counted. Then, the powder is placed on a clean surface of paper, porcelain, or glass and formed into a cake with a spatula. The cake should be approximately ¼ to ⅓ the height of the capsule body. The body of the capsule is then punched into the cake repeatedly until the capsule is full (Figure 8.7). The cap is then placed snugly over the body. Granules are generally poured into the capsule body from a piece of paper. Sometimes, hand-operated capsule-filling machines are used.

Most hard-shell capsules are meant to be swallowed whole, but a few are meant only as conveyances for granules or powders to be sprinkled on food or in drink. Capsules should only be used in this manner when specifically intended for this purpose, because opening the capsule can adversely affect the capsule's controlled-release properties.

Labeling, Record Keeping, and Cleanup

After the compounding operation, the product must be labeled with a prescription label (i.e., medication container label) containing all information required by the governing laws and regulations of the state in which the compounding is done. (For more information on proper labeling, see Chapter 7.) The ingredients of the compound and the amounts of these ingredients should be clearly stated on the label, and, in lieu of an expiration date from a manufacturer, the date of the compounding should also appear on the label. A careful record of the compounding operation, including ingredients and amounts of ingredients used, the preparer of the compound, and the name of the supervising pharmacist should be kept. Master formula sheets, such as the one shown in Figure 8.1, provide a means for keeping such a record.

Figure 8.7

The Punch Method for Extemporaneous Filling of Capsules
(a) The body of the capsule is filled by "punching" into a cake of the powder. (b) The filled capsule is then weighed to verify the dose.

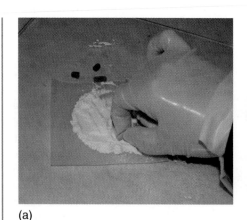
(a)

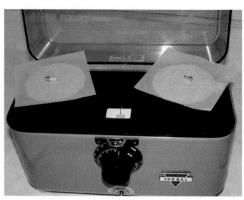
(b)

Once the compounding operation is finished, equipment and the work area should be thoroughly cleaned, and ingredients should be returned to their proper places in storage. The prescription balance, when not in use, should be placed in the locked position and covered, and weights must be placed back in their original container.

REFERENCE SOURCES FOR THE COMPOUNDING PHARMACY

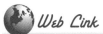

Web Link

For information about these resources, as well as others, visit this book's Internet Resource Center at **www.emcp.com** and visit Resources in the Pharmacy Library.

Web Link

Visit International Academy of Compounding Pharmacists **www.iacprx.com**

See the *Secundum Artem* article in the publications section at **www.paddock labs.com**

Visit Professional Compounding Centers of America (PCCA) **www.pccarx.com**

A thorough instruction in the complex art of extemporaneous compounding is beyond the scope of this text. The pharmacy technician can refer to a standard reference work on the subject, such as *Remington: The Science and Practice of Pharmacy* by Gennaro, as well as to the following Web sites:

- International Academy of Compounding Pharmacists
- *Secundum Artem: Current and Practical Compounding Information for the Pharmacist*
- Professional Compounding Centers of America (PCCA)

The PCCA holds national and regional seminars in extemporaneous compounding for pharmacists and pharmacy technicians. Membership also entitles one to the master formulas that have been developed and proven safe and effective over the years. Another helpful source of information is a hospital pharmacy, especially a pediatrics hospital, where pharmacists have experience in compounding formulations (especially for neonates, infants, and pediatric patients).

Chapter Terms

blending act of combining two substances

Class III prescription balance two-pan balance used to weigh small amounts of material (120 g or less) with a sensitivity rating of 6 mg

comminution act of reducing a substance to small, fine particles

compounding slab flat, hard, nonabsorbent surface used for mixing compounds; also known as *ointment slab*

counterbalance two-pan balance used for weighing material up to 5 kg, with a sensitivity rating of 100 mg

extemporaneous compounding production of medication in an appropriate quantity and dose form from several pharmaceutical ingredients in response to a prescription written by a physician

forceps instrument used to pick up small objects

geometric dilution method combining drugs using a mortar and pestle

good manufacturing practice (GMP) laboratory and industry guidelines to ensure a suitable work environment to prepare high-quality medications

graduates flasks used for measuring liquids

levigation process reducing the particle size of a solid during the preparation of an ointment

master formula sheet list of ingredients needed and procedures to follow when compounding; also called a *compounding log*

meniscus moon-shaped or concave appearance of a liquid in a graduate cylinder used in measurement

mortar and pestle instruments used for mixing and grinding pharmaceutical ingredients

percentage of error acceptable range of variation above and below the target measurement; used in compounding and manufacturing

pipette long, thin, calibrated hollow tube used for measuring liquids having a volume of less than 1.5 mL

powder finely divided combination or admixture of drugs and/or chemicals ranging in size from extremely fine (1 micron or less) to very coarse (about 10 mm)

pulverization process to reduce a solid tablet into a fine powder

punch method method for filling capsules in which the body of a capsule is repeatedly punched into a cake of medication until the capsule is full

spatulas stainless steel, plastic, or hard rubber instruments used for transferring or mixing solid pharmaceutical ingredients

spatulation process used to blend ingredients, often used in the preparation of creams and ointments

trituration process of rubbing, grinding, or pulverizing a substance to create fine particles, generally by means of a mortar and pestle

Chapter Summary

- Extemporaneous compounding is still used today to prepare medications in strengths, combinations, or dose forms not commercially available.
- Compounding is used to prepare solutions, suspensions, ointments, creams, powders, suppositories, and capsules according to formulas on master formula sheets.
- Instruments for extemporaneous compounding include the Class III prescription balance, weights, forceps, spatulas, weighing papers, the compounding or ointment slab, parchment paper, the mortar and pestle, graduates, and pipettes.
- Mortars and pestles come in glass, Wedgwood, and porcelain varieties. Graduates come in conical and cylindrical shapes, the latter being the more accurate.
- Proper technique and using the correct measuring devices is crucial when weighing pharmaceutical ingredients.
- Extemporaneous compounding is an art to be learned under the tutelage of an experienced pharmacist.

Chapter Review

Knowledge Inventory

Choose the best answer from those provided.

1. A large amount of material, such as 2 kg of Epsom salts, would be weighed using a
   a. Class III prescription balance.
   b. Class A prescription balance.
   c. counterbalance.
   d. Any of the above

2. Two pharmaceutical ingredients are combined, one a solid and the other a soluble, volatile liquid. The mixture is pulverized to reduce the particle size of the solid, and the liquid is allowed to evaporate in a process known as
   a. levigation.
   b. trituration.
   c. spatulation.
   d. pulverization by intervention.

3. An alternative to the ointment slab is
   a. weighing paper.
   b. parchment paper.
   c. a graduate.
   d. a pipette.

4. A prescription balance is unlocked, temporarily, when the technician
   a. adds weighing papers to the trays.
   b. adds pharmaceutical ingredients to the trays.
   c. moves the balance from one place to another.
   d. checks a measurement.

5. When measuring the amount of liquid in a graduate, one should place the eyes at the level of the liquid and measure the level of the meniscus from the
   a. top.
   b. bottom.
   c. back.
   d. front.

6. When using the geometric dilution method, the most potent ingredient, usually the one that occurs in the smallest amount, is placed into the mortar
   a. half at the beginning and half at the end.
   b. in stages throughout the compounding process.
   c. last.
   d. first.

7. An ingredient dissolved in a solution is known as a
    a. suspension.
    b. precipitate.
    c. solute.
    d. solvent.

8. A suppository mold is chilled immediately after filling to
    a. solidify the compound before its volatile components evaporate.
    b. reduce the possibility of spoilage.
    c. prevent contamination of the compound.
    d. solidify the compound before suspended ingredients have time to settle.

9. The punch method is used for filling
    a. hypodermics.
    b. capsules.
    c. graduates.
    d. unit dose containers.

10. An appropriate auxiliary label for a liquid suspension is
    a. "Take with food."
    b. "For topical use only; do not swallow."
    c. "Shake well before using."
    d. "May cause drowsiness."

Pharmacy in Practice

1. Practice using a Class III prescription balance and a mortar and pestle to prepare the following amounts of ingredients. Combine the ingredients and use the punch method to fill capsules with this "pumpkin pie spice" compound.
    a. 2.75 g of ground cinnamon
    b. 8.5 g of sugar
    c. 75 g of ground nutmeg
    d. 1.5 g of allspice
    e. 2.5 g of triturated anise seed or clove

2. Explain why using proper techniques and weighing ingredients with accuracy are important while preparing special compounds in the pharmacy.

3. Select the most appropriate size graduate to measure the following volumes. You have the following available in the pharmacy: 1 fl oz (30 mL), 2 fl oz (60 mL), 4 fl oz (120 mL), 8 fl oz (240 mL), 500 mL, and 1000 mL.
    a. 45 mL
    b. 75 mL
    c. 125 mL
    d. 450 mL
    e. 550 mL
    f. 890 mL

4. You are to dispense 453 mg of a powder. The original measurement is 453 mg. When you double-check the amount using a more accurate scale, the actual amount is 438 mg. What is the percentage of error of the first measurement?

5. You are instructed to weigh 80 g of a cream base for a topical compound. Your error range is 3%. What will be the least acceptable amount and the largest acceptable amount?

Improving Communication Skills

1. The art of compounding uses a whole different language, and you have been asked to describe the following terms to a pharmacy student who is visiting your pharmacy. Use simple terms.
   a. levigate
   b. punch method
   c. triturate
   d. spatulation
   e. diluent
   f. tumbling
   g. solute
   h. solvent
   i. geometric dilution
   j. comminution

2. A patient has arrived at the retail pharmacy where you work. She has a prescription for a compound that your store often makes. You are very busy and will not be able to get to this compound for at least 1 hour. The patient, frustrated from waiting so long at the physician's office, is now frustrated that you will not prepare her prescription immediately. What will you tell this patient? Explain why special compounded prescriptions take longer than other prescriptions. Write out your responses.

Internet Research

1. Visit the Web site for *Secundum Artem: Current and Practical Compounding Information for the Pharmacist* at www.paddocklabs.com, and choose articles that discuss three of the following topics. Use the information in the articles to write, in your own words, a summary of the issues involved in compounding the products you selected.
   good compounding practices
   compounding ointments
   topical antibiotics
   oral suspensions
   suppositories
   emulsions
   capsules

2. Visit the United States Pharmacopeia (USP) Web site at www.usp.org, and describe the resources available to assist in compounding prescriptions. Which ones would you choose to rely on?

3. Visit the Web site for your state board of pharmacy, and research rules for extemporaneous compounding by the pharmacy technician. Select a neighboring state, and compare how laws and regulations differ.

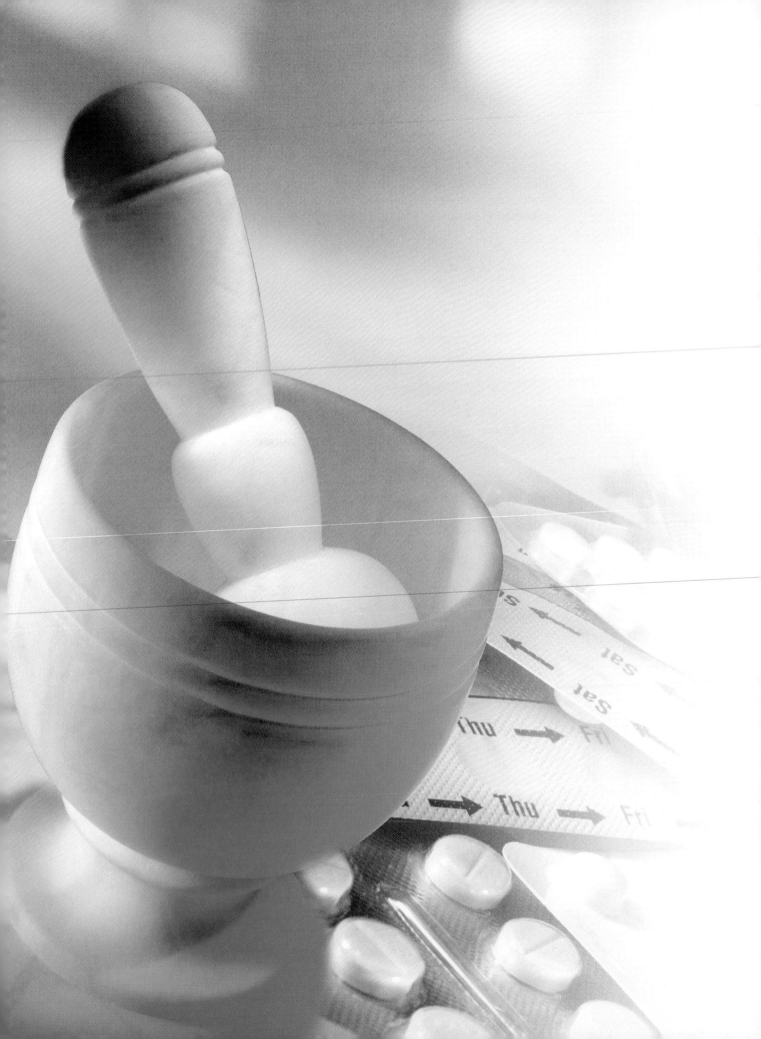

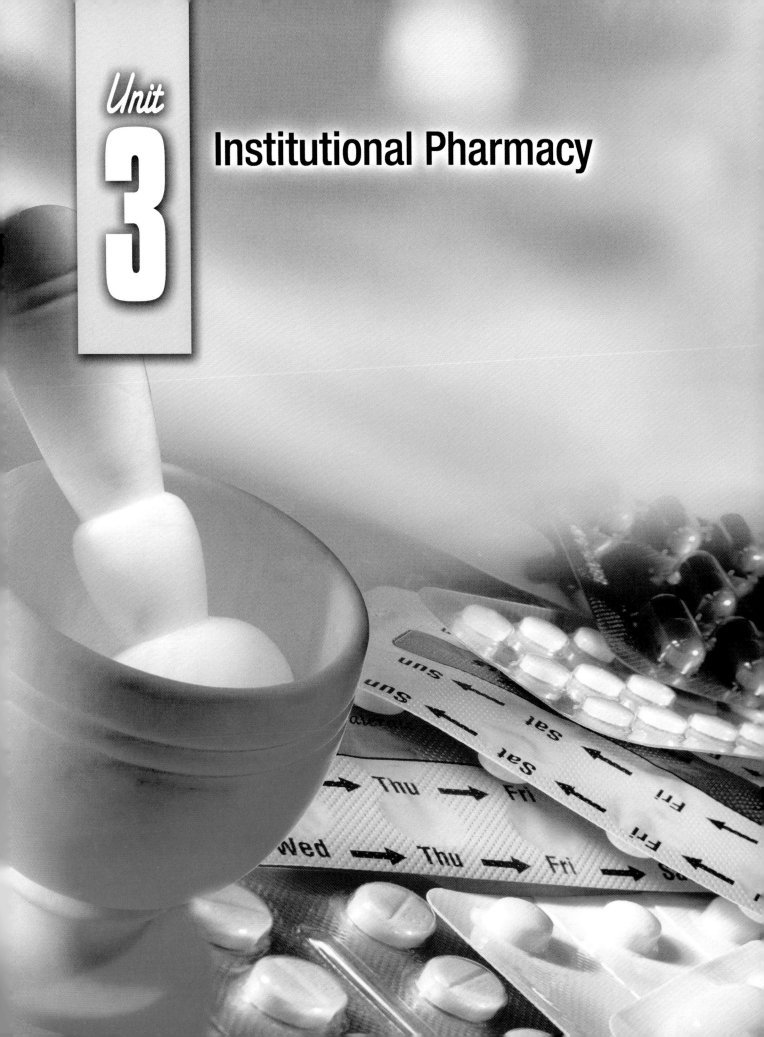

Unit
3
Institutional Pharmacy

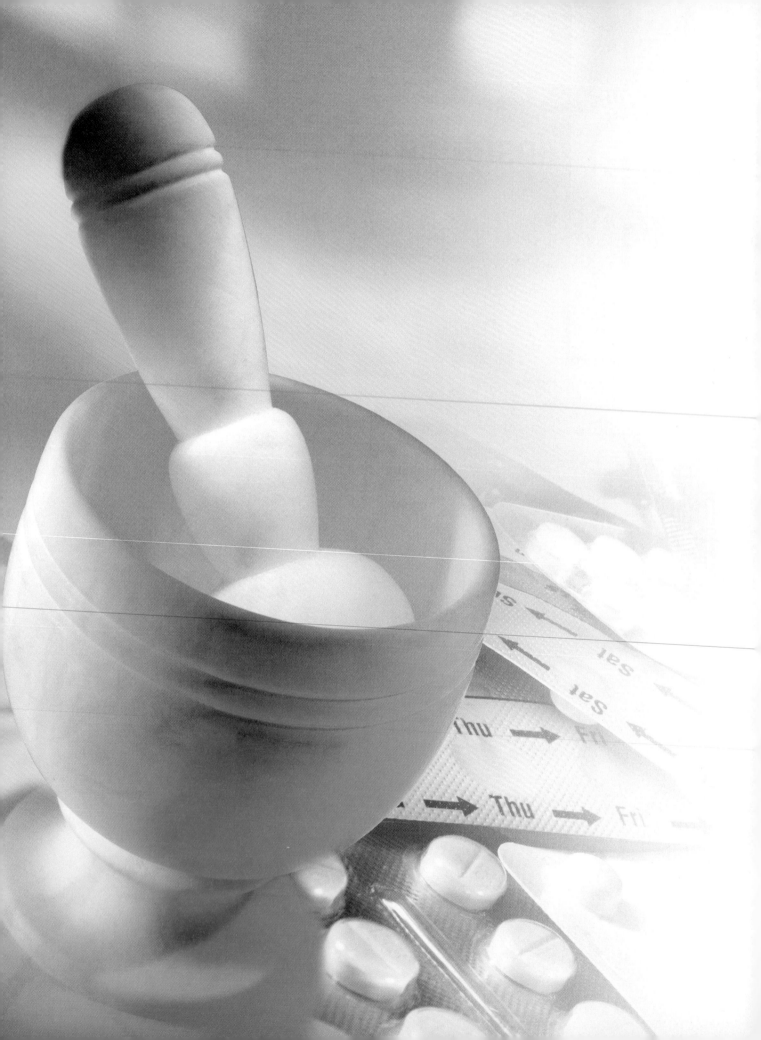

Hospital Pharmacy Practice

Chapter 9

Learning Objectives

- Describe the various inpatient drug distribution systems.
- Explain the proper procedure for repackaging of medications.
- Identify the process of medication dispensing.
- Describe specialty services such as intravenous admixtures and total parenteral nutrition.
- Identify the various roles of clinically trained pharmacists in the hospital.
- Describe the functions of a drug information center.
- Discuss the origins and purpose of the hospital formulary.
- Discuss the role of automation and inventory control in the hospital.
- Describe the classifications and functions of a hospital.
- Identify the roles of major hospital committees.
- List common universal precautions to protect hospital employees.

This chapter provides an overview of services offered by a hospital pharmacy with a special emphasis on understanding drug distribution systems such as unit dose, floor stock, repackaging intravenous admixture, and total parenteral nutrition. Chapter 10, *Infection Control and Safe Handling of Hazardous Agents*, will discuss the use of aseptic technique and the proper handling and disposal of hazardous agents. Chapter 11, *Preparing Sterile Intravenous Products*, will discuss the techniques and procedures used in the preparation of parenterals.

HOSPITAL PHARMACY SERVICES

The hospital is a complex organization that provides needed emergency, trauma, surgical, and medical services to the community. Hospitals employ hundreds if not thousands of employees, including pharmacy technicians. In fact, pharmacy technicians have been heavily used in this setting since the 1960s. Hospitals are often described according to bed capacity; in addition, they may be classified in several ways, including the following:

- type of service such as general and specialized hospitals
- university (i.e., teaching) and private (i.e., nonteaching) hospitals
- lengths of stay into short-term-care (i.e., under 30 days) and long-term-care (i.e., 30 days or more) hospitals
- governmental (i.e., Veterans Administration [VA]) and nongovernmental hospitals
- for-profit and nonprofit hospitals

Some of the functions of a hospital are listed in Table 9.1.

Table 9.1 Functions of a Hospital

- diagnosis and testing
- treatment and therapy
- patient processing (including admissions, record keeping, billing, and planning for post-release patient care)
- public health education and promotion, done through a variety of programs, including smoking cessation programs, weight loss programs, support group programs, and screenings of community members (including mammographies and testing of blood pressure and cholesterol)
- teaching (i.e., training health professionals)
- research (i.e., carrying out programs that add to the sum of medical knowledge)

Regardless of type, function, and size of hospital, nearly all will contain a hospital pharmacy. Many of the functions carried out in the community pharmacy are also carried out in hospital pharmacy settings. With the exception of insulin, most prescriptions dispensed in the typical community pharmacy are for oral medications or prepackaged specialty medications such as ophthalmics for the eye, otics for the ear, and topicals for the skin. The hospital pharmacy dispenses not only these types of medications but also parenteral and potentially hazardous medications.

As you learned in Chapter 1, pharmacists and pharmacy technicians work in a wide variety of practice settings. Some similarities exist between the functions of a hospital pharmacy and those of a community pharmacy. These similarities, as well as the services unique to a hospital pharmacy, are listed in Table 9.2. This section will focus on inpatient drug distribution services, clinical services, drug information services, and outpatient services unique to the hospital pharmacy.

Inpatient Drug Distribution Systems

Medication orders are processed differently in the hospital than in the community pharmacy. For example, the hospital pharmacy supports an inpatient drug distribution system where a 24-hour supply of individual doses for nearly all medications are prepackaged or specially prepared and sent to each nursing station. Selected drugs (mostly over-the-counter [OTC] medications) are available as floor stock and may be individualized to the medication needs of each floor in the hospital. The hospital pharmacy staff manages this floor stock and other medications.

Unit Dose Packaging Beginning in the 1960s, hospitals typically have made use of a unit dose system for dispensing medications. A **unit dose** is an amount of a drug prepackaged for a single administration. In other words, it is an amount of medication in a dose form ready for administration to a particular patient at a particular time. Unit dose preparation increases efficiency by making the drug form as ready to administer as possible, rather than requiring nurses to prepare doses from multiple-dose containers. Tablets and capsules are labeled, liquids are premeasured, injections are diluted as ordered and accurately measured into syringes, parenteral admixtures are compounded or mixed, and oral powders and other dose forms are prepared appropriately.

Safety Note

Only unopened unit doses can be returned to stock.

A unit dose system saves time and money. It provides increased security for medications, reducing medication errors; reducing nursing time; and making administration, charging, and crediting easier. Unit doses returned in their original unopened package may be returned to drug stock for reuse, thus minimizing wastage. A unit dose drug distribution system also ensures that proper hospital and departmental policies will be followed. A unit dose drug distribution system is more likely to get the right drug to the right patient at the right time.

Table 9.2 Hospital Pharmacy Services

Services Similar to Community Pharmacy Services
- maintaining drug treatment records
- ordering and stocking medications and medical supplies
- repackaging medications
- dispensing medications
- providing information about the proper use of medications
- collecting and evaluating information about adverse drug reactions and interactions
- preparing medications in various dose forms for dispensing
- educating and counseling patients about their drug therapies
- preventing, identifying, and resolving medication-related problems

Services Provided by a Hospital Pharmacy
- preparing and maintaining a formulary
- conducting drug use evaluations
- following universal precautions
- preparing products using aseptic techniques
- ensuring that hazardous agents are handled and disposed of properly
- filling medication orders (as opposed to prescriptions)
- routinely preparing 24-hour supplies of patient medications in a form appropriate for a single administration to a patient (as opposed to a 30- or 90-day supply)
- stocking nursing stations with medications and supplies
- delivering medications to patients' rooms
- maintaining a drug information service, and providing drug information to the other healthcare professionals in the institution
- educating and counseling inpatients and outpatients about their drug therapies
- monitoring patient outcomes
- preventing, identifying, and resolving medication-related problems
- participating in clinical drug investigations and research
- providing in-service drug-related education
- reviewing or auditing prescription services for evaluation of service accuracy and quality
- providing expert consultations in such areas as pediatric pharmacology, nutritional support, and pharmacokinetics

Repackaging Medications Because manufacturers do not prepare all drugs in a single or unit dose form, and because individual medication orders may call for nonstandard doses, preparing unit doses often involves repackaging. Oral medication specials (preparations made for a particular patient), intravenous (IV) specials, intramuscular (IM) injections, and suppositories are examples of drug forms typically provided in unit dose form.

Repackaging may involve the use of a variety of equipment, such as counting trays, automated packaging machines, and liquid-filling apparatus. Typical unit dose packaging includes heat-sealed zip-lock bags, adhesive-sealed bottles, blister packs, and heat-sealed strip packages for oral solids, as well as plastic or glass cups, heat-sealable aluminum cups, and plastic syringes labeled "For Oral Use Only" for liquid orals. Ointments, creams, eardrops, and eyedrops are not unit dose; these are bulk items that are supplied as floor stock (see following) at bedside or only on request.

Pharmacy technicians play an important role in repackaging medications for inpatient administration. However, like in all pharmacies, the pharmacy technician works under the direction of the pharmacist, and the pharmacist must always check the pharmacy technician's repackaging. When repackaging, a record is kept of what is done to track each dose for purposes of a drug recall and quality assurance. This type of record is known as a *repackaging control log* and contains the following information:

Safety Note

As in the community pharmacy, in the hospital pharmacy the technician works under the direct supervision of the pharmacist.

- internal control or lot number
- drug, strength, dose form
- manufacturer's name
- manufacturer's lot number and expiration date
- assigned expiration date
- resulting concentration
- quantity of units
- initials of the repackager
- initials of the pharmacist who has checked the repackaging

Additional information may be required, depending on hospital policy and state guidelines. (An example of such a log appears in Figure 9.1.)

Figure 9.1

Repackaging Control Log

REPACKAGING CONTROL LOG

DEPARTMENT OF PHARMACEUTICAL SERVICES

PHARMACY LOT NUMBER	DRUG-STRENGTH DOSE FORM	MANUFACTURER AND LOT NUMBER	EXP. DATE MANUF. MTC	RESULTING CONC.	QUANTITY	PREP. BY / CK'D

Medication Orders In the hospital pharmacy, prescriptions are in the form of medication orders. Figure 9.2 shows an example of a medication order for a patient being discharged to home healthcare. Figure 9.3 shows examples of medication orders for hospital patients..

Each day the hospital pharmacy's computer generates a **medication fill list**. This complete list records all current medications for all hospital patients. From this list, a unit dose profile is prepared. The **unit dose profile** provides the information necessary to prepare the unit doses and includes patient name and location, medication and strength, frequency or schedule of administration, and quantity for each order (Figure 9.4, page 208). Based on the information in the medication fill list, doses are prepared, labeled, and placed in patient drawers on carts that are taken to the wards or nursing stations. To comply with regulations, Schedule II drugs would not be dispensed during cart fill. Instead, they are obtained from the "narc cabinet" by the nurse at the time of administration to the patient. To control diversion, Schedule III–V drugs are also not dispensed during cart fill.

Unit dose labels include the following information:
- nonproprietary (i.e., generic) name or proprietary (i.e., brand) name of the drug
- dose form (if special or other than oral)
- strength of the dose and the total contents delivered (e.g., the number of tablets and their total dose)
- any special notes (e.g., "refrigerate")
- internal expiration date
- internal control number

A fill list is needed to stock patient drawers in a medication cart. This list is used to check medications left in the drawers and to provide needed medications. Most commonly a 24-hour supply is stocked. If some meds are left in the drawer, then these are subtracted from the 24-hour supply, and the difference is placed in the drawer. So, for example, if the fill list called for (and the medication drawer had) one 300 mg Tagamet tablet from the previous day, two tablets would be added to the drawer as shown below:

Medication	Sch	Daily Quantity	Post/Add
Tagamet	q8h	300 mg	3/2

Some pharmacy departments use the *meds remaining* in the patient drawer as a quality assurance tool to determine why a missed dose occurred.

Floor Stock The **floor stock** system provides medications including narcotics for each nursing unit. Floor stock distribution deals with those medications that are dispensed frequently on a prn (*pro re nata,* or as needed) basis. Typical floor stock consists of emergency medications and bulk items such as antacids, cough syrup, acetaminophen elixir or drops, ointments, creams, inhalers, and narcotics.

Figure 9.2

Medication Orders for Home Healthcare Discharge

(✓)	START HERE	DATE 10/16/XX	TIME	A.M. 1500 P.M.		(1) Doe, Jane 588123 1035 10 East
			Continue home meds:			
			1) enalapril 20 mg po bid			
			2) nystatin cream to affected area tid			
			3) digoxin 0.125 mg po q24h			
			4) nafcillin 1 g IV q6h			
			5) enteric-coated aspirin gr X po q24h			
			Smith, MD			

Figure 9.3

Medication Orders
(1 of 3)

NAME	ROOM #	ADMIT TIME
Barbara Ruth	825	
labetalol 200 mg IV q8h		
Emete-Con IM q2-3h prn nausea		
D5 ½NS 20 mEq KCl at 50 mL/hr		
npo after 12M		
John H. Jones	235	
naproxen 375 mg po q8h		
Benadryl elixir 5 mL po hs		
Mucomyst 10% 10 mL on call		
Billy Martin	821	
MOM 30 mL po prn hs		
lithium carbonate 300 mg po tid		
ASA gr X po q4h		
Hilda Hornblower	822	
Vistaril 25 mg po q4h		
Zantac 150 mg po bid		
acetaminophen 650 mg po q6h		
Vera Long	121	
Elixophyllin 250 mg po bid give 1 now		
ascorbic acid po daily		
albuterol 2 puffs q6h prn		
John Henry	432	
gentamicin 20 mg IV tid		
baby powder		
ASA gr V po q6h		
Casey Jones	333	
Haldol 10 mg bid		
Nitrostat SL prn		
Trental 10 mg po tid		
Dolly Madison	242	
amoxicillin 500 mg po bid 1 now		
hydrochlorothiazide 50 mg po bid		
Senokot po hs and bid		
Neil Buckner	383	
Colace 100 mg po bid		
Decadron 0.75 mg po		
Motrin 600 mg po q6h		
Darla Molari	422	
Prozac 20 mg po qam		
Folvite po daily		
Feosol po daily		
Larry Brindle	246	
Dilantin 30 mg po qid 1 now		
Allegra 180 mg po bid		
furosemide 40 mg po qam		

continues

Figure 9.3

Medication Orders–Continued
(2 of 3)

NAME	ROOM #	ADMIT TIME
Oscar Wilder	503	
Nitrostat SL prn		
Capoten 25 mg po stat, then bid		
Susan Anthony	610	
Catapres 0.3 mg po tid		
Coumadin 5 mg po q24h		
MOM 20 mL po prn hs		
Raul Garcia	111	
Zaroxolyn 5 mg po bid		
potassium chloride 10 mEq po tid pc		
prednisone 10 mg po qam with food		
Tom Smith	230	
ascorbic acid po daily		
Basaljel po prn ac and hs		
Toradol 10 mg po q4-6h		
Tim Turner	407	
10,000 units heparin IV now		
gentamicin 60 mg IVPB tid		
Bentyl 10 mg po tid prn		
Rick Bono	606	
Compazine 25 mg rectal prn		
Benylin Cough Syrup 2 tsp po q4h		
V-Cillin K 500 mg po q6h		
Marc Janzen	414	
Singulair 10 mg po daily		
erythromycin 250 mg po qid with food		
Aldactone 25 mg po bid		
Julia Shriver	409	
glyburide 5 mg po bid ac		
prednisone 15 mg po daily 8 AM		
Antivert 12.5 mg po tid		
Marian Carter	520	
PPD test with syringe		
Plavix 75 mg po qam		
Naprosyn 500 mg po q12h		
Natalie Wang	311	
Ambien 10 mg po		
Zyrtec 1 tsp qam		
MOM 30 mL po prn		
Ray Stevens	230	
Nitro-Dur patch 0.4 mg/hr apply qam and remove hs		
Aldactone 100 mg po tid		
Lasix 40 mg po bid		

continues

Figure 9.3

Medication
Orders–Continued
(3 of 3)

NAME	ROOM #	ADMIT TIME
Deborah Gunther	143	
acetaminophen elixir 160 mg po q6h		
Nexium 40 mg qam ac		
George Milar	502	
hydrochlorothiazide 25 mg po bid 1 now		
potassium chloride 10 mEq po daily		
Claritin-D 60 mg q12h		
Kathy Sooner	402	
Lipitor 40 mg po qam		
Dulcolax 5 mg po qd		
hydrocodone 5/650 1-2 tablets q6h prn pain		
Gloria Kramer	433	
Augmentin 375 mg po q6h		
Tylenol #3 1 tab q6h prn		
MOM 30 mL po hs		
Wesley Adams	321	
atenolol 100 mg qam		
MOM 10 mL po q pc		
Colace 150 mg po hs		
Jennie Conners	401	
Minitran 0.2 mg/hr apply qam		
Fleet prep kit		
ASA 650 mg po q4h		
Jeffrey Hart	213	
Ceftin 250 mg po q6h		
baby oil		
hydrochlorothiazide 25 mg po qam		
Jennifer Hightower	334	
Darvocet-N 100 mg po q6h		
Mylanta 60 mL po ac & hs		
Motrin 800 mg po q6h if react to Darvon		
Serena Sarles	416	
levodopa 1 g qid pc		
lisinopril 10 mg po bid		
Tylenol 650 mg po q4h		

Figure 9.4

Unit Dose Profile

R_x

John Doe	Room 535	
ampicillin 250 mg		
q6h	5P 11P 5A 11A	
Joanne Riggs	Room 532	
Nalfon 300 mg		
q8h	8A 4P 12A	

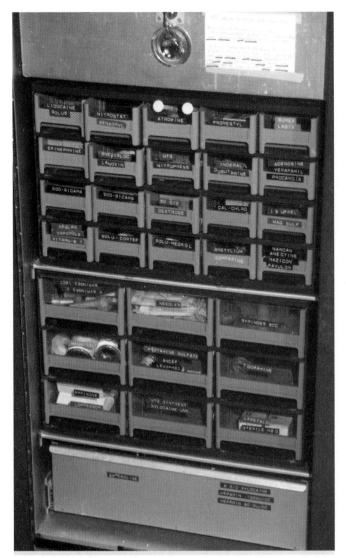

This automated dispensing machine dispenses stock items on the hospital floor.

Advantages of the floor stock system are a quick turnaround time from the writing of the order to the administration of the medication and the convenience of immediate availability of medications to the nursing staff. Disadvantages include increased diversion, increased risk of medication errors, and expense as a result of lost charges and revenue. The cost of floor stock may be covered by the nursing unit or may be included as a portion of the hospital overhead.

The pharmacy assumes responsibility for maintaining inventory through a floor stock replacement system. Pharmacy personnel maintain the inventory according to predetermined levels. As with any distribution system, checks are necessary to determine use and levels of remaining supply as well as expiration dates.

Floor stock must be inspected regularly by the pharmacy tech. When checking floor stock, it is important to check for expired drugs, to remove excess inventory, to see that all medications are stored properly including items requiring refrigeration, and to ensure that the refrigerator temperature is correct. A pharmacist may also be responsible for checking and reconciling the narcotic inventory records on each nursing unit.

In many institutions, floor stock items are kept in automated dispensing machines rather than in a stock room or on shelf space on the patient care unit. Automated dispensing machines keep an electronic record of bulk, floor stock, and items used for each patient.

Intravenous Admixture Service Nearly all hospital pharmacies provide an intravenous (IV) admixture or an IV additive service. This service involves the compounding of medications and IV solutions in a sterile "germ-free" work environment in the central pharmacy by specially trained pharmacists and pharmacy technicians. In addition to maintaining sterility, these medications can be more accurately prepared and labeled, resulting in fewer medication errors. Many medications ordered in the hospital are to be reconstituted or dissolved and then added to an IV solution or minibag. In the past, nurses would be required to add some medications (e.g., electrolytes) to IV solutions without benefit of a sterile work environment. Some potentially hazardous drugs must be prepared using specialized equipment. Chapters 10 and 11 will explore germ theory, aseptic technique, handling and disposal of hazardous drugs, and preparation of IV fluids in much more detail.

Total parenteral nutrition (TPN) is a specially formulated parenteral solution that provides for the entire nutritional needs intravenously (IV) when a patient cannot or will not eat. It is also used in patients with certain inflammatory diseases of the gastrointestinal (GI) tract that may prevent the absorption of nutrients. TPN is

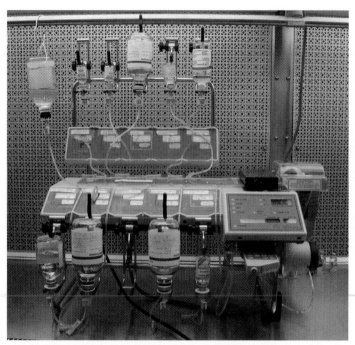
This micromix admixture machine adds micronutrients to IV TPN solutions. This procedure is done within a laminar airflow hood.

valuable because if a patient does not receive adequate caloric intake, the patient's immune system becomes suppressed and he or she is more susceptible to infection. TPN solutions are used in patients of all ages in both the hospital and home healthcare environments.

It is important for the technician to understand the importance of having the pharmacist conduct an end product evaluation before any drug added to an IV is sent to the nursing unit. The pharmacist will observe any IV product for particulate matter or physical incompatibility of the drugs under special lighting. If a defective IV product is administered, then it could cause a severe adverse reaction in the patient.

Clinical Services

A hospital pharmacy typically carries out numerous clinical functions that involve dispensing information as opposed to drugs. These clinical functions include providing drug information to healthcare professionals, monitoring drug therapy profiles, educating and counseling patients about their drug therapies, conducting drug use evaluations, evaluating information about adverse drug reactions, coordinating and participating in clinical drug investigations and research, providing in-service drug-related education, and auditing for quality assurance. In a teaching hospital, the pharmacist is often responsible for providing education to the medical or pharmacy residents in training.

In some smaller hospitals the pharmacy staff oversees both the dispensing and clinical functions. In larger hospitals pharmacists and pharmacy techs may function together in a satellite pharmacy. A **satellite pharmacy** is a minipharmacy located on the nursing unit of the hospital.

Often a specialty trained clinical pharmacist in the hospital may provide expert consultation in one or more areas such as neonatology/pediatrics (the effects of drugs on babies and children), critical care, surgery, internal medicine, transplant, infectious disease, oncology (cancer), and psychiatry (mental health). A typical day would involve the pharmacist accompanying the physician or medical/surgical teams on rounds or visits to each patient on that medical service. The pharmacist is responsible for reviewing all medication orders and doses, as well as preventing any drug-drug interactions or adverse drug reactions from occurring. After rounds, the pharmacist may need to review lab test results, counsel the patient on new or discharged drug therapies, or research drug-related questions for the medical team.

The clinically trained pharmacist may also provide consultant services in the areas of nutritional support and pharmacokinetics. A nutritional support pharmacist may make rounds with a nutritional support team to visit patients of all ages on all medical services that have nutritional needs. Medication orders are written for TPNs, which are individualized to the needs of each patient. The pharmacist may be responsible for making all the necessary calculations and writing the orders under a physician-approved **protocol**, which is a list of drugs and doses developed and approved by a physician for use by a nurse or pharmacist in the absence of the physician.

A hospital pharmacy will often provide a pharmacokinetics consult service. This service is responsible for individualizing the dose of selected medications based on patient factors (e.g., body weight, kidney function). Many drugs have a narrow margin of safety between the amount of drug in the bloodstream needed for its therapeutic effect or when it may cause toxicity. This service makes precise calculations to estimate the dose needed for patients of all ages. Examples of drugs that might require a pharmacokinetics consult service include drugs used for the heart, asthma, seizures, and many antibiotics.

Without the pharmacy tech providing some of the dispensing functions, it would be impossible for the pharmacist to perform these clinical functions.

Drug Information Services

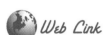

Web Link

For a list of the types of references that might be kept in the drug information center, visit the Resources list in the Pharmacy Library section of this book's Internet Resource Center (IRC) at **www.emcp .com**

To fulfill its clinical functions, a hospital pharmacy may maintain a drug information center, which is basically a small library containing reference works, including books, periodicals, microfilm, compact disks (CDs), digital versatile disks (DVDs), and access to computerized or Internet databases providing information about drugs and their uses. The purpose of the drug information center or service is to collect and provide information and literature about drugs and their effects.

Since ancient times one of the functions of the "healer" has been to compile a list or formulary of medications (e.g., plants, mineral substances) that are efficacious, or useful, for treating particular conditions. One of the earliest known formularies was listed in the *Papyrus Ebers,* a scroll from ancient Egypt. In the modern world one of the major functions of a drug information pharmacist is the development and maintenance of a formulary. A **formulary** is the official list of medications approved for use in a particular institution. Unlike the community pharmacy, which may need to stock multiple brands of medication, the hospital pharmacy has a restricted amount of medications that it stocks. For each product, a formulary lists the product name, dose form, concentration, and package size. The formulary is usually available on-line to all health professionals.

Considerations in preparing and maintaining a formulary include the latest technical information regarding the risks and benefits of a drug; information about the costs, risks, and benefits of new drugs; ongoing drug use evaluations that provide information about drug use patterns and costs within the institution; and ongoing new drug research within the institution. The drug information center is usually responsible for evaluating adverse drug reactions and reporting them to the appropriate hospital committee.

In addition to researching drugs for the formulary, the drug information pharmacist is also responsible for providing drug information to all health professionals in the hospital. This may include patient-specific questions from physicians, pharmacists, or nurses, and providing information on investigational drugs to nurses. The drug information center may be involved in comparing the equivalency of similar drugs in the annual bid process.

The pharmacy technician working in a hospital's drug information center may be responsible for maintaining and filing correspondence and pharmacy-related literature, including abstracts, catalogs, correspondence, journals, microfilm, and newsletters; for logging information requests and compiling statistics about those requests; and for collating data on drug use and adverse reactions.

Outpatient Pharmacy Services

In addition to caring for patients within the hospital, many large hospitals operate an outpatient pharmacy to serve the medication needs of patients discharged from the hospital, as well as for those patients who are seen in the emergency room or other ambulatory clinics adjoining the hospital. If the hospital pharmacy has clinically trained pharmacists on each unit of the hospital, then the pharmacists may provide some of the necessary patient counseling when the patients are being prepared for discharge from the hospital. Such a pharmacy operates much like a community pharmacy but within the guidelines of the hospital formulary. Some hospitals may elect to "outsource" or rent available space to a local pharmacy to provide these services.

AUTOMATION IN THE HOSPITAL PHARMACY

Technology is used in the hospital pharmacy to increase accuracy and improve efficiency and quality of pharmacy services. A computer system within a hospital is most often networked with other departments such as nursing, laboratory, and administration. These provide the opportunity for transmitting and sharing of information, including patient data, laboratory results, medication orders, pharmacy literature, and adverse reaction reports.

In many hospital pharmacies, automated pharmacy services are replacing some of the routine, time-consuming filling procedures. Automation has the capability to improve medication safety. Automation in almost every hospital pharmacy includes computerized generation of prescription orders and repackaging of bulk items into unit dose packaging. Larger pharmacies have installed robotic equipment to make IV admixtures and TPNs and to fill outpatient prescriptions. Narcotic distribution services use automation to enhance record keeping and minimize administration errors. Many hospital pharmacies have computerized inventory systems with their wholesaler to maintain an adequate drug supply. Both pharmacists and technicians are responsible for operating the equipment and maintaining supplies used in the automation process. Although human error is minimized with automation, technical errors must also be monitored.

Prescription orders that have been keyed into the computer are often filled on a regular 24-hour basis until the patient is released from the hospital or an order for a change in the medication is received. A pharmacist or technician will pull the medication fill list from the computer database once daily (usually in early morning) and begin the fill process for the upcoming day. As new orders arrive in the pharmacy they are keyed into the computer system, and the first day's medications are prepared. Orders for **stat medications** are filled immediately according to protocol and sent to the nursing station. Maintenance medications are then included in the following day's automated report.

Pharmacies may use a variety of different time- and cost-saving devices to assist in the preparation of medications. As mentioned earlier, most medications in the pharmacy are purchased in unit dose packaging. However, some medications are not available or are cost prohibitive in this packaging. Pharmacies may purchase the product in bulk and use a machine in the pharmacy to place the individual doses into a single-dose, heat-sealed package. This process is labor intensive and is often the responsibility of a pharmacy technician. Repackaging and labeling of medications must be performed according to set guidelines regarding the record keeping and new labeling that must be printed on the unit dose. Expiration dating must be on each label.

Larger automated robots are being used to perform some of the filling procedures with near 100% accuracy. Patients are assigned a bar code with their patient identification, and the computer matches the needed prescription medications with

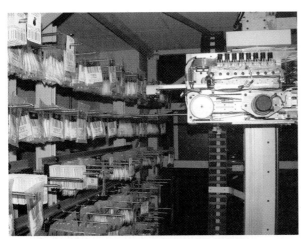

A robotic device fills prescriptions using the downloaded prescription orders and bar-coded unit-dose-packaged medications.

the patient. All of the unit dose medications are packaged with an identifying bar code and placed on pegs. Both solid and liquid oral medications, as well as prefilled syringes and vials, are packaged in the bar-coded plastic devices. The arm of the robotic device uses suction devices and pneumatic air to pull the medication from a peg on the wall and transfer it to a collection area.

Patients' individualized prescription orders may be collected by the robot and placed in an envelope or plastic tray for delivery. By using technology such as this, the pharmacist is able to spend more time reviewing and monitoring the patient's medical progress. The technician's responsibilities are also changed in that much time will be spent keeping the robotic area well stocked with medications. Using technology such as this has allowed the pharmacy to operate more efficiently and significantly reduces the amount of inventory.

INVENTORY MANAGEMENT

Pharmacists must ensure that their patients receive the highest quality pharmaceuticals at the lowest cost. With the assistance of the drug information pharmacist and the inventory control pharmacist, criteria are developed based on projected use. These criteria are used as the basis for a confidential, sealed competitive bid process, which includes suppliers and manufacturers of drugs and IV solutions. These bids are very competitive, especially in large hospitals where hundreds of thousands of dose units of some products may be used each year.

Most accepted bids will lock in the medication cost for 1 year; however, some contracts for IV solutions may be for a longer period of time. Bids on IV solutions and sets are often under the purview of the hospital pharmacy. Why are IV solutions different? Changing IV solutions and IV sets and educating all nurses every year on the changes is not feasible or cost-effective and may increase medication administration errors.

The bid process will determine the source of approved drug products listed in the hospital formulary. Will the brand name drug win the bid, or will one of many generic drugs be selected? Changing brands of oral or parenteral medication may cause confusion to the pharmacist, nurse, and physician, because the color, shape, or packaging may differ from previously stocked medication. To minimize confusion and medication errors, changing the source of drug products is infrequent unless major economic incentives exist. The American Society of Health-System Pharmacists (ASHP) recommends these "best practice" guidelines for a hospital pharmacy purchasing pharmaceuticals:

- Invitations to bid should be mailed to the pharmaceutical company's home office with a copy to the local sales representative.
- Potential bidders should be given a minimum of 3 weeks to respond to the bid.
- Opening date of the bid should be specified and honored.
- The bid should contain complete specifications with respect to products, packaging, and quantities desired.
- Quantities in the bid should be reasonable estimates of what will actually be purchased.

Web Link

The American Society of Health-System Pharmacist's Web site provides standards for information technology and automation in the hospital pharmacy. Visit **www.ashp.org /bestpractices**

- Adequate space on the bidding form should be provided.
- The winner should be notified in writing; unsuccessful bidders may be informed who made the winning bid if they request the information.
- With a group purchase bid, each hospital pharmacy should honor the winning bid.

Pharmacy technicians may be responsible for collecting information for the drug-bidding process. Many states require a separate bidding process and a separate physician inventory if the hospital operates an outpatient community pharmacy. Similar to the community pharmacy, the hospital pharmacists and technicians will usually perform a physical inventory of their drugs on an annual basis.

An important part of the technician's position is the receipt, storage, and ordering of pharmaceuticals; discrepancies in the order from the wholesaler or pharmaceutical manufacturer should be resolved. Automation from the pharmacy wholesalers is making inventory management more accurate and less costly. Computerized handheld systems such as Pyxis ParAssist help manage inventory in each area of the hospital by collecting data using bar code scanning devices and sending this information to the hospital pharmacy. Inventory and labor costs are reduced with the efficiencies of this technology.

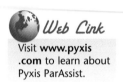

Web Link

Visit **www.pyxis .com** to learn about Pyxis ParAssist.

Two types of pharmaceuticals require special consideration: (1) controlled substances and (2) investigational drugs. The Controlled Substances Act (CSA) defines ordering and inventory requirements for controlled substances. Purchase of Schedule II controlled substances must be authorized by a pharmacist and executed on the Drug Enforcement Administration (DEA) 222 form as discussed in Chapter 7. A physical inventory of Schedule II substances is required every 2 years. **Investigational drugs**—ones that are being used in clinical trials and have not yet been approved by the Food and Drug Administration (FDA) for use in the general population—also require special ordering, handling, and record-keeping procedures.

At times a hospital pharmacy may need to "borrow" a medication from a local hospital or community pharmacy; the policy and procedure manual should outline the process, and the "borrowed" drug should be returned when received from the wholesaler. Another important area of responsibility for the tech is the storage and return of expired drugs (or drugs subject to FDA or drug manufacturer recalls) for credit.

ORGANIZATION OF THE HOSPITAL

The hospital pharmacy exists as part of a much larger and more complex organization called the *hospital*. An overview of this structure is important to better understand the roles and responsibilities of the hospital pharmacy. Traditionally, a president or director who reports to a board of directors runs a hospital. Reporting to the president or to an executive vice president, in a typical hospital, are the vice presidents of various departments. The vice president for professional services usually oversees the departments responsible for anesthesiology, clinical services, laboratory testing, medical records, psychiatry, radiology, rehabilitation, respiratory care, social services, and pharmacy.

Web Link

Visit **www.hca healthcare.com** to see an example of the vision and mission of a large hospital corporation. Note the emphasis on patient safety.

The director of pharmacy generally reports to the vice president for professional services (or similar title). If a corporation owns several hospitals in the region, then there may be a position like chief executive director of pharmacy that is responsible for all hospital pharmacy activities; the directors of pharmacy function as chief operating officer of each hospital pharmacy and report to this individual. The director of pharmacy works closely with the director of nursing and the chief of staff in medicine to provide quality patient care.

An extensive committee structure is needed to support the functions of the hospital. The main committees relating to pharmacy include pharmacy and therapeutics (P&T), infection control, and institutional review board (IRB). These are all discussed in more detail in the following sections.

Pharmacy Administration

The director of pharmacy is the *pharmacist-in-charge*, with overall responsibility for the hospital's pharmacy services. This includes managing the budget, hiring and firing personnel, developing a strategic vision, complying with all federal and state regulations and laws, and developing policy and procedures to comply with hospital policy and accreditation standards. Depending on the hospital size, additional assistant or associate directors with more specific responsibilities within the hospital may work under the director of pharmacy. In a small rural hospital, only one or two pharmacists may make up the pharmacy staff, yet the responsibilities are the same.

The pharmacy director is responsible for submitting a budget and complying with that budget. Unfortunately, nearly 70% of the budget relates to medications prescribed by physicians, and this is not under the direct control of the pharmacy director. Drug budgets can be difficult to predict, especially 1 to 2 years in advance; newer more expensive drugs may come into the marketplace to replace lower-cost alternatives, or a new transplant service may be implemented in the hospital requiring the use of expensive immune-suppressing drugs.

The hospital's human resources department will generally advertise for personnel positions and screen candidates; however, the director of pharmacy makes the final decision when pharmacy staff is hired. It is common for the hospital to request criminal background checks for all its personnel before they are hired. Many pharmacy technicians may be hired on a contingency basis (i.e., their performance will be re-evaluated after 3 or 6 months). Applicants with prior hospital experience or formalized training are considered to be more qualified than other applicants without such experience or training.

In addition to providing oversight on the day-to-day operations, the director of pharmacy is responsible for developing and justifying a strategic vision for the department to hospital administration. Where will the department be in 5 years? What new services are needed to maintain patient safety and quality of care? The director is also responsible for developing adequate and consistent written policies and procedures for every aspect of the operation including state and federal laws. Importantly, pharmacy technicians must study this manual; often it may take a technician 1 to 2 months to function in the hospital pharmacy adequately.

The director of pharmacy also determines the level and scope of services that will be offered by the hospital pharmacy. Examples include the following:
- type of medication distribution systems
- services available 24 hours, 7 days a week
- presence of IV admixture and TPN service
- satellite pharmacies on the hospital floor
- outpatient pharmacy services or outsourcing
- pharmacy participation in emergency codes
- clinical pharmacists making rounds with physician and monitoring patients
- clinical services offered in nutritional support, pharmacokinetics
- drug information center or service provided by staff

Because of budget or staffing restrictions, some hospital pharmacies may elect to "outsource" their services. Outsourcing is contracting with a pharmacy outside the hospital to provide services. For example, an IV admixture or nutrition service may be located off-premises and delivered to the hospital, or a hospital may contract with a local community pharmacy to lease space and provide outpatient pharmacy services in the hospital. In any case, safety and quality of care must not be compromised.

Joint Commission on Accreditation of Healthcare Organizations

The **Joint Commission on Accreditation of Healthcare Organizations** (**JCAHO**) is an independent, not-for-profit group that sets the standards by which quality of healthcare is measured. The mission of JCAHO is to continuously improve both safety and the quality of care provided to patients. As part of this mission, JCAHO awards hospitals **accreditation**, or a stamp of approval, if a hospital meets the specific standards defined by JCAHO. Nearly 80% of hospitals have JCAHO accreditation, which is often needed for Medicare and other third-party insurance reimbursement.

JCAHO evaluates the level of quality and safety of care for more than 15,000 healthcare organizations. In addition to hospitals, it accredits assisted living facilities, nursing homes, urgent care centers, surgical centers, mental health/substance abuse facilities, laboratories, and many outpatient clinics. JCAHO sets standards and evaluates the organization's performance in those areas. These standards are developed in consultation with healthcare experts, providers, and researchers.

The JCAHO accreditation process is rather extensive, requires a multiday on-site visit (often called a *survey*), and is completed every 3 years. The process requires a thorough review of each department's policy and procedure manual to be sure that it meets JCAHO safety and quality standards. The process is not meant to be punitive but to ensure patients that standards have been met. Many hospital personnel fear "failing" an accreditation, and occasionally it does occur. However, if the pharmacy department, for example, has received multiple budget cuts that have compromised safety or quality, JCAHO has the authority to require prompt corrective action.

The objective of the on-site survey is not only to evaluate the hospital but also to provide education and guidance that will help staff continue to improve the hospital's performance. The survey team includes healthcare professionals who are extensively trained and certified and who receive continuing education to keep them informed about advances in quality-related performance evaluation. The survey team generally provides a summary report to the hospital administrative staff and employees.

The accreditation report for all healthcare facilities is available for review on the Web site by any consumer or healthcare professional.

Safety-Related Standards Almost 50% of JCAHO standards are *directly* related to safety. The standards involving the hospital pharmacy include medication use, infection control, staffing and staff competence, medical equipment, and security. These standards address a number of significant patient safety issues, including the implementation of patient safety programs, the response to adverse events when they occur, the prevention of accidental harm through the prospective analysis and redesign of vulnerable patient systems (e.g., the ordering, preparation, and dispensing of medications), and the organization's responsibility to tell a patient about the outcomes of the care provided to the patient—whether good or bad.

Quality of Care Standards JCAHO has National Quality Improvement Goals, which provide standards for quality of patient care in select patient populations. It allows hospitals to report on the key indicators of quality of care in three of four treatment areas: heart attack, heart failure, community-acquired pneumonia, and pregnancy and related conditions. Algorithms are used to determine whether an organization's performance is above, similar to, or below the performance of other JCAHO-accredited organizations. Comparative analysis is performed at a state level and nationwide, and it is made available to employers and patients. Appropriate medication use is an important part of the quality of care standard.

For example, in assessing the hospital performance for the care of the heart attack patient, the following medication-related issues will be evaluated, measured, and compared with other JCAHO-accredited hospitals:

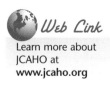

Web Link

Learn more about JCAHO at www.jcaho.org

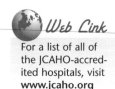

Web Link

For a list of all of the JCAHO-accredited hospitals, visit www.jcaho.org

Safety Note

Almost 50% of JCAHO standards relate directly to safety.

- use of aspirin prescribed at discharge because it decreases the risk of recurrent blood clots and improves survival
- use of certain heart drugs called *beta blockers* within the first 24 hours and at discharge to minimize damage to the heart
- timely use of thrombolytic or clot buster therapy to reduce stroke
- prescribing another class of heart drugs called *angiotensin-converting enzyme inhibitors* (ACEI) at discharge if heart failure is present
- documentation that the physician discussed smoking cessation programs with patients who smoke

Pharmacy and Therapeutics Committee

In the hospital setting, the **pharmacy and therapeutics (P&T) committee** reviews, approves, and revises the hospital's formulary. The P&T committee routinely meets on a monthly basis and usually consists of multiple members from the medical staff, as well as representatives from the hospital and nursing administration. The director of pharmacy and the drug information center pharmacist often represent the pharmacy department. The director of pharmacy is often the secretary of this committee and is responsible for taking and disseminating the minutes of the meeting; the drug information pharmacist is responsible for researching and making unbiased recommendations to the committee.

If a medical staff member would like the P&T committee to consider a new drug to be added to the hospital formulary, then he or she must complete and submit an extensive medication application form. The drug information pharmacist then reviews this initial information and completes a research of the medical literature. The cost, advantages, and disadvantages of the new drug will then be compared with an existing formulary drug, and these findings will then be presented to the entire committee for approval.

Formulary status is usually available at the time the medication is ordered and entered into the hospital's computer system. At times, formulary approval may be restricted to a certain medical service. For example, a new, high-cost antibiotic with limited indications and high resistance patterns may be restricted to the *infectious disease service*. A physician not on this service would not be allowed to write for this prescription (and the pharmacy cannot fill the order) unless it is approved and signed by an infectious disease physician.

If a physician writes for a *nonformulary* drug—one not on the approved list—then it is his or her responsibility to justify to the chairperson of the P&T committee the reasons such a drug is necessary for this patient. The formulary system is based on providing effective medications while limiting patient and hospital costs. The concept of a drug formulary has been adopted by managed care and most third-party insurance carriers.

Infection Control Committee

Infection control is the responsibility of all healthcare workers. Patients and employees are only safe from infectious processes when everyone follows good infection control techniques. The **infection control committee (ICC)** provides leadership and acts as a clearinghouse of information for the hospital.

The ICC is generally made up of physicians, nursing staff, infection control practitioners, quality assurance personnel, and risk management personnel, as well as representatives from microbiology, surgery, central sterilization, and environmental services. A pharmacist with an interest and expertise in antibiotics is also a member of the team. The goal of this interdisciplinary team is to bring together individuals with expertise in different areas of healthcare.

The primary role of the ICC is to prevent, identify, and control nosocomial infections, as well as infections from the community brought into the hospital. A **nosocomial infection** occurs when bacteria found in the hospital from any source cause a patient to develop an infectious disease. Some nosocomial infections are resistant to antibiotic treatment and can be life threatening. This committee sets infection control policy and is involved in planning, monitoring, evaluating, updating, and educating. This is accomplished by the following:

- surveillance of nosocomial infections
- antibiotic and other product evaluations
- investigation of infection outbreaks and infection clusters
- development of infection control procedures for all departments and staff
- patient education concerning medical waste management

The committee may be involved in evaluating which disinfectant should be used in the surgical operating room or which kind of sterilization is best for medical instruments. If resistance to microorganisms is increasing, then the committee may review if the antibiotic is being used inappropriately or in too small a dose. If an outbreak should occur, then it undertakes an epidemiologic investigation to determine the cause of the problem and recommends the necessary education or changes in protocols. Annual educational programs are conducted for all hospital employees on general infection control guidelines and mechanisms to update and disseminate new information to staff are designed. Another policy of importance to the pharmacy technician may include the handling and disposal of medical waste, as well as the proper discarding of **sharps**, or used needles, into a special and appropriately labeled container.

In addition to preventing hospital workers from spreading infectious disease to patients, the hospital is also responsible for preventing workers from contracting infectious disease from patients. The ICC is responsible for educating all hospital employees about the importance of following necessary procedures to minimize employee exposure.

Bacteria or viruses may be carried in the blood and other bodily fluids such as saliva, semen, gastrointestinal (GI) fluid, lymphatic fluid, sebum, mucus, and excrement. Examples of diseases that can be spread by means of bodily fluids include human immune deficiency virus (HIV) and hepatitis B. Procedures followed in all healthcare settings to prevent such infection as a result of exposure to blood or other bodily fluids are known as **universal precautions**, and Table 9.3 provides a list of the general guidelines that make up the universal precautions. It is important for all hospital workers to be fully up to date on their immunizations.

Pharmacy personnel generally do not have the kind of direct patient contact as described previously but should be cautious and cover an open wound or cut. Universal precautions are applied more by those healthcare workers with direct patient contact or by those who handle patient body fluids and tissues such as physicians, nurses, laboratory staff, and respiratory care technicians. Instead, pharmacy personnel are very concerned about exposure to toxic drugs. Handling and disposal of toxic materials will be described in Chapter 10.

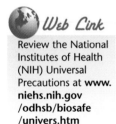

Web Link

Review the National Institutes of Health (NIH) Universal Precautions at **www. niehs.nih.gov /odhsb/biosafe /univers.htm**

Institutional Review Board

The **institutional review board (IRB)** is a committee that ensures that appropriate protection is provided to a patient in terms of investigational drugs or procedures. Another name for the IRB is the *human use committee*. Any hospital conducting any clinical research must have such a committee in place. This committee consists of

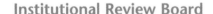

Table 9.3   Universal Precaution Guidelines

- Universal precautions apply to all persons within the hospital.
- Universal precautions apply to all contact or potential contact with blood, other bodily fluids, or body substances.
- Disposable latex gloves must be worn when contact with blood or other bodily fluids is anticipated or possible.
- Hands must be washed thoroughly after removing the latex gloves.
- Blood-soaked or contaminated materials, such as gloves, towels, or bandages, must be disposed of in a wastebasket lined with a plastic bag.
- Properly trained custodial personnel must be called if cleanup or removal of contaminated waste is necessary.
- Contaminated materials such as needles, syringes, swabs, and catheters must be placed into red plastic containers labeled for disposal of biohazardous materials. Proper institutional procedures generally involve incineration.
- A first-aid kit must be kept on hand in any area in which contact with blood or other bodily fluids is possible. The kit should contain, at minimum, the following items:
  - adhesive bandages for covering small wounds
  - alcohol
  - antiseptic/disinfectant
  - bottle of bleach, which will be diluted at time of use to create a solution containing 1 part bleach to 10 parts water, for use in cleaning up blood spills
  - box of disposable latex gloves
  - disposable towels
  - medical tape
  - plastic bag or container for contaminated waste disposal
  - sterile gauze for covering large wounds

representatives from medicine, pharmacy, nursing, hospital administration, as well as a consumer member. Most committees meet every month.

Protection for the patient generally consists of adequate knowledge of the risks for investigational drugs or procedures and confidentiality of medical information. Any investigational study requires approval by the IRB before enrollment can begin. The investigator usually submits an application outlining the study, including number of subjects, age of subjects, and type of subjects (i.e., patients versus healthy volunteers), as well as an informed consent form. An **informed consent** is a document written about the study in terms understandable to the lay public. The patient must initial and date each page of the informed consent.

In the informed consent the study must specify the risks versus the benefits, reimbursement (if any), and follow-up responsibilities and procedures should an adverse event occur. All such adverse events must be reported to the IRB, which will re-evaluate the approval of the study if necessary. Special procedures exist for neonates, pediatrics, underage women of childbearing age, and mental health patients. The investigator and the IRB must also meet regulations at the state level.

The IRB also protects patient confidentiality for participation in investigational studies. Besides the physician, who will see the medical data? The answer to this question must be specified in the application and protocol. Most commonly, patients are assigned a number (separate from their hospital number) to maintain anonymity. Investigational data may be collected, collated, and sent outside the hospital to a government agency or private company; however, the individual patient's identity and medical data remain protected. Patient confidentiality in the pharmacy will be discussed in more detail in Chapter 13, *Human Relations and Communications*.

Because many investigational studies involve pharmaceuticals, the pharmacy and pharmacy technician have major responsibilities in the receipt, storage, inventorying, and record keeping of these studies. Most hospitals do not allow physicians to dispense investigational drugs; they must be maintained in a secure area of the pharmacy until a medication order is received. In most of these studies the drug is not labeled with a name or strength. The drug information pharmacist is responsible for disseminating appropriate information to the nursing staff so that nurses can assist in monitoring the patient for an adverse reaction.

Chapter Terms

accreditation stamp of approval of the quality of services of a hospital by JCAHO

floor stock medications stocked on each nursing unit

formulary a list of approved drugs available through a hospital pharmacy

infection control committee (ICC) a committee of the hospital that provides leadership in relation to infection control techniques

informed consent a document written about a study in terms understandable to the lay public

institutional review board (IRB) a committee of the hospital that ensures the appropriate protection is provided to patients using investigational drugs or procedures

investigational drugs drugs being used in clinical trials that have not yet been approved by the FDA for use in the general population or drugs used for non-approved indications

Joint Commission on Accreditation of Healthcare Organizations (JCAHO) an independent, not-for-profit group that sets the standards by which quality of healthcare is measured and accredits hospitals according to those standards

medication fill list a complete list of all current medications for all hospital patients; used to create a unit dose profile

nosocomial infection an infection acquired by patients when they are in the hospital

pharmacy and therapeutics (P&T) committee a committee of the hospital that reviews, approves, and revises the hospital's formulary

protocol a list of drugs and doses developed and approved by a physician for use by a nurse or pharmacist in the absence of the physician; similar to "standing orders"

satellite pharmacy a minipharmacy located on a nursing unit of the hospital

sharps used needles; a potential source of infection

stat medications medications that are to be administered immediately

total parenteral nutrition (TPN) specially formulated parenteral solution that provides for the nutritional needs intravenously (IV) when a patient cannot or will not eat; also known as hyperalimentation solutions

unit dose an amount of a drug prepackaged for a single administration to a particular patient at a particular time

unit dose profile documentation that provides the information necessary to prepare the unit doses and includes patient name and location, medication and strength, frequency or schedule of administration, and quantity for each order

universal precautions procedures followed in healthcare settings to prevent infection as a result of exposure to blood or other bodily fluids

Chapter Summary

- Hospital pharmacies carry out a number of unique activities such as unit dose drug distribution system, repackaging, floor stock, and an IV admixture/TPN service.
- A unit dose drug distribution system saves money and reduces the chance of medication errors.
- Many hospitals offer clinical and consultative services such as nutrition support, pharmacokinetics, critical care, and other specialties.
- Most hospitals have a drug information service that is primarily responsible for making recommendations on a drug formulary.
- The primary mission of JCAHO is to ensure quality care and patient safety in the hospitals that are accredited.
- The P&T committee is primarily responsible for making the final decision on drug formulary decisions.
- The major role of the infection control committee (ICC) is the prevention of nosocomial infections in the hospital.
- Universal precautions are used to prevent infection when a hospital worker comes into contact with blood or other bodily fluids.
- The IRB is responsible for protecting the patient in investigational studies undertaken in the hospital.

Chapter Review

Knowledge Inventory

Choose the best answer from those provided.

1. A formulary is a
   a. list of approved drugs available through a hospital pharmacy.
   b. description of the contents and pharmacological characteristics of manufactured drugs.
   c. set of formulae for extemporaneous compounding.
   d. set of formulae for preparation of common parenteral admixtures.

2. Patient confidentiality for participation in investigational studies is a function of
   a. the P&T committee.
   b. the infection control committee (ICC).
   c. the institutional review board (IRB).
   d. JCAHO.

3. A unit dose is
   a. a supply prepared for a hospital ward or unit.
   b. an amount and dose form appropriate for a single administration to a single patient.
   c. the average recommended dose for an adult male.
   d. the dose recommended by the United States Pharmacopeia (USP).

4. A function unique to a hospital pharmacy, compared to a community pharmacy, would include
   a. maintaining drug treatment records.
   b. ordering and stocking medications and medical supplies.
   c. dispensing and repackaging medications.
   d. handling sterile parenteral hazardous drugs.

5. JCAHO is primarily interested in patient safety and
   a. quality of care.
   b. patient satisfaction.
   c. decreasing hospital costs.
   d. drug information services.

6. Universal precautions deal with infections by disease-causing microorganisms found in
   a. tap water and other liquid sources.
   b. blood and other bodily fluids.
   c. emergency rooms.
   d. pharmacies.

7. The primary role of the infection control committee (ICC) is to

a. approve antibiotics for the hospital formulary.
b. provide pharmacokinetic consultations on antibiotics.
c. verify correct doses on all medication orders for antibiotics.
d. prevent nosocomial infections.

8. When the pharmacy technician receives a *stat* order, the medication should be sent to the nurse
   a. immediately.
   b. within the next 1 to 2 hours.
   c. at the next shift change.
   d. the next morning.

9. Physical inventory of drugs in the hospital pharmacy is usually done every
   a. month.
   b. 6 months.
   c. year (annually).
   d. 2 years.

10. The provision of the entire nutritional needs of a patient by means of intravenous (IV) infusion is known as
    a. Pyxis ParAssist.
    b. prn.
    c. JCAHO.
    d. TPN.

Pharmacy in Practice

Write out a complete description, not using abbreviations, of the medication orders given in Figure 9.2 and Figure 9.3.

Improving Communication Skills

1. Communicating in the hospital setting often means working with a wide variety of other healthcare providers. Understanding what role they play in the patients' healthcare is essential to effective communication. What duties do each of the following have?
   a. primary care physician
   b. anesthesiologist
   c. registered nurse
   d. practical nurse
   e. nurse's aide
   f. housekeeping aide
   g. social services aide or worker
   h. respiratory therapist
   i. phlebotomist
   j. medical lab technician
   k. pharmacist
   l. pharmacy technician

Internet Research

1. Visit the ASHP Web site.
    a. What types of training does ASHP offer?
    b. What are the benefits of technician membership?
    c. How do you become a member?
    d. Go to www.ashp.org/bestpractices/medtherapy/Specific_St
        _Infection.pdf
        List ways that the pharmacy department can provide support for
        hospital infection control policies.

2. Go to the www.cdc.gov Web site and see what immunizations are
    recommended for you if you start to work in a hospital pharmacy.

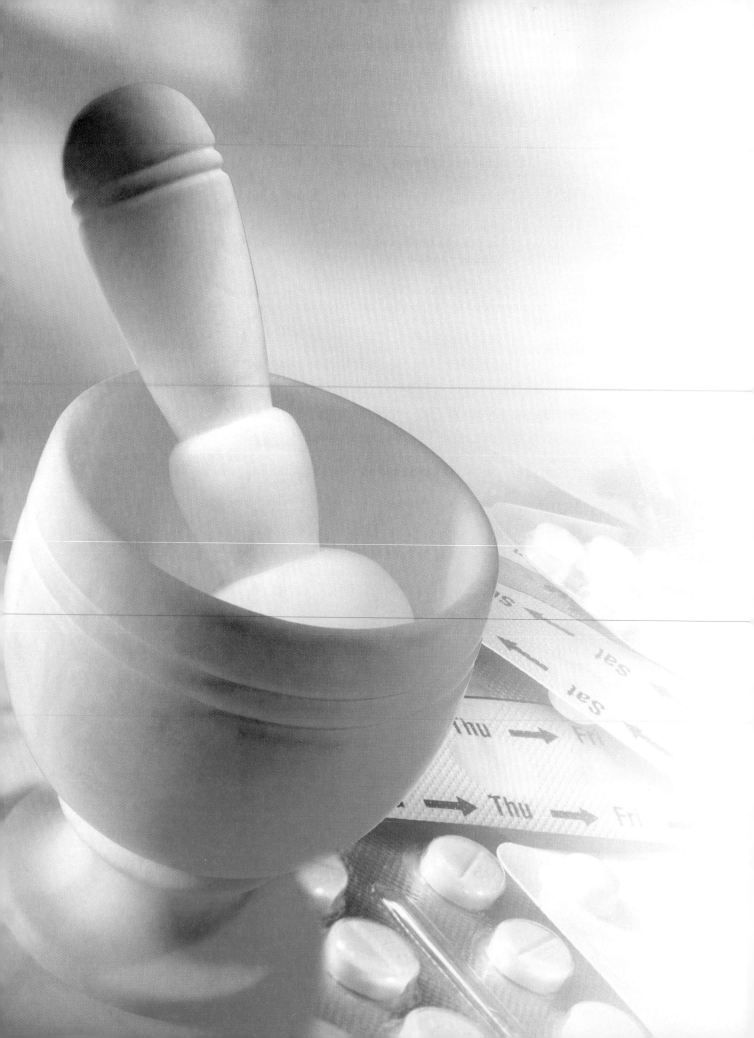

Infection Control and Safe Handling of Hazardous Agents

Chapter **10**

Learning Objectives

- Explain the germ theory of disease—the role of pathogenic organisms in causing disease.

- Distinguish among viruses, bacteria, fungi, and protozoa.

- Discuss the advantages and disadvantages of various forms of sterilization.

- Identify sources and prevention of common causes of contamination.

- Describe proper aseptic technique, including the use of horizontal and vertical laminar airflow hoods and the new United States Pharmacopeia requirements.

- Discuss the importance of and techniques for handling and disposing of hazardous agents.

Infection control is critical in a hospital setting. Patients with severe disease may have a compromised immune system and thus be more susceptible to serious and sometimes life-threatening infections. Microorganisms have a greater ability to adapt and become resistant to potent antibiotics in the hospital than in the community setting. Aseptic technique must be carefully followed throughout the hospital. Compared with community pharmacies, hospital pharmacies carry out additional unique activities such as routine preparation of parenteral intravenous (IV) admixtures using sterile aseptic techniques. Handling of hazardous agents also occurs in hospital pharmacies. In this chapter the student learns the importance of following correct technique in both preparing IV solutions free from microorganisms and preparing, handling, and disposing of hazardous drugs.

INFECTION CONTROL

Hospitals and home healthcare pharmacies commonly make use of "sterile" preparations. To understand what a sterile preparation is, one needs to know something of microbiology and the germ theory of disease. The comprehension of the potential dangers of contaminants will make the processes of sterilization and aseptic technique more easily understood.

Development of the Germ Theory of Disease

Until recently, the causes of illness—especially infectious diseases—were not understood. Disease was attributed to evil influences, and knowledge of the actual causes of infectious disease progressed slowly over the centuries. In the seventeenth century, the Dutch merchant Anton van Leeuwenhoek made the first crude microscope. In 1673 he wrote the first of a series of letters to the Royal Society of London describing the "animalcules" that he observed through his microscope, which we would today call microorganisms. Although van Leeuwenhoek observed microbes, the Englishman Robert Hooke used a microscope to observe thin slices of cork, which is composed of the walls of dead plant cells. Hooke called the pores between the walls "little cells." His discovery of this structure marked the beginning of a cell theory.

Until the second half of the nineteenth century, it was generally believed that some forms of life could arise spontaneously from matter. This process was known as spontaneous generation. People thought that toads, snakes, and mice could be born from moist soil, that flies could emerge from manure, and that maggots could arise from decaying flesh. In 1668 the Italian physician Francesco Redi demonstrated that maggots could not arise spontaneously from decaying meat by conducting a simple experiment in which jars containing meat were left open, sealed, or covered with a fine net. Redi showed that maggots appeared only when the jars were left open, allowing flies to enter to lay eggs.

In 1798 Edward Jenner discovered the principle of immunization against disease. He noticed that milkmaids who had caught cowpox from cows were then immune to contracting smallpox from humans. By infecting healthy persons with cowpox, Jenner successfully inoculated them against smallpox. However, because microorganisms had not yet been identified as disease-causing agents, the reasons behind the success of Jenner's immunizations were not fully understood.

In 1861, Louis Pasteur demonstrated that microorganisms are present in the air and that they can contaminate seemingly sterile solutions, but that the air itself does not give rise, spontaneously, to microbial life. Pasteur filled several short-necked flasks with beef broth and boiled ham. Some flasks were left open and allowed to cool. In a few days, these flasks were contaminated with microbes. The other flasks, sealed after boiling, remained free of microorganisms.

In Pasteur's time, the quality of wine making was very inconsistent. One year the wine would be sweet, and next year it would be sour. No uniform method had been discovered to ensure the same quality year after year. While experimenting along the lines used in his broth experiment, Pasteur discovered that if grape juice was heated to a certain temperature, cooled, and then treated with specific yeast, the wine would be more consistent year after year. This procedure established the basis for pasteurization of milk and the development of the aseptic technique.

The realization that yeasts play a crucial role in fermentation led people to link the activity of microorganisms with physical and chemical changes in organic materials. This discovery alerted scientists to the possibility that microorganisms might affect plants and animals. The idea that microorganisms cause diseases came to be known as the **germ theory of disease**. Pasteur, the originator of the theory, designed experiments to prove it. In one experiment, he successfully immunized chickens against chicken cholera.

Joseph Lister, an English surgeon, built upon Pasteur's work and applied it to human medicine. Lister knew that carbolic acid (or phenol) kills the bacteria, so he began soaking surgical dressings in a mild carbolic acid solution. This practice reduced surgical infections and was widely and quickly adopted. In 1876 Robert Koch defined a series of steps, known as *Koch's postulates*, which could be taken to prove that a certain disease was caused by a specific microorganism. Koch discovered rod-shaped bacteria in cattle that had died from anthrax. He cultured the bacteria in artificial media and used them to infect healthy animals. When these animals became sick and died, Koch isolated the bacteria in their blood, compared them with the bacteria originally isolated, and found them to be the same.

Microorganisms and Disease

Since the days of Pasteur, Lister, and Koch, thousands of pathogenic, or disease-causing, microorganisms have been identified. Not all microorganisms cause disease. Some, in fact, perform essential functions, such as creating byproducts that are used

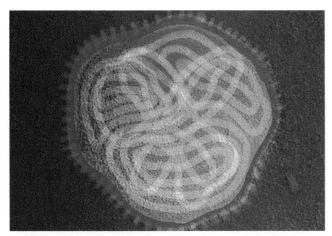

An electron micrograph of a virus. The virus is much smaller than a bacterium and can only be viewed with an electron microscope. It does not have all the components of a cell and requires other living cells to replicate itself. This virus that infects bacteria is called a *bacteriophage*.

as medicines, fermenting wine, fixing nitrogen in the soil, or helping the body to break down various food substances. For example, yogurt consists of "good bacteria" that can re-establish normal flora in the gastrointestinal (GI) tract and reduce diarrhea. However, some organisms of each of the following types are pathogenic.

Viruses **Viruses** are very small microorganisms, each of which consists of little more than a bit of genetic material enclosed by a casing of protein. Viruses need a living host in which to reproduce, and they cause a wide variety of diseases, including colds, mumps, measles, chickenpox, influenza, and human immune deficiency virus (HIV).

Bacteria **Bacteria** are small, single-celled microorganisms that exist in three main forms: spherical (i.e., cocci), rod shaped (i.e., bacilli), and spiral (i.e., spirilla) (Figure 10.1). Bacteria cause a wide variety of illnesses, such as food poisoning, strep throat, rheumatic fever, meningitis, pneumonia, pinkeye, and acne.

Fungi **Fungi** are parasites on living organisms (or they feed on dead organic material) and reproduce by means of spores. Spores and some fungi are microscopic and travel through the air. Fungi are microscopic plants that can occur as molds, mildews, or mushrooms. Some molds are the source of antibiotics such as penicillin. Others are implicated in mild conditions such as athlete's foot and ringworm or systemic fungal infections in the hospital, which are very serious and potentially life threatening.

Protozoa **Protozoa** are microscopic organisms made up of a single cell or of a group of more or less identical cells; they live in water or as parasites inside other creatures. Examples of protozoa include paramecia and amoebae. Amoebic dysentery, malaria, and sleeping sickness are examples of illnesses caused by protozoa.

Asepsis and Sterilization

The scientific control of harmful microorganisms began only about 100 years ago. Before that time, epidemics or pandemics caused by microorganisms (e.g., smallpox or cholera) killed millions of people. Three different bubonic plagues killed 137 million people in Europe (fleas spreading the bacteria from diseased black rats was the cause). In addition, European diseases such as smallpox and syphilis decimated the native population of the Americas. Before the modern era, in some hospitals, 25% of delivering mothers died of infections carried by the hands and instruments

Figure 10.1

Characteristic Bacterial Shapes
(a) Round cocci. (b) Rodlike bacilli. (c) Spiral-shaped spirochetes.

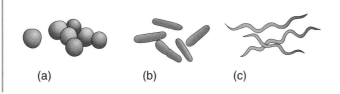

(a)   (b)   (c)

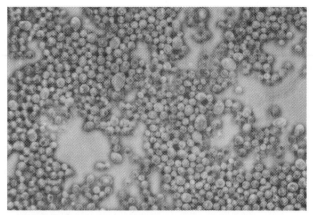
A photomicrograph of a fungus. Fungi are multicellular organisms, unlike bacteria or viruses.

of attending nurses and physicians. During the American Civil War, surgeons sometimes cleaned their scalpels on their boot soles between incisions. The "flu epidemic" of 1918 killed over 25 million people worldwide including 650,000 in the United States. The source of this epidemic was a bird virus that was transmitted to humans. There are concerns today that a reactivation of this "avian flu" would cause a pandemic and high mortality. Developing an efficacious vaccine is a global major health priority.

Asepsis is the absence of disease-causing microorganisms. The condition of asepsis is brought about by **sterilization**—any process that destroys the microorganisms in a substance. When an object like a medical instrument is sterilized, no need exists to identify the species of microbes on it, because sterilization kills even the most resistant microbial life forms present. Many types of sterilization exist: heat, dry heat, mechanical, gas, and chemical. A brief overview is provided for the pharmacy technician.

Heat Sterilization One traditional method for killing microbes is heat sterilization or boiling. Heat is available, effective, economical, and easily controlled. Boiling kills vegetative forms, many viruses, and fungi in about 10 minutes, but more time is required to kill some organisms, such as fungus spores and the hepatitis viruses. If water supply in the home is compromised, the recommendation is to boil water before drinking. Automatic dishwashers loosely borrow from the concept of heat sterilization during their drying cycle.

Heat sterilization uses an **autoclave**, a device that generates heat and pressure to sterilize. When moist heat of 121° C or 270° F under pressure of 15 psi (pounds per square inch) is applied to instruments, solutions, or powders, most known organisms—including spores and viruses—will be killed in about 15 minutes. At home, pressure cookers use the concept of heat and pressure to sterilize vegetables. Heat sterilization is being used less frequently in the hospital setting due in part to space requirements, equipment expense, and personnel training issues.

Dry-Heat Sterilization Dry heat, such as direct flaming, also destroys all microorganisms. Dry heat is impractical for many substances but is practical as a means for disposal of contaminated objects, which are often incinerated. For proper sterilization using hot, dry air, a temperature of 170° C must be maintained for nearly 2 hours. Note that a higher temperature is necessary for dry heat, because a heated liquid more readily transfers heat to a cool object.

Mechanical Sterilization Mechanical sterilization is achieved by means of filtration, which is the passage of a liquid or gas through a screenlike material with pores small enough to block microorganisms. This method of sterilization is used for heat-sensitive materials such as culture media (used for growing colonies of bacteria or other microorganisms), enzymes, vaccines, and antibiotic solutions. Filter pore sizes are 0.22 micron for bacteria and 0.01 micron for viruses and some large proteins. Filters are discussed more in Chapter 11, *Preparing Sterile Intravenous Products*.

Gas Sterilization Gas sterilization makes use of the gas ethylene oxide and is used for objects that are liable, or subject, to destruction by heat. Gas sterilization requires special equipment and aeration of materials after application of the gas. This gas is highly flammable and is used only in large institutions and manufacturing facilities that have adequate equipment to handle the gas. Many prepackaged IV products and bandages are manufactured and sterilized using this type of sterilization. Ethylene oxide will leave a slight nonharmful residue that can be detected as an odor, such as the odor present on simple adhesive bandages or IV bags.

Chemical Sterilization Chemical sterilization is the destruction of microorganisms on inanimate objects by chemical means. Few chemicals produce complete sterility, but many reduce microbial numbers to safe levels. A chemical applied to an object or topically to the body for sterilization purposes is known as a *disinfectant*. Alcohol, chlorinated bleach, and iodine are often used as topical disinfectants.

Contamination

Harmful microorganisms, especially bacteria, are everywhere in large numbers. For example, the Harvard biologist, E.O. Wilson, estimates that as many as 30 billion bacteria are to be found in a single cubic gram of soil. It is extremely easy to introduce bacteria or other contaminants onto a sterile object or device or into a sterile solution.

For the pharmacy technician working in the preparation of sterile IV products, the prevention of contamination is crucial. The introduction of contamination of an IV solution into a patient at surgery or with a compromised immune system can cause serious infection or even death. In a pharmacy it can occur by three primary means: (1) touch, (2) air, and (3) water.

Touch Millions of bacteria live on our skin, in our hair, and under our nails. Proper scrubbing for at least 30 seconds is very important to reduce the numbers of bacteria on the hands before handling sterile materials. Touching is the most common method of contamination, and it is the easiest to prevent. In addition to washing, the use of latex gloves and cap or hair nets can minimize touch contamination.

Air Microorganisms are commonly found in the air, in dust particles, and in moisture droplets. It is important to prepare sterile materials in a special area in which the numbers of possible contaminants are maintained at a low level. Special equipment called *laminar flow hoods* can control airflow and minimize contamination. They are discussed later in this chapter.

Water Tap water is not free of microorganisms. Moisture droplets in the air, especially after a sneeze or cough, often contain harmful microbes. It is important not to contaminate sterile materials by exposure to droplets of tap water or other sources of contaminated moisture. A pharmacy technician with a common cold should notify the pharmacist supervisor; often a change in work functions for that day will be recommended. Protective plastic shields on equipment and use of masks minimize moisture contamination.

ASEPTIC TECHNIQUE AND USP CHAPTER 797

Aseptic technique is the manipulation of sterile products and devices in such a way as to avoid introducing pathogens, or disease-causing microorganisms. Sterile products include fluids and medications stored in vials, ampules, prefilled syringes, and other

Table 10.1   Aseptic Technique

1. Remove all jewelry (e.g., watches, rings, bracelets, necklaces).
2. Put on non-shedding coats, gowns, or coveralls (hospital scrubs); head and facial hair covers; face masks; and shoe covers. Note that it is important to follow the sequence of items indicated in this step.
3. Scrub hands and arms to the elbows thoroughly with an antiseptic cleanser (e.g., povidone-iodine or chlorhexidine gluconate).
4. Clean the laminar flow hood with isopropyl alcohol. The alcohol must remain in contact with the surface for 30 seconds prior to compounding any sterile product.
5. Place only essential materials under the airflow hood—no paper, pens, or labels. Remove the selected syringe(s) from its overwrap, attach a needle, then discard the waste.
6. Scrub again and glove.
7. Swab or spray needle-penetration closures on vials, injection ports, and other materials.
8. Prepare the sterile product by withdrawing the medication from vials or ampules and introducing it into the IV container.
9. Complete a quality check of the product for container integrity and leaks, solution cloudiness, particulates, color of solution, and proper preparation of product.
10. Present the product, the containers and devices used, and the label to a pharmacist for verification of the product preparation.

Safety Note

When working in the pharmacy lab clean room, it is important to wear appropriate sterile gear, including face mask, full head covering, scrubs or gown with back closure, and gloves.

Web Link

Learn more about hand-washing techniques at **www.cdc.gov /handhygiene/**

Safety Note

Coughing and talking should be directed away from the hood.

containers for parenteral administration. Ophthalmic solutions and suspensions are also examples of sterile products. Sterile devices include syringes, needles, and IV sets.

Aseptic technique is used for the preparation of parenteral admixtures, combinations of fluids and/or medications or nutrients, which are administered using bolus (i.e., push) or other intravenous (IV) methods. Aseptic technique is treated in this chapter because of the frequency with which parenterals are prepared in the hospital pharmacy, though it is also used in home healthcare, long-term care, and some community pharmacies. Table 10.1 summarizes the steps for preparing parenterals using aseptic technique, and the sections that follow explain the procedure in more detail.

When preparing a product in a sterile environment in the pharmacy, it is necessary to work in an environment using a laminar airflow hood. Such an instrument produces parallel layers of highly filtered air that flow across a work area enclosed on all but one side. It is important to note that the clean area created within the hood will provide a very clean environment, but it will not prevent all means of contamination, especially those caused by human error and human touch. Two types of airflow hoods exist: (1) horizontal and (2) vertical.

In a **horizontal laminar airflow hood** (Figure 10.2), air from the room is pulled into the back of the hood where it is prefiltered with an air-conditioner-like filter to remove large particles. The air then passes through a **high-efficiency particulate air (HEPA) filter**, where 99.97% of all particles 0.3 micron or larger are removed. The air flows from the back of the hood, across the work surface, and out into the room. It is necessary to work at least 6 inches into the hood to avoid the mix of filtered and room air at the front of the hood. Blockage from objects placed between the HEPA filter and sterile objects creates an air disturbance that is three times the diameter of the object. Placed next to the side of that hood, it is six times the diameter. Coughing and talking should always be directed away from the hood.

Most IV solutions, nutritional products, and compounded ophthalmic medications prepared in the hospital (as well as other pharmacy settings) use this type of hood. More discussion on proper procedures for preparing IV solutions in laminar flow hoods is contained in Chapter 11.

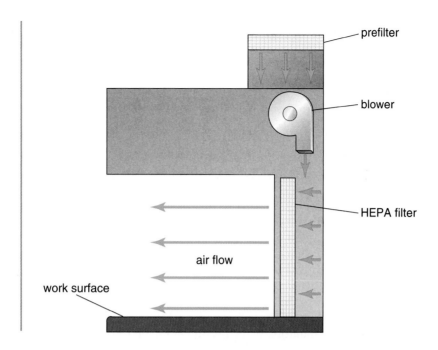

Figure 10.2

Horizontal Airflow Hood

prefilter

blower

HEPA filter

air flow

work surface

In a **vertical laminar airflow hood** (Figure 10.3), the air flows from the top of the hood down, through a prefilter and a HEPA filter, and onto the work area. The air is then recirculated through another HEPA filter and out into the room. The front of the hood is partially blocked by a glass shield. Because of the extra protection that it provides to the employee, this type of hood is used to prepare hazardous substances, such as parenteral IV chemotherapy solutions used for treating cancers. These hoods are vented to outside air to minimize human exposure.

At the start of each shift, the laminar airflow hood should receive a thorough cleaning with an agent that acts both as a detergent (for cleaning) and as a germicide, fungicide, and virucide. A commonly used agent for cleaning the hood is 70%

Figure 10.3

Vertical Airflow Hood

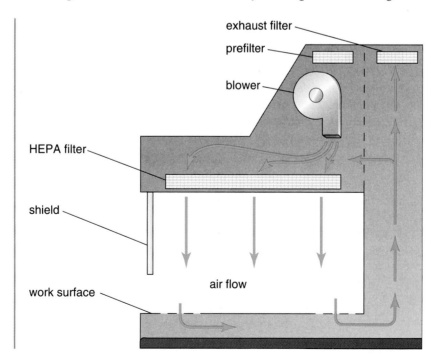

exhaust filter

prefilter

blower

HEPA filter

shield

work surface

air flow

isopropyl alcohol. The hood should be cleaned several times during a shift or as needed (e.g., after a spill) with the alcohol. The clear Plexiglas protective sides should be cleaned with sterile water and then with 70% isopropyl alcohol. The hood should be cleaned in such a way as to work contamination from the back out toward the room. The cleaning motion should be a side-to-side motion, with each stroke farther out than the previous stroke. The parts of the hood should be cleaned in this order: top, back, sides (top to bottom), and work area or bench (back to front).

The hospital pharmacy technician working in the IV sterile area is often responsible for checking and documenting the status of the HEPA air filters for the laminar flow hoods. These air filters should be changed to comply with requirements from the manufacturer of the horizontal or vertical laminar flow hoods.

How does the pharmacist or pharmacy technician know whether or not the sterile IV product he or she prepared, labeled, checked, and sent to the nurse for the patient was accurate or free from microorganisms? Each hospital pharmacy must have a **quality assurance (QA) program** in its policy and procedure manual to check for medication errors or contamination. The Joint Commission on Accreditation of Healthcare Organizations (JCAHO) (which accredits hospitals) requires such programs with oversight provided by the infection control committee (ICC). If breakdowns in accuracy or sterility are identified, existing procedures must be reviewed and all pharmacy personnel may need refresher training. A breakdown in sterility in the pharmacy could lead to a serious breakout of nosocomial infections in the hospital.

As of January 1, 2004, the United States Pharmacopeia (USP) developed the first official and enforceable requirements for sterile preparation compounding to improve the quality of sterile preparations made in the pharmacy. JCAHO has adopted these guidelines and will evaluate their compliance in hospital pharmacies on future accreditation visits.

The standard, known as **USP Chapter 797**, focuses on assessing the risk level of microbial contamination, physical contamination, and chemical contamination of **compounded sterile products (CSPs)**. Risk levels are defined as low, medium, and high.

- Low risk includes sterile products and devices that have been manipulated for a single transfer, such as the transfer of a sterile solution withdrawn from an ampule. This level also includes manually prepared TPN containing three or fewer ingredients.
- Medium risk includes multiple or small doses of sterile products combined using automated devices or transferred from multiple sterile containers into a final sterile container. Examples include TPN containing electrolytes and batch syringes or batch antibiotics without preservatives.
- High risk includes products compounded from nonsterile ingredients and sterile products and devices exposed to inferior air quality. Examples include sterile ingredients that have been measured and mixed using nonsterile devices before final sterilization.

The environmental quality control requirements are provided for sterile "clean" room, equipment, and protective clothing. **Beyond-use dating** is the date after which a CSP should not be used. The main factors in defining such dating include chemical stability and sterility of the solution. Beyond-use dating is determined by risk of contamination and storage conditions (e.g., room temperature, refrigeration, freezer).

Formalized didactic and experiential training on aseptic technique must be documented and repeated on a regular basis. The department's policy and procedure manual should incorporate these new requirements.

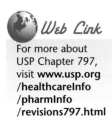

Web Link

For more about USP Chapter 797, visit **www.usp.org /healthcareInfo /pharmInfo /revisions797.html**

HANDLING AND DISPOSAL OF HAZARDOUS AGENTS

In all pharmacy settings, but particularly in the hospital setting, workers bear the risk of coming into contact with potentially hazardous medications and other chemicals. Many kinds of dangerous drugs and chemicals are encountered in pharmacy, including corrosive materials (i.e., acids that can dissolve or eat away at bodily tissues) and **cytotoxic materials** (i.e., materials that are poisonous to cells), as is the case with **antineoplastic drugs** (i.e., used in the treatment of cancer). These materials require special handling and preparation.

Four routes of exposure to hazardous substances include (1) trauma, (2) inhalation, (3) direct skin contact, and (4) ingestion, illustrated by the following examples:

- trauma or injury (A technician using a syringe to add a drug to an IV bag might accidentally prick himself or herself with the needle or receive a cut from a broken container of the substance.)
- inhalation, or breathing in, of the hazardous substance (A technician might drop and break a bottle containing a volatile substance, or poor manipulation technique may release a fine mist of the medication from the container.)
- direct skin contact (A technician might accidentally spill a medication when pouring it from a large container into a smaller container or flask. Direct contact with some cancer drugs can cause immediate reactions.)
  - Asparaginase may cause skin irritation.
  - Doxorubicin can cause tissue death and sloughing if introduced into a skin abrasion. Nitrogen mustards can cause irritation of the eyes, mucous membranes, and skin.
  - Streptozocin is a potential carcinogen when it is exposed to skin. Accidental exposures in the pharmacy may result in trauma, direct skin contact, and inhalation.
- ingestion (A technician might ingest dust when crushing an oral tablet or cleaning a counting tray.)

In any of these acute exposure examples, the exposure incident may produce symptoms or signs of sensitivity, eye irritation, lesions on the skin, coughing, headache, and dizziness. Continual exposure and improper technique could result in chronic long-term effects. Any pharmacy worker who is pregnant, breast-feeding, or trying to conceive should notify his or her supervisor so that extra precautions can be taken to minimize contact with hazardous substances or to schedule a change in work responsibilities.

All personnel in the hospital should have proper training in procedures involving identification, containment, collection, segregation, and disposal of cytotoxic and other hazardous drugs. Any organization involved with cytotoxic or other hazardous drugs should have written procedures for proper handling and disposal of such drugs and should provide access to medical care and methods for documentation in the case of incidents of exposure. All pharmacy personnel involved should have documented specialized training on policies and procedures, individual instruction, and check-off on competencies of technique and proper use of equipment.

Receipt and Storage of Hazardous Agents

Hazardous drugs should be delivered directly to the storage area, inventoried, and, if necessary, refrigerated. The inventory should be separated to reduce the potential error of pulling a look-alike container from an adjacent shelf or bin. Equipment for storage and transport should minimize container breakage. For example, storage shelves should have a barrier at the front, carts should have rims, and hazardous

Table 10.2 Commonly Used Cytotoxic and Hazardous Drugs

asparaginase	doxorubicin	mercaptopurine
bleomycin	estramustine	methotrexate
busulfan	etoposide	mitomycin
carboplatin	floxuridine	mitotane
carmustine	fluorouracil	mitoxantrone
chlorambucil	ganciclovir	plicamycin
cisplatin	hydroxyurea	procarbazine
cyclophosphamide	idarubicin	streptozocin
cytarabine	ifosfamide	thioguanine
dacarbazine	lomustine	thiotepa
dactinomycin	mechlorethamine	vinblastine
daunorubicin	melphalan	vincristine

drugs should be stored at eye level or lower. Hazardous drugs requiring refrigeration should be stored separately from other drugs in bins that prevent breakage and to contain leakage, should it occur. The person checking a shipment should wear gloves in case drug containers were broken in transit. Damaged packages should be inspected in an insulated area, such as a vertical airflow hood. Broken vials of unreconstituted drugs should be treated as drug spills.

A list of cytotoxic and otherwise hazardous drugs should be compiled and posted in appropriate locations in the workplace. Table 10.2 lists some commonly used cytotoxic and hazardous drugs. Storage areas, such as drug cartons, shelves, bins, counters, and trays should carry appropriate brightly colored warning labels and should be designed in such a way as to minimize the possibility of falling and breakage. Access to storage areas and work areas for hazardous materials should be limited to specified trained personnel.

Protective Clothing

A disposable, lint-free, nonabsorbent, closed-front gown with cuffed sleeves should be worn. Hair covers and shoe covers should be worn to reduce the potential for particulate contamination. Other protective clothing would include eye protection, mask, and use of latex gloves when disposing of damaged packages.

Double gloves should be put on after a thorough washing of the hands. Factors that influence glove permeability are thickness of the glove and time of exposure. All glove sizes should be available so that each worker has a good fit. The first pair of gloves should be tucked under the sleeve cuff, whereas the second pair should be placed over the top of the cuff. Gloved hands should then be washed to remove any powder that may be present to prevent unnecessary particles in the hood. Gloves should be changed every 20 to 30 minutes with continuous use or immediately when contamination or puncture occurs. Gloves should be turned inside out as they are removed and discarded.

After exposure to cytotoxic or hazardous drugs, no protective clothing should be taken outside the area where the exposure occurred. Caution should be taken, including warning others, so as not to contaminate other persons or objects. In case of an accidental exposure or skin contact, the area should be thoroughly washed with soap and large amounts of water. Report any exposure incident to a supervisor, and complete an incident report (Figure 10.4).

Technique for Handling Hazardous Agents

Rapid movements should be avoided to minimize airflow disturbances. Cytotoxic drugs should be prepared in a vertical laminar airflow hood (also called a *biologic*

Figure 10.4

Cytotoxic and
Hazardous
Materials Incident
Report Form

MT. HOPE HOSPITAL
CYTOTOXIC AND HAZARDOUS MATERIALS INCIDENT REPORT

Date: Time   Dept.

Person/persons Involved   Sex   Date of birth
Name:

Home Address   Phone

Name: Sex   Date of birth

Home Address   Phone

Witness:

Description of Incident:

Agent and Amount of Spill:

Actions Taken:

Was Medical Treatment Necessary?
If Yes, Physician Name and Address.

Diagnosis:

Follow-up:

Suggestions for Prevention of Future Incidences:

Signature: _____
Title: Date:

safety cabinet). The construction and operation of a vertical laminar airflow hood was introduced earlier in this chapter. This instrument should be cleaned and disinfected on a regular basis, at least every 8 hours or immediately when a spill is visible.

During cleaning, the blower in the laminar flow hood should be left on, and the area underneath the tray and the spillage trough should also be thoroughly cleaned. The technician should wear eye protection, a mask, and proper apparel—gown, gloves, and hair cover—even when cleaning the vertical laminar airflow hood. Avoid excessive use of alcohol to disinfect the work surface to avoid buildup of alcohol vapors in the cabinet. Allow the disinfectant to dry before medication preparation. Often, a lint-free, plastic-lined pad will be used to absorb small particles or spills in the hood.

When adding a diluent like sterile water for injection or normal saline to a vial, one should do so slowly, allowing pressure in the vial and syringe to equalize. The needle should be kept in the vial while gently swirling the vial until the contents are dissolved. The vial is inverted, and the drug solution is gradually withdrawn. The vial is then inverted into an upright position, and a small amount of air is drawn from the needle and syringe hub before the needle is drawn out of the vial.

When preparing cytotoxic agents, the technician should follow proper aseptic technique. All syringes and IV containers should be labeled according to institutional guidelines. Syringes should be large enough so that they will not be full when the full dose is drawn into them. Therefore when syringes are prefilled with the full dose, the plunger will not separate from the barrel. Because drugs in vials may build up pressure, causing the drug to spray out around the needle, a slight negative pressure should be maintained. To prevent excessive negative pressure, inject into the vial enough air to equal about 75% of the volume of drug to be withdrawn. Do not inject a volume of air that is equal to or greater than the amount of drug to be withdrawn. Excessive negative pressure may cause leakage from the needle or splash back when it is withdrawn, causing a safety concern to the pharmacy technician. For example, if you are to withdraw 4 mL of a cytotoxic drug in a multidose vial, you should inject no more than 3 mL of air (75%) before withdrawing the drug in your syringe. The use of a *chemo venting pin* will also equalize air pressure in the vial. Vials should not be vented unless one is using a filter device.

When opening an ampule, one should tap the drug from the top of the ampule, wrap a pad around the ampule, and hold the ampule away from the face before breaking off the top. A 5-micron filter needle should be placed on the syringe to withdraw the solution from the ampule. The fluid should be drawn through the syringe hub. A regular needle is placed on the syringe. Excess drug and any air are ejected into the sterile vial until the correct volume is left.

If the medication is to be dispensed from the syringe, then the solution should be cleared from the needle and hub and the needle replaced with a locking cap. The syringe should be wiped with a moistened wipe and then labeled. If the medication is to be added to an IV bag, care should be used to prevent a puncture of the bag. The injection port and the bag should be wiped with a moistened alcohol wipe. The bag should be placed in a sealable container, a bag, to contain leakage.

Priming of IV administration sets should be done in the vertical laminar airflow hood where the cytotoxic agent can be captured in an appropriate container. If the set is not primed in the cabinet, then other priming techniques should be followed:

1. Retrograde priming, with the fluid from the primary IV solution (without the cytotoxic drug), is used to fill the tubing of the set.
2. The set is attached to the drug container.
3. The priming fluid is run through the set into the port of the drug container.
4. Gauze is placed in a sealable container, and fluid is run through the set onto the gauze to prevent splashing.

IV sets will be discussed in more detail in Chapter 11.

Hazardous Agent Spills

The goal for the containment of a cytotoxic or hazardous material spill is to ensure that the healthcare setting, staff, patients, visitors, and environment (both inside and outside of the medical facility) are not contaminated. Similar precautions to those described previously in the discussion of receiving damaged hazardous drugs should be followed.

All spills should be dealt with immediately. Cleanup and decontamination should be done with a spill kit. Spill kits will contain materials to control and clean up spills of up to 1000 mL. A commercially available spill kit may be used or one may be assembled with the following contents:

- nonabsorbent, lint-free gown
- gloves, two pair
- respirator mask
- goggles, one pair
- absorbent towels
- chemo hazard labels
- incident report form (see Figure 10.4)
- spill control pillows or towels folded to work as pillows
- scoop and brush (for collecting glass fragments)
- plastic disposal bags labeled "Chemo Waste"
- "CAUTION: Chemo Spill" sign

A spill outside the airflow hood should be posted with a warning sign. Proper attire should be worn, including gown, double gloves, goggles, and a mask or respirator. Broken glass should be placed in the appropriate container but never with the hands. When cleaning up the spill, one should start from the edge of the spill and work inward, using absorbent sheets, spill pads, or pillows for the liquids or damp cloths or towels for solids. Use spill pads and water to rinse the area. Detergent should be used to remove residue.

Spills in the laminar airflow hood require additional steps. The spill is removed as previously described. The drain trough should be thoroughly cleaned and the cabinet decontaminated. All contaminated materials from a spill should be sealed in hazardous waste containers and placed in leak-resistant containers. The spill and cleanup must be documented.

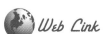

Web Link

For more specific information on the handling of cytotoxic and hazardous agents, visit the American Society of Health-System Pharmacists' (ASHP's) Web site at **www.ashp.org /bestpractices/**

Procedures in Case of Exposure

Any body area exposed should be flooded with water and thoroughly cleansed with soap and water. The exposed person should be sent or escorted to the employee health or emergency room. If the substance comes in contact with the skin, wash the skin thoroughly with soap and water and seek appropriate medical attention. If the substance comes in contact with the eyes, flush the affected eyes with large amounts of water or use an eye flush kit and seek appropriate medical attention. Remove contaminated garments and/or gloves, and wash hands after removing the gloves. Dispose of contaminated garments appropriately in specially designated biohazard materials containers.

Hazardous Oral Dose Forms

During routine handling of hazardous oral drugs, workers should wear one pair of gloves of good quality and thickness, as well as a gown and respirator. The counting and pouring of these drugs should be done carefully, and contaminated equipment such as counting trays should be immediately cleaned with detergent and rinsed. Tablet and capsule forms of hazardous materials should not be placed in any automated counting or packaging machine. When one is crushing a hazardous drug in a unit-of-use package, the package should be placed in a small, sealable plastic bag and crushed with a spoon or pestle, using caution not to break the plastic bag. Compounding with any of these drugs should be done in a protected area away from drafts and traffic.

Chapter Terms

antineoplastic drugs another name for cancer-fighting drugs that are considered cytotoxic materials

asepsis absence of disease-causing microorganisms

aseptic technique manipulation of sterile products and devices in such a way as to avoid introducing pathogens or disease-causing organisms

autoclave device that generates heat and pressure to sterilize

bacteria small, single-celled microorganisms that exist in three main forms: spherical (i.e., focci), rod shaped (i.e., bacilli), and spiral (i.e., spirilla)

beyond-use dating date after which a compounded sterile product should not be used

compounded sterile products (CSPs) sterile products that are prepared outside of the pharmaceutical manufacturer's facility

cytotoxic materials hazardous chemicals or drugs that must be handled and prepared with extra precautions

fungi parasites that feed on living organisms (or on dead organic material) and reproduce by means of spores

germ theory of disease idea that microorganisms cause diseases

high-efficiency particulate air (HEPA) filter used with laminar flow hoods to filter out most particulate matter (0.3 micron and larger) to prepare parenteral products safely and aseptically

horizontal laminar airflow hood special biological safety cabinet used to aseptically prepare IV drug admixtures, nutrition solutions, and other parenteral products

protozoa single-cell organisms that inhabit water and soil

quality assurance (QA) program feedback system to improve care

sterilization process that destroys the microorganisms in a substance, resulting in asepsis

USP Chapter 797 guidelines on parenteral product preparation developed by the United States Pharmacopeia (USP) that have become standards for hospital accreditation

vertical laminar airflow hood special biological safety cabinet used to aseptically prepare hazardous drugs, especially cytotoxic drugs

viruses minute infectious agents that do not have all of the components of a cell and thus can replicate only within a living host cell

contents, whereas other packaging has an opaque package with a diagram of the enclosed set printed on the outside. A damaged package cannot ensure sterility. It is best to discard sets that are found in unoriginal, opened, or damaged packages.

Flanges (i.e., Y-sites) and other rigid parts of an IV set are molded from tough plastic. Most of the length of the tubing is molded from a pliable polyvinyl chloride (PVC). PVC sets should not be used for nitroglycerin, which is absorbed by the tubing, nor for IV fat emulsions, which may leach out of the tubing. Special types of plastic sets are required for such infusions.

The length of sets varies from 6-inch extensions up to 110- to 120-inch sets used in surgery. The priming of tubing depends on the length of the set, from 3 mL for the short extension up to 15 mL for longer sets. Standard sets have a lumen diameter of 0.28 cm. Varying the size of the lumen diameter achieves different flow rates. Regulation of flow rates is especially critical in neonates and infants but may also be useful in limiting fluid flow to any patient.

The tubing's interior lumen generally contains particles that flush out when fluid is run through the set. Use of final filtration, a filter in the set (discussed later in this chapter), has reduced the need for flushing the line with the IV fluid before attaching the set to the patient.

Regardless of manufacturer, sets have certain basic components (Figure 11.3), which include a spike to pierce the rubber stopper or port on the IV container, a drip chamber for trapping air and adjusting flow rate, a control clamp for adjusting flow rate or shutting down the flow, flexible tubing to convey the fluid, and a needle adapter for attaching a needle or a catheter. A catheter, or tube, may be implanted into the patient and fixed with tape to avoid having to repuncture the patient each time an infusion is given. In addition to these parts, most IV sets contain a **Y-site**, or injection port, a rigid piece of plastic with one arm terminating in a resealable port that is used for adding medication to the IV. Some IV sets also contain resealable in-line filters that offer protection for the patient against particulates, including bacteria and emboli. IV infusions may use any of a variety of IV pumps to regulate amount, rate, and timing of flow.

The spike is a rigid, sharpened plastic piece used proximal to the IV fluid container. The spike is covered with a protective unit to maintain sterility and is removed only when ready for insertion into the IV container. The spike generally has a rigid area to grip while it is inserted into the IV container.

If an air vent is present on a set, it is located below the spike. The air vent points downward and has a bacterial filter covering. The vent allows air to enter the bottle as fluid flows out of it. Some glass bottles do not have an air tube. For these, a vented set is necessary.

A transparent, hollow chamber, the drip chamber, is located below the set's spike. Drops of fluid fall into the chamber from an opening at the uppermost end, closest to the spike. The number of drops it takes to make 1 mL identifies an IV set. This calibration is referred to as a *drop set*. The most common IV drop sets are 10,

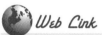

Safety Note
Do not use PVC IV sets for nitroglycerin or fat emulsions.

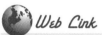
Web Link
Go to **www.baxter.com** to see IV tubing products from a major manufacturer.

Figure 11.2

Components of a Needle

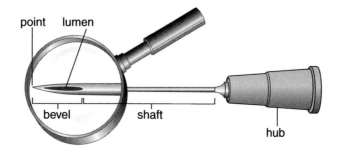

point   lumen

bevel   shaft

hub

Figure 11.3

**Basic Components
of an IV Set**

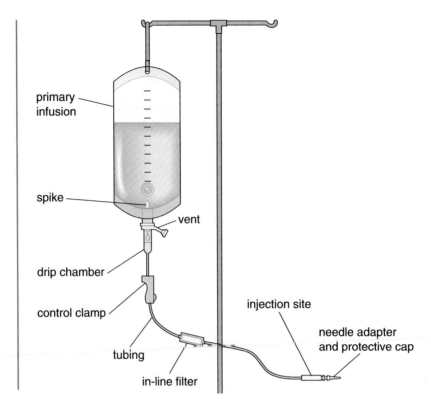

15, 20, and 60, meaning 10 gtt/mL, 15 gtt/mL, 20 gtt/mL, and 60 gtt/mL, respectively (Figure 11.4). An opening that provides 10, 15, or 20 gtt/mL is commonly used for adults. An opening that provides 60 gtt/mL is used for pediatric patients and is called a mini-drip set. The drip chamber serves to prevent air bubbles from entering the tubing. Air bubbles generally rise to the top of the fluid if they do form and will not enter the patient. The chamber allows the attending nurse or pharmacist to set the flow rate by counting the drops.

The person administering the fluid starts the flow by filling the chamber with fluid from an attached inverted IV container. The chamber sides are squeezed and released. Then fluid flows into the chamber. The procedure is repeated until an indicated level is reached or approximately half the chamber is filled. The entering drops are then counted for 15 seconds. Adjustments are made until the approximate number of drops desired is obtained. The rate should be checked five times, at 30-second intervals, and again for a last count of 1 minute.

Clamps allow for adjusting the rate of the flow and for shutting down the flow. Clamps may be located at any position along the flexible tubing. Usually a clamp moves freely, allowing its location to be changed to one that is convenient for the health professional administering the medication.

Three types of clamps are commonly used for IV solutions: (1) slide clamp, (2) screw clamp, and (3) roller clamp.

- A slide clamp has an increasingly narrow channel that constricts IV tubing as it is pressed farther into the narrowed area. Slide clamps do not allow for accurate adjustment of flow rate but may be used to shut off flow while a more accurate clamp is regulated.
- A screw clamp consists of a thumbscrew that is tightened or loosened to speed or slow the flow.

Figure 11.4

Drop Sets

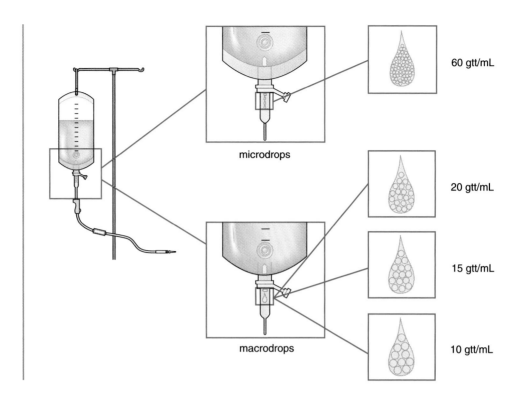

microdrops

60 gtt/mL

20 gtt/mL

15 gtt/mL

macrodrops

10 gtt/mL

- A roller clamp is a small roller that is pushed along an incline. The roller, when moved down the incline, constricts the tubing and reduces the fluid flow. Moving the roller up the incline, in contrast, increases the flow.

"Creep" or cold flow can affect clamp accuracy. Creep is a tendency of some clamps to slowly return to a more open position with increased fluid flow. Cold flow is the tendency of PVC tubing to return to its previous position. Tubing clamps are open during packaging and shipping. As a result, the tube tends to expand when the clamp constricts it. If, on the other hand, the tubing clamp has previously constricted the tubing, then as it is adjusted open, it tends to constrict with the reduced fluid flow, moving in the direction of its original position.

A needle adapter is usually located at the distal end of the IV set, close to the patient. A needle or catheter may be attached to the adapter. The adapter has a standard taper to fit all needles or catheters and is covered by a sterile cover before removal for connection.

A set may have a built-in or in-line filter, which provides a final filtration of the fluid before it enters the patient. Final filtration should protect the patient against particulate matter, bacteria, air emboli, and phlebitis. A 0.22-micron filter is optimal. A 5-micron filter removes particles that block pulmonary microcirculation but will not ensure sterility.

As mentioned, Y-site is an injection port found on most sets. The *Y* is a rigid plastic piece with one arm terminating in a resealable port. The port, once disinfected with alcohol, is ready for the insertion of a needle and the injection of medication.

Filters

Filters are devices used to remove contaminants such as glass, paint, fibers, and rubber cores. Filters will not remove virus particles or toxins. A filter will occasionally become clogged, thus slowing expected flow rates. Filter sizes are as follows:

- 5.0 microns—random path membrane (RPM) filter, removes large particulate matter
- 0.45 micron—in-line filter for IV suspension drug
- 0.22 micron—removes bacteria and produces a sterile solution

Catheters

IV administration for fluids and drug therapy can be accomplished through needle-like devices called *catheters*. **Catheters** are devices that are inserted into veins for direct access to the blood vascular system and are used in two primary ways: (1) close to the surface, peripheral venous catheters, and (2) deeper in the body, central venous catheters.

Peripheral Venous Catheters   A **peripheral venous catheter** is inserted into veins close to the surface of the skin and used for up to 72 hours. The unit is inserted into a vein, the needle portion is withdrawn, and a flexible, Teflon catheter is left in place. Peripheral catheters are easy to insert, and most nurses can do this at a patient's bedside. Although various brand names of catheters are available, the brand name Jelco is commonly used and is accepted terminology when referring to a peripheral venous catheter. Peripheral venous catheters are usually inserted in sites on the arms or hands but can also be inserted in the feet and scalp if the nurse or physician cannot locate "good" veins in the arms or hands. A good vein is one that allows access to the bloodstream and does not collapse.

Peripheral venous catheters will likely cause problems such as pain and irritation for 20 to 50% of patients. Some drugs cause vein irritation because of their inherent drug properties. Because the blood flow in peripheral veins is slow, the drug and fluid stay in contact with the vessel wall longer, thus causing irritation. Another problem is infiltration. **Infiltration** is a breakdown or collapse of a vein that allows the drug to leak into tissues surrounding the catheter site, causing edema and/or tissue damage.

Central Venous Catheters   A **central venous catheter** is used to dilute hypertonic solutions such as total parenteral nutrition (TPN) solutions or potentially toxic drugs such as cancer chemotherapeutic agents. This type of catheter is also used for administering phenytoin, a drug used for seizures or heart arrhythmias. These catheters are placed deeper in the body; they are more complicated to place, and are inserted by a physician to minimize the risk of infection. Central catheters are commonly used for therapy of 1 to 2 weeks, or even longer in some cases.

The most common sites of insertion are the **subclavian vein**, lying below the clavicle, and the jugular vein, in the neck. The femoral vein, in the groin area, is also used but is the least desirable site because of the risk of infection. Subclavian catheters are placed deep in the vein so that the end enters the superior vena cava close to the heart where the blood flow is the greatest. Problems with subclavian catheters are the possibility of subclavian vein laceration (i.e., missing the vein and puncturing a lung), and a greater risk of infection because the procedure is more invasive.

A larger blood flow in the subclavian vein will dilute a more concentrated solution such as TPN. These TPN solutions provide needed calories in the form of amino acids (the building blocks for protein) and dextrose (for carbohydrates), as well as vitamins, minerals, trace elements, and electrolytes. Many large hospitals will use an automated and programmable compounder to prepare multiple TPN solutions.

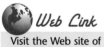

Web Link

Visit the Web site of the American Society of Enteral and Parenteral Nutrition, a good source for information and networking, at **www. nutritioncare.org**

Instances occur when several physically incompatible drugs must be given. A **multiple-lumen catheter** can be used to administer these drugs together. Central venous catheters come with one, two, three, or four lumens. The triple and quad catheters will be used with patients who are more ill. Each lumen exits the catheter at a different location, so no opportunity exists for the drugs to mix before being diluted in the bloodstream.

Other Types of Catheters   Midline catheters are longer peripheral catheters that go from insertion site into a deep vein. These catheters are designed to stay in place 1 week or longer. The **peripherally inserted central (PIC) line** is a very fine line that is threaded through the peripheral vein into the subclavian vein. This catheter has the same characteristics as a central line; however, a skilled nurse can insert it at the bedside.

Some patients may be on TPN therapy for months or even years in the hospital or at home. Infusion devices are surgically implanted to provide long-term therapy and also reduce the risk of infection. Implantable infusion devices include the Hickman and Broviac external catheters, also called *tunnel catheters*. The surgeon inserts the catheter below the breast and tunnels it under the skin into the sub-clavian vein. The catheter has a cuff to which the body's connective tissue heals, thus sealing off bacterial entry into the surgical area. The lower point of body insertion makes the catheter easier for the patient to see and clean. Another form of implantable device is the internal port, such as the Port-A-Cath Life Port. When implanted the only evidence is a bump in the skin. Drugs, especially cancer chemotherapeutic drugs, are administered by a small needle through the skin in an injection port in this device.

Pumps and Controllers

Fluids and drugs are often delivered to catheters by some form of device, including electronic devices, to control the infusion rate. These devices are the pumps and controllers.

The first system to deliver a drug intravenously was the syringe system. The patient must have an IV line or direct entry into a vein. The drug is injected in a port, and it goes directly into the vein. One of the problems with this system is safety. Care must be taken when administering drugs that have to be diluted or given very slowly. The syringe system is very nurse labor-intensive, because a nurse has to stand by the bedside and push the drug in. This system is also pharmacy labor-intensive, because the pharmacy has to fill, label, and deliver the syringe with drugs to the nursing station.

The Buretrol or the Soluset has a built-in graduated cylinder. Fluid is run into the cylinder, and the nurse can add a drug in the top of the cylinder injection port for dilution and mixing of the drug before it is infused. The Buretrol or the Soluset was in use before infusion pumps and replaced the syringe system. This is a better system than the syringe system, because the drug is being diluted in the cylinder and it can be infused over a long period of time. A problem with the use of this system is that all drugs have to be drawn up in syringes, and it is very labor intensive. Another problem in using this system is potential drug incompatibility, and a drug cannot be identified once it is injected into the cylinder. A good reference for physical drug incompatibility is *Trissel's Stability of Compounded Formulations*, which is found in most hospital pharmacies.

Controllers are low-pressure devices of 2 to 3 psi (pounds per square inch). The pressure of the controller is generated by gravity. Flow rate is controlled by the rate of fluid drops falling through a counting chamber. Maximum flow rate is 400 mL/hr. The low pressure of controllers is less likely to cause vein breakdown or infiltration. A problem with controllers is alarms. An alarm will sound with a kink in a line or even the interruption of blood flow when the patient bends an elbow. These devices are infrequently used today.

More popular devices are the infusion pumps used in institutional and home therapy. These devices produce a positive pressure of 10 to 25 psi, are more accurate than controllers, and have fewer flow interruptions, which causes both nurses and physicians to prefer them. Maximum flow is 999 mL/hr, therefore providing a higher rate of infusion; higher pressure, however, presents the problem of infiltration.

As mentioned in Chapter 3, another type of medication delivery that uses a parenteral route is the patient-controlled analgesia (PCA) device. The PCA device allows the patient, and only the patient, to administer analgesics by pressing a button. The device controls the medication so that the patient cannot overdose or give the medication too soon after the previous dose. Often, after surgery or severe injuries, a physician will order a PCA for the patient for 24 to 72 hours, after which time the patient may be treated adequately with oral analgesics.

PREPARING IVS

Pharmacists and technicians prepare drugs and IV solutions in a form ready to be administered to a patient. Solutions and drug products are delivered to the patient; however, other health professionals, generally a nurse or physician, administer the therapy.

IV push (i.e., bolus) and IV infusion dose forms should be prepared in laminar airflow hoods using aseptic techniques as discussed in Chapter 10. Products used during the preparation must always be sterile and handled in such a manner as to prevent contamination. Preparation should always be done under the supervision of a licensed pharmacist.

IV Preparation Guidelines

Begin any IV preparation by washing your hands thoroughly using a germicidal agent such as chlorhexidine gluconate or povidone-iodine. Wear gloves during the procedure. Laminar airflow hoods are normally kept running. Should the hood be turned off for installation, repair, maintenance, or relocation, it should be operated at least 30 minutes before being used to prepare sterile products. It is the responsibility of the institution to ensure proper positioning of the hood away from high-traffic areas, doorways, air vents, or other locations that could produce air currents contaminating the hood working area. Eating, drinking, talking, or coughing is prohibited in the laminar airflow hood. Working in the laminar flow hood should be free from interruptions to maintain a sterile environment and to stay mentally focused on IV preparation tasks to minimize medication errors.

Before making the product, thoroughly clean all interior working surfaces. Also make sure that the inside of the airflow hood has been thoroughly cleaned with disinfectant. All jewelry should be removed from the hands and wrists before scrubbing and while making a sterile product. To ensure topical antimicrobial action of chlorhexidine, iodine, or other acceptable scrubs, use 3 to 5 mL and scrub the hands, nails, wrists, and forearms vigorously for at least 30 seconds.

Gather all the necessary materials for the operation, and check these to make sure they are not expired and are free from particulate matter such as dust. Only essential objects and materials necessary for product preparation should be placed in the airflow hood. If you are using plastic solution containers, then check for leaks by squeezing them. Work in the center of the work area within the laminar airflow hood, at least 6 inches inside the edge of the hood. Make sure that nothing obstructs the flow of air from the high-efficiency particulate air (HEPA) filter over the preparation area. Nothing should pass behind a sterile object and the HEPA filter in a horizontal airflow hood or above a sterile object in a vertical airflow hood.

Follow proper procedure for handling sterile devices and medication containers to ensure an accurate microbial-free product. Remember that the plunger and tip of the syringe are sterile and must not be touched. For greatest accuracy, use the smallest syringe that can hold the desired amount of solution. In any case the syringe should not be larger than twice the volume to be measured. A syringe is considered accurate to half the smallest measurement mark on its barrel. To get an accurate dose, observe closely the calibrations on the syringe barrel. Count the number of marks between labeled measurement units. If 10 marks are seen, then each mark measures off one tenth of the unit. If 5 marks are seen, then each mark measures two tenths of the unit. The volume of solution drawn into a syringe is measured at the point of contact between the rubber piston and the side of the syringe barrel. The measurement is not read at the tip of the piston.

Electrolytes, vitamins, and minerals, are commonly added to IV solutions. These medications may be packaged in vials or ampules. Some products come from the manufacturer ready to use; others (for stability reasons) come in dry powders that must be reconstituted before they can be added to the IV admixture. Proper technique in using vials and ampules is an important skill for the pharmacy technician to learn.

Safety Note

With the exception of cytotoxic drugs, inject an equal amount of air into the vial with the syringe and needle before withdrawing the medication.

Vials   Reconstituting a powder by introducing a diluent (similar to sterile water for injection) produces a positive pressure inside the vial. Vials are closed systems; therefore the amount of air introduced should be equal to the volume of fluid removed. An exception to this guideline is the withdrawal of cytotoxic drugs from vials where a volume of air less than the solution volume is introduced, producing a vacuum and preventing an aspirate when the needle is withdrawn from the rubber closure (see Chapter 10).

Table 11.2 details the procedures generally followed for using a syringe to draw liquid from a vial. Begin by first swabbing the rubber stopper with an alcohol swab using firm strokes, in the same direction, or by spraying with 70% alcohol prior to entering the laminar airflow hood. The needle bevel tip should penetrate the rubber closure at an angle, which is then straightened to 90 degrees so that as additional pressure is applied to the syringe, the bevel heel enters the closure at the same point as the tip. This technique prevents **coring**, or introducing a small chunk of the rubber closure into the solution.

Ampules   An **ampule** is a *single-dose-only* drug container. The glass ampule offers another challenge because one must first break the top off the ampule before withdrawing the medication. The contents in the top of the ampule must be moved into the body by swirling the ampule in an upright position, inverting it quickly, and then turning it back upright, or by tapping the top with a finger. Clean the neck with an alcohol swab; then grasp the ampule between the thumb and index finger at the neck with the swab still in place. The glass around the top is scored to make such breaking easy and clean. Use a quick motion to snap off the top (Figure 11.6). The ampule will generally snap at the neck. Do not break in the direction of the HEPA filter. Tilt the ampule, place the needle bevel of a filter needle or tip of a filter straw

Table 11.2   Using a Syringe to Draw Liquid from a Vial

1. Choose the smallest gauge needle appropriate for the task, and avoid coring the rubber top of the vial and thus introducing particulate into the liquid within it.
2. Attach the needle to the syringe.
3. Draw into the syringe an amount of air equal to the amount of drug to be drawn from the vial.
4. Swab or spray the top of the vial with alcohol before entering the laminar flow hood; allow the alcohol to dry. Puncture the rubber top of the vial with the needle bevel up. Then bring the syringe and needle straight up, penetrate the stopper, and depress the plunger of the syringe, emptying the air into the vial (Figure 11.5, *a*).
5. Invert the vial with the attached syringe.
6. Draw up from the vial the amount of liquid required (Figure 11.5, *b*).
7. Withdraw the needle from the vial. In the case of a multidose vial, the rubber cap will close, sealing the contents of the vial.
8. Remove and properly dispose of the needle, and cap the syringe. A new needle will be attached at the time of injection into a patient.

in the corner near the opening, and withdraw the medication. Use a needle equipped with a filter for filtering out any tiny glass particles, fibers, or paint chips that may have fallen into the ampule. Before injecting the contents of a syringe into an IV, the needle must be changed to avoid introducing glass or particles into the admixture. A standard needle could be used to withdraw the drug from the ampule; it is then replaced with a filter device before the drug is pushed out of the syringe. Filter needles are for one directional use only.

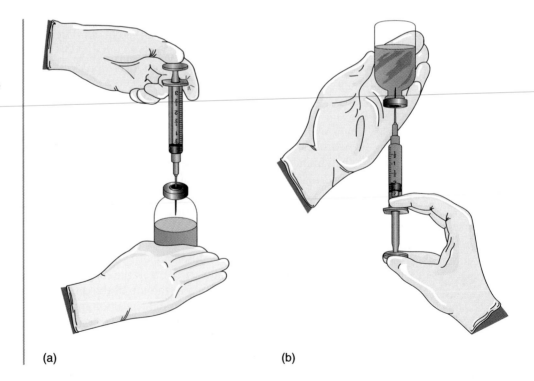

Figure 11.5

Withdrawing Medication from a Vial
(a) Inject air into the vial, equal to the volume of liquid needed.
(b) Withdraw the desired amount of medication into the syringe from the inverted vial.

(a)   (b)

Figure 11.6

Opening an Ampule

(a) Gently tap the top of the ampule to bring the medication to the lower portion of the ampule. (b) Wrap gauze around the neck and top of the ampule. (c) Forcefully snap the neck away from you.

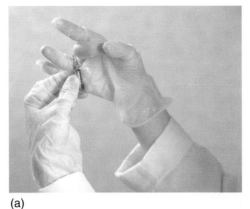

(a)

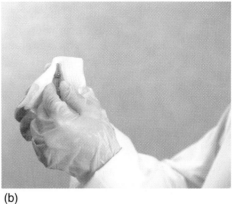

(b)

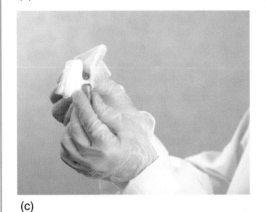

(c)

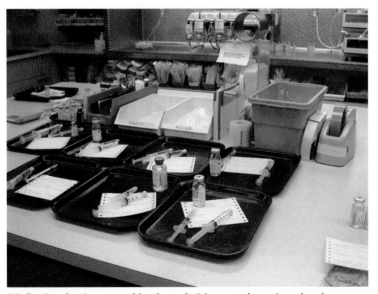

Medication that is prepared by the technician must be reviewed and approved by the pharmacist.

IV Solutions

Most IV, intrathecal, intra-arterial, and intracardiac injections will be solutions, and preservative-free sterile water for injection (SWFI) or normal saline (NS) will be used as the diluent. A **diluent** is the sterile fluid to be added to a powder to reconstitute or dissolve the medication. Another common diluent is bacteriostatic water for injection (BWFI), which contains preservatives for multiple uses. Check the medication package insert to verify which diluent and what volume should be added to the medication vial to make a sterile solution. These alternative routes of administration may also require special preparation, storage, and needles, so it is best to check with the pharmacist if such a medication order is received.

The vehicles most commonly used for IV infusions are dextrose in water, NS solution, or dextrose in saline solution. The two main types of IV solutions are **small-volume parenterals (SVPs)** of 50 or 100 mL and large-volume parenterals (LVPs) of more than 100 mL. SVPs are typically used for delivering medications at a controlled infusion rate. **Large-volume parenterals (LVPs)** are used to replenish fluids, to provide electrolytes (i.e., essential minerals), and to provide nutrients such as vitamins and glucose. LVPs are commonly available in 250 mL, 500 mL, and 1000 mL sizes. Figure 11.7 illustrates types of IV containers and their components.

In some cases an infusion is prepared specifically to deliver a medication. In other cases a medication is "piggybacked" onto a running IV. A **piggyback** involves the preparation of a small amount of solution, usually 50 to 100 mL, in a minibag or bottle. Some IV piggybacks are prepared in 250 mL solution because they contain a medication that is irritating to the veins and thus requires a larger volume of solution. The piggybacked solution is infused into the tubing of the running IV, usually over a short time, from 30 minutes to 1 hour. In some cases, syringes are used instead of piggyback containers to deliver medication into a running IV.

An LVP usually contains one or more electrolytes that are "added" to the IV solution. Potassium chloride is the most common additive, but other salts of potassium, magnesium, or sodium can be added based on the requirements of the individual patient. An IV solution that contains some electrolytes is called *lactated Ringer's solution* and may be used alone or in combination with a dextrose or NS solution. Additives to IV solutions are multivitamins or trace elements as in the case of TPN solutions. Figure 11.8 shows some typical physician's orders for IV infusions.

Preparing a Label for an IV Admixture

When making an IV admixture, a label must also be prepared. The label should contain the following information:
- patient's name and identification number
- room number

Figure 11.7

Different Types of IV Containers

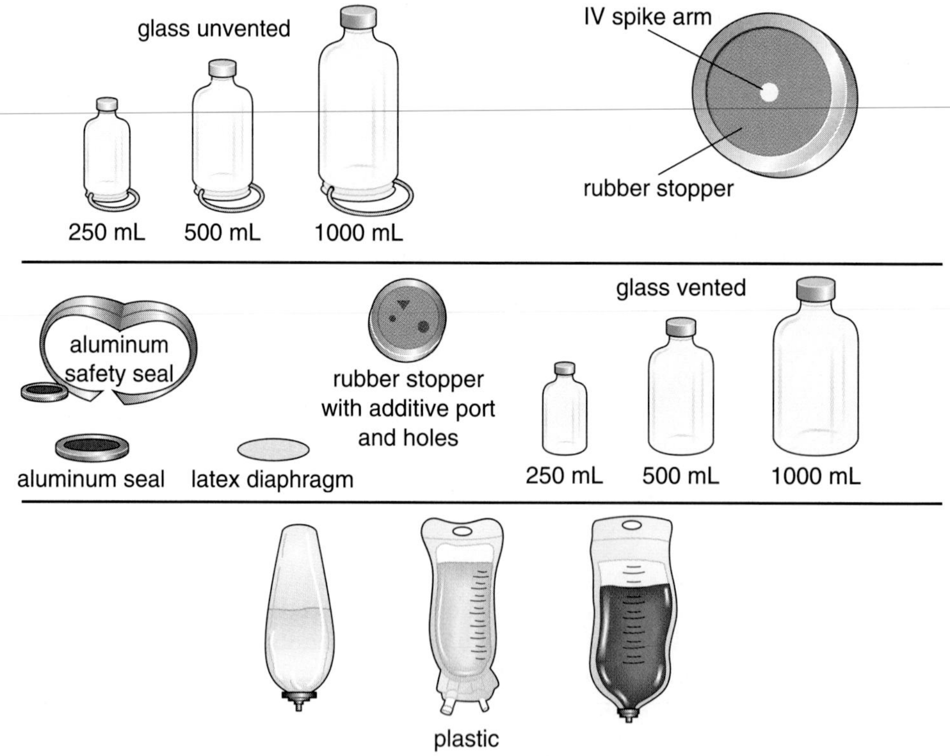

Figure 11.8

Physician's Orders for IV Infusions

R$_x$ Mefoxin 1 g IV q6h

R$_x$ nafcillin 1 g IV q4h

R$_x$ PCN 2 million units q4h

R$_x$ add 100 units Humulin Regular Insulin to D$_5$W 500 mL @ 20 mL/hr (label concentration 0.2 units/mL)

R$_x$ begin magnesium sulfate 5 g in 500 mL NS to run over 5 hours × 1 dose only

R$_x$ Δ fluids to 0.45 NS with 20 mEq KCl @ 125 mL/hr

- fluid and amount
- drug name and strength (if appropriate)
- infusion period
- flow rate (e.g., 100 mL/hr or infuse over 30 min)
- expiration date and time
- additional information as required by the institution or by state or federal guidelines, including auxiliary labeling, storage requirements, and device-specific information

Figure 11.9 shows an example of a label prepared for a large-volume parenteral (LVP).

Figure 11.9

Large-Volume Parenteral (LVP) Label and Minibag Label

PATIENT NAME	ROOM NUMBER
IDENTIFICATION NUMBER	DATE
FLUID VOLUME	
DRUG DOSE	
INFUSION RATE (for minibags)	
SCHEDULE (times due)	
	RATE (for LVPs)
EXPIRATION DATE & TIME	

John Brown	815-2
04596875	10/10/XX
D5 0.45NS 1000 mL	
potassium chloride 20 mEq	
MVI-12 10 mL	
q13h 6P 7A/11	75 mL/hr
EXP: 10/11/XX 5P	

CALCULATIONS FOR THE HOSPITAL PHARMACY TECHNICIAN

To enable the pharmacy technician to prepare sterile IV preparations in the hospital or home healthcare setting, it is important to understand math skills somewhat unique to these environments. In particular, it is important to double- and triple-check calculations and flow rates for IV admixtures or TPN solutions for neonatal or pediatric patients. This section will focus on the basic math skills needed to perform calculations in the areas of reading time, temperature and temperature conversions, electrolyte replacement therapy, specific gravity, and IV infusion flow rates.

Time Conversions

In the hospital setting, medication orders are commonly time-stamped with international or military time. Dose administration schedules for unit dose and IV admixtures also use this method. This time is based on a 24-hour clock, with midnight being considered time 0000. The first two digits are the time in hours, and the second two digits are the time in minutes. No AM or PM are used, thus less confusion—and fewer medication errors—on whether a drug should be given at 4 AM or 4 PM. For example:

0000	Midnight
0600	6 AM
1200	Noon
1800	6 PM

Example 1

At 0125, you receive an order for gentamicin 80 mg IV every 8 hours. The order is due to be administered at 0200, 1000, and 1800. When was the order received, and when should doses be prepared and sent to the nursing unit?

The order was received at 1:25 AM. The first dose is to be given at 2:00 AM followed by doses at 10:00 AM and 6:00 PM.

Temperature Conversions

The United States is one of the few countries in the world that commonly uses Fahrenheit as its temperature scale. The **Fahrenheit temperature scale** uses 32° F as the temperature when ice freezes and 212° F as the temperature when water boils; the difference between these two extremes is 180° F.

In the 1700s a Swedish scientist with the last name of Celsius suggested a thermometer with a difference of 100 degrees between freezing and boiling. He used zero degrees (0° C) as the freezing point and 100° C as the boiling point. The **Celsius temperature scale** is commonly used in Europe and globally in science, and it is often the scale used in the pharmacy.

Storing unstable drugs under the proper refrigeration and maintaining refrigerated equipment at the appropriate temperature are very important responsibilities for the pharmacy technician. Most often the temperatures in the drug package inserts or in the policy and procedure manual will be in centigrade. Most refrigerators in the pharmacy need to maintain a temperature of 5° C to 10° C. Pharmacy technicians will need to know how to convert between the Celsius scale and the Fahrenheit scales.

Every 5° C change in temperature is equivalent to a 9° F change (as indicated in Table 11.3). In addition to using this chart, here are several mathematical methods for converting from Fahrenheit to centigrade and vice versa. One method uses the following equations:

$$°F = (1.8 \times °C) + 32$$

$$°C = (°F - 32) \div 1.8$$

An alternative method uses the following algebraic equation:

$$5F = 9C + 160$$

When calculating the conversion, the final temperature is usually rounded up to the closest whole number. The use of these equations is demonstrated in the following examples.

Example 2

Convert 75° F to degrees Celsius.

$°C = (°F - 32) \div 1.8$
$°C = (75 - 32) \div 1.8$
$°C = 43 \div 1.8$
$°C = 23.888$, rounded to 24

Example 3

Convert 75° C to degrees Fahrenheit.

$°F = (1.8 \times °C) + 32$
$°F = (1.8 \times 75) + 32$
$°F = 135 + 32$
$°F = 167$

Electrolytes

Many IV fluids used in pharmacy practice contain dissolved mineral salts; such fluids are known as **electrolytes**. They are so-named because they conduct an electrical charge through the solution when connected to electrodes. Electrolyte solutions and certain oral drugs, besides being measured in the usual metric units such as milliliters, are also measured in millimoles (mM) and milliequivalents (mEq). These measures are particularly important in working with IV solutions.

Table 11.3 **Temperature Equivalencies between Celsius and Fahrenheit**

Celsius	Fahrenheit
0° C	32° F
5° C	41° F
10° C	50° F
15° C	59° F
20° C	68° F

This section is challenging and requires some basic chemistry knowledge as well as mathematical prowess. It is designed for those pharmacy technicians who will be compounding sterile products in a hospital (or home healthcare) pharmacy setting. An understanding of electrolytes and milliequivalents will enhance the expertise of the pharmacy technician and may minimize calculation errors.

Understanding Millimoles and Milliequivalents Most electrolyte solutions are measured by milliequivalents (mEq), which are related to molecular weight. Molecular weights are based on the atomic weights of common elements. You may recall the *periodic elements table* posted on the wall in your chemistry class. The **atomic weight** of an element is the weight of a single atom of that element compared with the weight of one atom of hydrogen. The **molecular weight** of a compound is the sum of the atomic weights of all the atoms in one molecule of the compound. A **millimole (mM)** is the molecular weight expressed as milligrams.

The **valence** of an element is a number that represents its capacity to combine to form a molecule of a stable compound. An element can exist in various forms. Valence may vary depending on an elemental form. Table 11.4 lists the valences and atomic weights of common elements. For pharmaceutical calculations, atomic weights are usually rounded to the nearest tenth (i.e., one unit to the right of the decimal point), as shown in the fourth column of the table.

One **mole (M)** of an element is equal to its atomic weight in grams. Thus 1 mole of sodium (Na) is equal to 22.9898 g, or typically rounded to 23 g. Compounds are also measured in moles. For example, 1 mole of salt or sodium chloride (NaCl) would equal its grams, which is as follows:

atomic weight of sodium (23 g) + atomic weight of chlorine (35.5 g) = 58.5 g

As stated before, 1 mM is the molecular weight expressed in milligrams. Because 1 g equals 1000 mg, 1 mole equals 1000 mM. Thus 1 mM of sodium chloride equals 58.5 mg.

One **equivalent (Eq)** is equal to one mole divided by its valence or the number of grams of solute dissolved in 1 mL of solution, as shown in the following formula:

$$\text{equivalent weight} = \frac{\text{molecular weight (expressed in milligrams)}}{\text{valence}}$$

Table 11.4 Valences and Atomic Weights of Common Elements

Element	Valence	Atomic Weight	Rounded-off Value
hydrogen (H)	1	1.008 g	1 g
carbon (C)	2, 4	12.011 g	12 g
nitrogen (N)	3, 5	14.007 g	14 g
oxygen (O)	2	15.999 g	16 g
sodium (Na)	1	22.9898 g	23 g
sulphur (S)	2, 4, 6	32.064 g	32.1 g
chlorine (Cl)	1, 3, 5, 7	35.453 g	35.5 g
potassium (K)	1	39.102 g	39.1 g
calcium (Ca)	2	40.08 g	40.1 g

One **milliequivalent (mEq)** is equal to 1 mM divided by its valence. Thus as before, 1 equivalent equals 1000 mEq, or one thousandth of a gram equivalent.

Determining the Milliequivalents of Compounds   The first step in determining the number of milliequivalents of a compound is to identify the formula of the compound. The next step is to separate the formula into atoms. The atomic weight of each atom is then multiplied by the number of those atoms, the products are added together, and that sum is substituted into the formula for atomic weight.

$$mEq = \frac{molecular\ weight\ (expressed\ in\ milligrams)}{valence}$$

Example 4

The molecular weight of magnesium sulfate (Mg + +SO4– –) is 120 mg and its valence is 2. How many milligrams does 1 mEq of magnesium sulfate weigh?

$$1\ mEq = \frac{molecular\ weight\ (expressed\ in\ milligrams)}{valence}$$

$$1\ mEq = \frac{120\ mg}{2}$$

$$1\ mEq = 60\ mg$$

Example 5

Magnesium has an atomic weight of 24 g. What is the weight of 1 mM?

$$1\ mM = 24\ g \div 1000 = 0.024\ g = 24\ mg$$

Converting between Milligrams and Milliequivalents   To convert back and forth between milligrams and milliequivalents, use the following formula:

$$number\ of\ milliequivalents = \frac{weight\ of\ substance\ (expressed\ in\ milligrams)}{milliequivalent\ weight}$$

This equation will be demonstrated in the following example.

Example 6

Sodium has an atomic weight of 23 mg and a valence of 1. How many milliequivalents are in 92 mg of sodium?

Step 1. Determine the weight of 1 milliequivalent of sodium by dividing the molecular weight (from the atomic weight) by the valence.

$$1\ mEq = \frac{molecular\ weight}{valence} = \frac{23\ mg}{1} = 23\ mg$$

Step 2. Determine the number of milliequivalents in 92 mg of sodium.

$$mEq = \frac{weight\ of\ sodium}{weight\ of\ 1\ mEq} = \frac{92\ mg}{23\ mg} = 4\ mEq$$

Measuring Electrolytes   Milliequivalents (and sometimes millimoles) are used to measure electrolytes in the bloodstream and/or in an IV preparation.

Example 7

You are requested to add 44 mEq of sodium chloride (NaCl) to an IV bag. Sodium chloride is available as a 4 mEq/mL solution. How many milliliters will you add to the bag?

Set up a proportion (see Chapter 5), comparing the solution you will need to create to the available solution, and solve for the unknown.

$$\frac{x \text{ mL}}{44 \text{ mEq}} = \frac{1 \text{ mL}}{4 \text{ mEq}}$$

$$\frac{(44 \text{ mEq}) \; x \text{ mL}}{44 \text{ mEq}} = \frac{(44 \text{ mEq}) \; 1 \text{ mL}}{4 \text{ mEq}}$$

$$x \text{ mL} = \frac{44 \text{ mL}}{4}$$

$$x \text{ mL} = 11 \text{ mL}$$

Specific Gravity

Specific gravity can be defined as the ratio of the weight of a substance to the weight of an equal volume of water, the standard, when both have the same temperature. Final weight can be measured in grams, because 1 mL of water weighs 1 g.

> 1 mL, volume of water = 1 g, weight of water
> specific gravity of water = 1

Safety Note
Usually numbers are not written without units; however, no units exist for specific gravity.

The specific gravity represents the weight of 1 mL of the substance and has no units of measure. The ratio called *specific gravity* is in essence a comparison of the weight of a liquid to the weight of water when exactly 1 mL of each is measured out. Water is the standard that is used, and the specific gravity assigned to it is 1. The formula for determining specific gravity is as follows:

$$\text{specific gravity} = \frac{\text{weight of a substance}}{\text{weight of an equal volume of water}}$$

When the specific gravity is known, certain assumptions can be made regarding the physical properties of a liquid. Solutions that are viscous or have particles floating in them often have a specific gravity higher than 1. Solutions that contain volatile chemicals (or something that is prone to quick evaporation), such as alcohol, often have a specific gravity lower than 1.

Example 8   **If the weight of 100 mL of dextrose solution is 117 g, what is the specific gravity of the dextrose solution?**

$$\text{specific gravity} = \frac{\text{weight of a substance}}{\text{weight of an equal volume of water}}$$

$$= \frac{117 \text{ g}}{100 \text{ g}}$$

$$= 1.17$$

If the specific gravity is known, you can determine the weight of a volume of a liquid.

Example 9   **If a liquid has a specific gravity of 0.85, how much does 125 mL weigh?**

Because the specific gravity of the liquid is 0.85,

$$\text{specific gravity} = \frac{\text{weight of a substance}}{\text{weight of an equal volume of water}}$$

$$0.85 = \frac{85 \text{ g (weight of 100 mL of the liquid)}}{100 \text{ g (weight of 100 mL of water)}}$$

Now, set up a proportion to find the weight of 125 mL.

$$\frac{x \text{ g}}{125 \text{ mL}} = \frac{85 \text{ g}}{100 \text{ mL}}$$

$$\frac{(\cancel{125 \text{ mL}}) \, x \text{ g}}{\cancel{125 \text{ mL}}} = \frac{(125 \text{ mL}) \, 85 \text{ g}}{\cancel{100 \text{ mL}}}$$

$$x \text{ g} = \frac{10,625 \text{ g}}{100}$$

$$x \text{ g} = 106.25 \text{ g}$$

Calculation of IV Rate and Administration

Another common type of calculation in hospital pharmacy practice is the rate of flow for an IV infusion. IV flow rates are usually described as milliliters per hour or as drops per minute (expressed as gtt/min). The pharmacy usually uses the milliliters per hour method, whereas nurses generally prefer drops per minute.

The formula used to determine the rate in drops per minute is as follows:

$$x \text{ gtt/min} = \frac{(\text{volume of fluid} \div \text{delivery time in hrs}) \times (\text{drop rate of administration set})}{60 \text{ min/hr}}$$

The following examples will demonstrate the use of this equation.

Example 10

A physician orders 4000 mL of a 5% dextrose and normal saline (D5NS) IV over a 36-hour period. If the IV set will deliver 15 gtt/mL, then how many drops must be administered per minute?

Begin by identifying the amounts to insert into the equation.

$$\text{volume of fluid} = 4000 \text{ mL}$$

$$\text{fluid delivery time} = 36 \text{ hr}$$

$$\text{drop rate of the administration set} = 15 \text{ gtt/mL}$$

$$x \text{ gtt/min} = \frac{(\text{volume of fluid} \div \text{delivery time}) \times (\text{drop rate of administration set})}{60 \text{ min/hr}}$$

$$= \frac{(4000 \text{ mL} \div 36 \text{ hr}) \times (15 \text{ gtt/mL})}{60 \text{ min/hr}}$$

$$= \frac{(111 \text{ mL/hr}) \times (15 \text{ gtt/mL})}{60 \text{ min/hr}} = 27.75 \text{ gtt/min, rounded to } 28 \text{ gtt/min}$$

Example 11

If 500 mg of a drug is to be administered from a 50 mL minibag over 30 minutes using a 15-drop set, how many drops per minute is that?

Begin by identifying the amounts to insert into the equation.

$$\text{volume of fluid} = 50 \text{ mL}$$

$$\text{fluid delivery time} = 30 \text{ min or } 0.5 \text{ hr}$$

$$\text{drop rate of the administration set} = 15 \text{ gtt/mL}$$

$$x \text{ gtt/min} = \frac{(\text{volume of fluid} \div \text{delivery time}) \times (\text{drop rate per milliliter of set used})}{60 \text{ min/hr}}$$

$$= \frac{(50 \text{ mL} \div 0.5 \text{ hr}) \times (15 \text{ gtt/mL})}{60 \text{ min/hr}}$$

$$= \frac{(100 \text{ mL/hr}) \times (15 \text{ gtt/mL})}{60 \text{ min/hr}} = 25 \text{ gtt/min}$$

Example 12

You are to prepare 750 mg of medication in 75 mL for infusion over 30 minutes, using a 10-drop set. How many drops per minute will that be?

Begin by identifying the amounts to insert into the equation.

$$\text{volume of fluid} = 75 \text{ mL}$$

$$\text{fluid delivery time} = 30 \text{ min or } 0.5 \text{ hr}$$

$$\text{drop rate of the administration set} = 10 \text{ gtt/mL}$$

$$x \text{ gtt/min} = \frac{(\text{volume of fluid} \div \text{delivery time}) \times (\text{drop rate per milliliter of set used})}{60 \text{ min/hr}}$$

$$= \frac{(75 \text{ mL} \div 0.5 \text{ hr}) \times (10 \text{ gtt/mL})}{60 \text{ min/hr}}$$

$$= \frac{(150 \text{ mL/hr}) \times (10 \text{ gtt/mL})}{60 \text{ min/hr}} = 25 \text{ gtt/min}$$

The number of hours that the IV will last can be determined by dividing the volume of the IV bag (expressed in milliliters) by the flow rate (expressed in milliliters per hour). The following example will demonstrate this calculation.

Example 13

A 1 L IV is running at 125 mL/hr. How often will a new bag have to be administered?

Begin by converting 1 L to 1000 mL, and then divide the volume by the volume per hour rate.

$$\frac{\text{hours the IV will last}}{125 \text{ mL/hr}} = 1000 \text{ mL} = 8 \text{ hr}$$

Chapter Terms

ampule single-dose drug container

atomic weight the weight of a single atom of that element compared with the weight of one atom of hydrogen

catheters devices inserted into veins for direct access to the blood vascular system

Celsius temperature scale temperature scale that uses zero degrees (i.e., 0° C) as the temperature at which water freezes and 100° C as the temperature at which water boils

central venous catheter catheter placed deep into the body

coring introducing a small chunk of the rubber closure into the solution while removing medication from a vial

diluent sterile fluid added to a powder to reconstitute, dilute, or dissolve a medication

electrolytes dissolved mineral salts, commonly found in IV fluids

equivalent (Eq) mole divided by its valence, or the number of grams of solute dissolved in 1 mL of solution

Fahrenheit temperature scale temperature scale that uses 32° F as the temperature at which water freezes and 212° F as the temperature at which water boils

filters devices used to remove contaminants such as glass, paint, fibers, and rubber cores from IV fluids

hypertonic solution parenteral solution with a greater number of particles than blood cells

infiltration breakdown or collapse of a vein that allows the drug to leak into tissues surrounding the catheter site, causing edema or tissue damage or both

isotonic solution parenteral solution with an equal number of particles as blood cells

IV administration set sterile, pyrogen-free disposable device used to deliver IV fluids to patients

large-volume parenterals (LVPs) IV infusion of more than 100 mL

milliequivalent (mEq) millimole divided by its valence

millimole (mM) molecular weight, expressed as milligrams

mole (M) measurement of an element equal to its atomic weight in grams

molecular weight sum of the atomic weights of all the atoms in one molecule of a compound

multiple-lumen catheter catheters used to separately administer potentially physically incompatible drugs

osmolality amount of particulate per unit volume of a liquid preparation, measured in milliosmoles (mOsm)

osmotic pressure the osmotic pressure of red blood cells is 285 mOsm/L

peripheral venous catheter catheter inserted into a vein close to the surface of the skin

peripherally inserted central (PIC) line very fine catheter that is threaded through the peripheral vein into the subclavian vein; can be inserted by a skilled nurse

pH value degree of acidity or alkalinity of a solution; less than 7 is acidic and more than 7 is alkaline

piggyback small-volume parenteral (SVP) admixture often containing a medication that is attached to an existing IV line

small-volume parenterals (SVPs) an IV infusion of 100 mL or less, commonly used to administer drugs

subclavian vein vein in the neck, lying below the clavicle and jugular vein

valence number that represents an element's capacity to combine to form a molecule of a stable compound

Y-site injection port found on most IV administration sets

Chapter Summary

- Parenteral IV drugs can be administered by bolus injection or by infusion.
- Infusions have many characteristics including solubility, osmolality, and acid/base ratio or pH.
- IV infusions are used to deliver blood, water, other fluids, nutrients such as lipids and sugars, electrolytes, and drugs.
- A wide variety of equipment is used in the preparation and administration of medications for IV use such as syringes, IV sets, filters, catheters, and infusion pumps.
- Many vehicles exist for IV solutions that are individualized to the needs of the patient, such as dextrose in water, normal saline (NS), and dextrose in NS.
- In addition to fluids, IV solutions commonly contain vitamins, electrolytes, and medications.
- A pharmacy technician must become familiar with the components of each IV administration set including, controller clamps, drip chamber, and Y-sites.
- IV push (i.e., bolus) and IV infusion dose forms should be prepared in a laminar airflow hood using proper aseptic technique and under the supervision of a licensed pharmacist.
- A basic understanding of temperature conversions, milliequivalents, and specific gravity is necessary to practice in the IV admixture area.
- A technician must be able to compute drip and infusion rates for IV solutions.

Knowledge Inventory

Choose the best answer from those provided.

1. An example of an isotonic solution is
   a. 0.9% normal saline (NS).
   b. dextrose 50%.
   c. sodium chloride (NaCl) 3%.
   d. 0.45% normal saline (NS).

2. The pH of blood is considered to be slightly
   a. acidic.
   b. alkaline.
   c. neutral.
   d. hypotonic.

3. The laminar flow hood must be turned on for _____ before preparing IV products.
   a. 30 seconds
   b. 10 minutes
   c. 30 minutes
   d. 1 hour

4. An IV administration set commonly includes all the following *except* a
   a. peripheral catheter.
   b. drip chamber.
   c. clamp controller.
   d. Y-site.

5. For a pediatric patient the flow rate of an IV administration set is commonly
   a. 10 gtt/min.
   b. 15 gtt/min.
   c. 20 gtt/min.
   d. 60 gtt/min.

6. What size filter is needed to eliminate any bacteria in the IV solution?
   a. 0.22 micron
   b. 0.45 micron
   c. 5 microns
   d. none (bacteria cannot be filtered)

7. Due to their hypertonicity most TPN solutions will require administration via a
   a. peripheral venous catheter.
   b. central venous catheter.
   c. PIC line.
   d. midline venous catheter.

8. Potassium has an atomic weight of approximately 39 and a valence of 1. How many mEq are in 780 mg of potassium?
   a. 20 mEq
   b. 39 mEq
   c. 78 mEq
   d. 117 mEq

9. An IV solution has a specific gravity of 0.9. What is the weight of 1000 mL?
   a. 90 g
   b. 900 g
   c. 1000 g
   d. 1100 g

10. An IV order is received for $D_5\frac{1}{2}NS$ to be infused at a rate of 125 mL/hour. How many 1L bottles must be prepared for use over the next 24 hours?
    a. one
    b. two
    c. three
    d. five

Pharmacy in Practice

Using the following orders and the reconstitution chart in the workbook (workbook Table 9.1), answer the medication questions.

1.
   R aclovir 1 g q12h

   a. In what fluid is the drug mixed?
   b. What is the expiration time at room temperature?
   c. Can it be refrigerated?

2.
   R vancomycin 1.5 g q8h

   a. What size bag is used?
   b. What is the infusion time?
   c. What is the room temperature expiration?

3.
   R Primaxin 500 mg q6h × 3 days

   a. In what fluid is the drug mixed?
   b. What size bag is needed?
   c. How many bags will be needed?

4.

| R_x | oxacillin 1 g × 5 days |

a. What size bag is needed?
b. What fluid?
c. If all bags are prepared today, will the last one expire before the end of therapy?
d. What is the infusion rate?

5. Solve the following IV rate and administration problems.
a. A physician orders 3000 mL of a 10% dextrose and normal saline ($D_{10}NS$) IV over a 48-hour period. If the IV set will deliver 15 gtt/mL, then how many drops must be administered per minute?
b. A ½ L IV is running at a rate of 100 mL/hr. How long will the bag last?

6. Convert the following (round off to nearest whole number):
a. 32° F to degrees Celsius
b. 35° C to degrees Fahrenheit
c. 86° F to degrees Celsius
d. 100° C to degrees Fahrenheit

Improving Communication Skills

1. Communicating in the hospital setting often means working with a wide variety of other healthcare providers. Understanding what role they play in patient healthcare is essential to effective communication. What duties do each of the following have in IV and TPN therapy?
a. physicians
b. nurses
c. pharmacists
d. pharmacy techs

2. Interview an IV hospital pharmacist about the applications of milliequivalents into IV admixtures and TPN solutions. Report to the class.

Internet Research

1. Visit the ASHP Web site.
a. What types of training does ASHP offer?
b. What are the benefits of technician membership?
c. How do you become a member?

2. Visit the ASHP Web site again, and find the link to your state affiliate organization.
    a. Where is it located?
    b. What is the phone number to contact the state organization?
    c. What services are offered to members?

3. Check the infusion rates in adults and pediatrics for Intralipid or Liposyn II/III in the PDR or other reference.

4. Visit the following Web links for TPN forms. What are the advantages to using this form for preparing pediatric TPN solutions? Any there any disadvantages?
    • www.bms.jhmi.edu/CFI/inside/studies/CFI_IH_CaseStudies _TPNCalculator.asp
    • www.hopkinsmedicine.org/Press_releases/2004_05_04.html

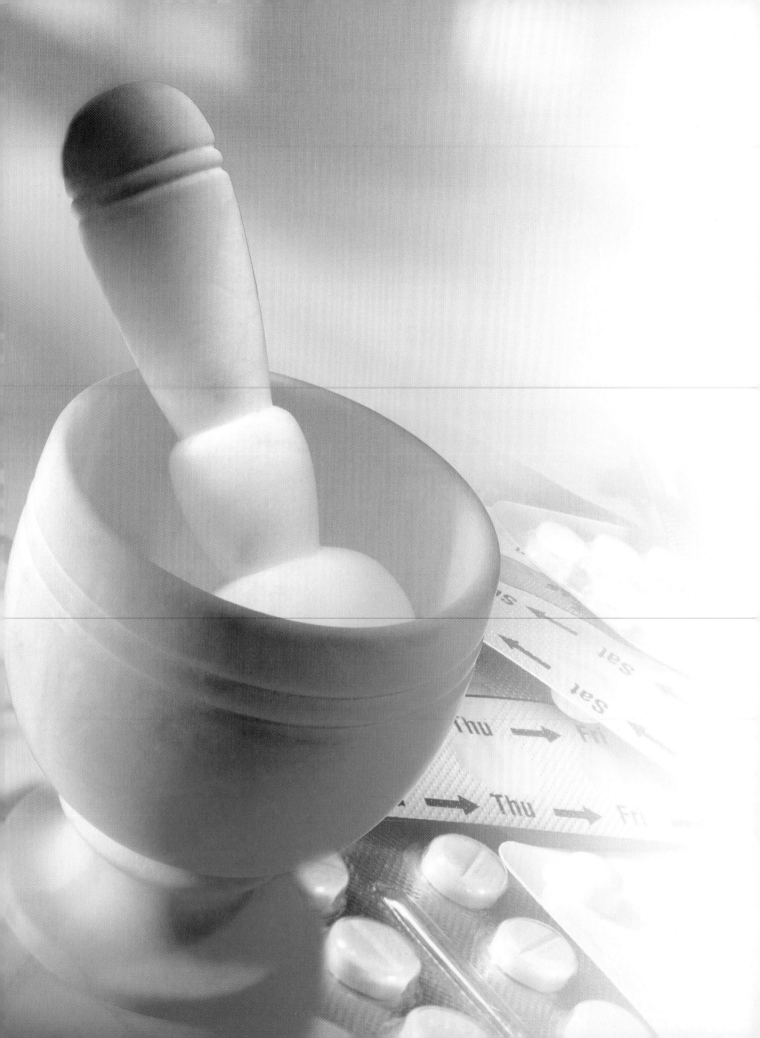

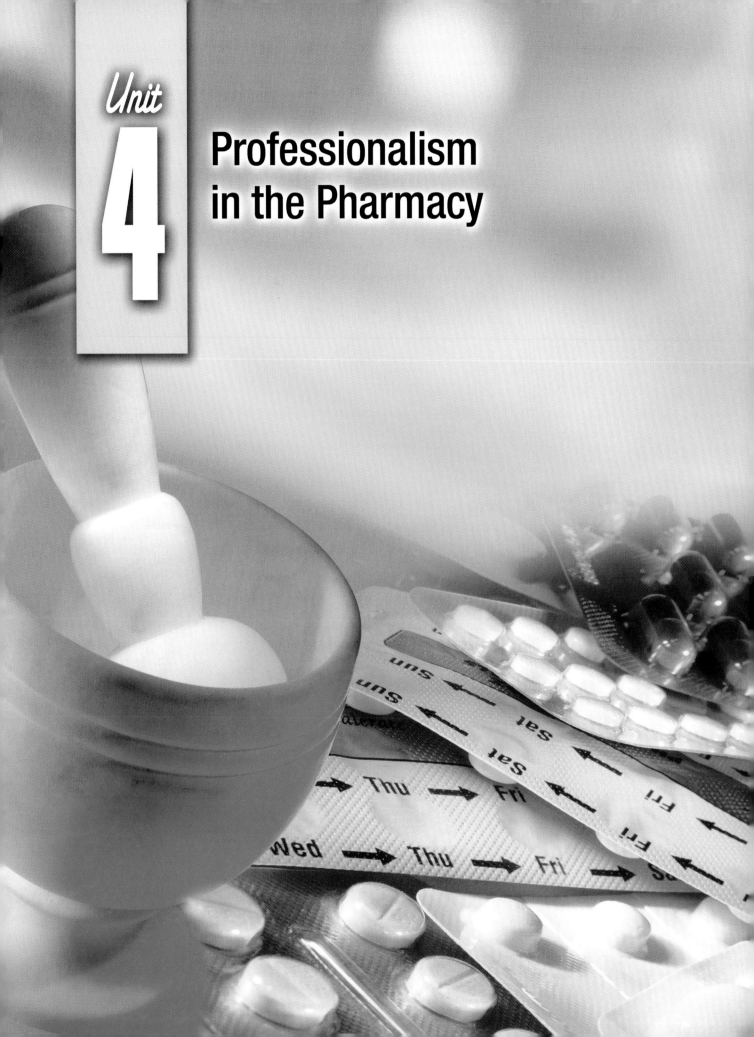

Unit 4

Professionalism in the Pharmacy

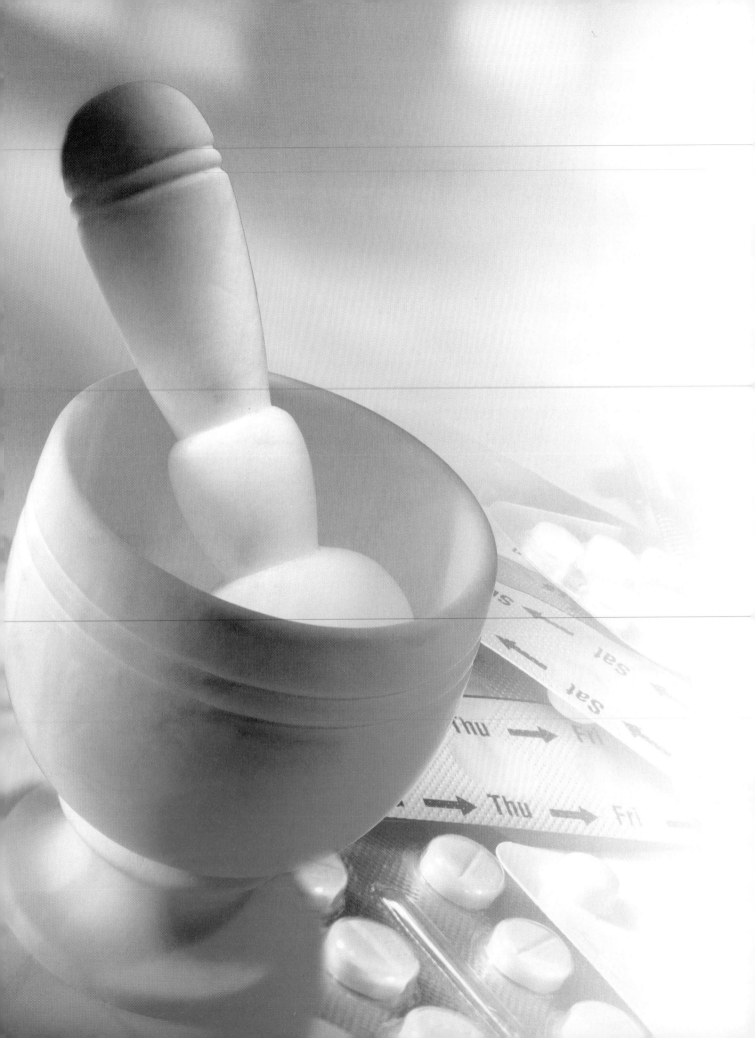

Medication Safety

Kimberly Vernachio, PharmD, RPh

Chapter 12

Learning Objectives

- Understand the extent and effect of medical errors on patient health and safety.
- Describe how and to what degree medication errors contribute to medical errors.
- List examples of medication errors commonly seen in practice settings.
- Apply a systematic evaluation of opportunities for medication error to a pharmacy practice model.
- Identify the common medication error–reporting systems available.

The pharmacy technician can play a crucial role in the prevention of medication errors in all pharmacy settings. Through categorizing types of medication errors and their common causes, pharmacy personnel work to establish practices to promote safety throughout the prescription-filling process. Hospitals, accrediting agencies, and several states provide reporting systems to help document events of medication errors to study their cause and to prevent future ones from occurring. The Food and Drug Administration (FDA) and the United States Pharmacopeia (USP) have developed other reporting systems to detect adverse reactions to drugs on the market.

MEDICAL ERRORS

A **medical error** is any circumstance, action, inaction, or decision related to health-care that contributes to an unintended health result. A medical error can be as simple as a lab test drawn at the wrong time, resulting in an inaccurate result, to a major surgical error that ends in death. A majority of what is known about medical errors comes from information collected in the hospital setting; however, hospital data make up only a part of a much larger picture. Generally, medical errors are difficult to define, because the circumstances that cause them are infinite.

Most healthcare is administered in the outpatient, office-based, or clinic setting. Although medical errors are more difficult to measure in these settings, one has only to look at the number of medical-related lawsuits to get a sense of the real scope of medical errors in the United States.

Several studies have attempted to measure the number and common causes of medical errors. These studies provide estimates on how many people die from medical errors. Examining only medical errors during hospitalization, one large government study suggested that as many as 98,000 people in the United States may die each year as a result of medical errors. This risk is greater than the risk of death from accident, diabetes, homicide, or human immunodeficiency virus (HIV) and acquired immunodeficiency syndrome (AIDS). It is important to remember that on the continuum of healthcare delivery, multiple sources for potential medical errors exist. Pharmacy technicians are an important part of the healthcare team, and therefore should be constantly on the "lookout" for possible sources of medical errors and adopt patient-safety-oriented work practices. When pharmacy technicians take steps to protect the safety of patients, they become an important barrier against an adverse patient outcome.

MEDICATION ERRORS

Medication errors are considered to be one of the many types of medical errors. Like medical errors, medication errors have no specific definition, because the possible causes can be endless; however, **medication errors** can generally be described as a medical error in which the source of error or harm includes a drug. Again, like medical errors, the information on the effect of medication errors comes mostly from studies done in the hospital setting. From these studies, medication-related deaths are estimated at about 7000 per year. Far fewer studies of medication errors in community practice exist; however, a few studies do give a sense of just how large an issue medication errors can be in community practice. An estimated 1.7% of all prescriptions dispensed in a community practice setting contain a medication error. That means 4 of every 250 prescriptions contain a medication error of some type. Although not all medication errors result in harm to a patient, the same study estimated that 65% of the medication errors detected had an adverse effect on the patient's health.[1]

The results of medication errors cannot be easily measured. Lives are lost daily, patients are disabled or lose valuable time from work or school, and the direct and indirect cost to the healthcare system is in the billions of dollars annually. These costs go to additional hospitalizations, admissions to long-term care, physician visits, emergency room visits, and continuation of disease.

Healthcare Professional's Responsibility

Working in healthcare means making a commitment to "first do no harm." This means that healthcare workers must put safety first. As discussed in Chapter 1, the profession of pharmacy exists to safeguard the health of the public. Because the effect of a potential medication error on the patient cannot be predicted, all professionals working in the healthcare system must focus on treating the patient to the best possible outcome by the safest possible means. As a result, no "acceptable" level of medication error exists, and each step in the task of filling medication orders should be reviewed with a 100% error-free goal in mind.

Safety Note
The only acceptable level of medication errors is zero.

Pharmacists are ultimately responsible for the accuracy of the medication-filling process, but technicians working in hospital and community pharmacy settings can assist in ensuring safety. By following some basic safe-practice guidelines listed in Table 12.1, pharmacists and pharmacy technicians can work together to create a larger margin of safety.

Additionally, proper packaging and instruction on medication use is essential to facilitate correct administration by a patient. Through careful listening and observation during a patient or medical staff interaction, a pharmacy technician can identify these potential patient sources of medication error and actively prevent the error by notifying the pharmacist. By constant surveillance for potential sources of medication error, pharmacy technicians become vital assistants to pharmacists and make a significant contribution to patient safety beyond the borders of the pharmacy.

Patient Response

Most patients will have the intended therapeutic response a physician expects from the medication selected; however, an individual's unique physical and social circumstances make it impossible to predict which medication errors may result in no substantial harm and which may result in death.

[1] Flynn, E.A., et al., "National Observational Study of Prescription Dispensing Accuracy and Safety in 50 Pharmacies." *Journal of American Pharmaceutical Association* 43 (2003): 191–200.

Table 12.1 General Tips for Reducing Medication Errors

General Tips	• Always keep the prescription and the label together during the fill process. • Know the common look-alike and sound-alike drugs, and keep them stored in different areas. • Keep dangerous or high-alert medications in a separate storage area of the pharmacy. • Always question bad handwriting. • Prescriptions/orders should be correctly spelled with drug name, strength, appropriate dosing, quantity or duration of therapy, dose form, and route. Missing information should be obtained from the prescriber. • Use the metric system. A leading zero should always be present in decimal values less than one. • Question the prescription/order that uses uncommon abbreviations. Avoid using abbreviations that have more than one meaning, and verify with the prescriber those of which you are unsure. • Be aware of insulin mistakes. Insulin brands should be clearly separated from one another. Educate patients to always verify their insulin purchase. • Keep the work area clean and uncluttered. Only keep drugs that are needed for immediate use in the work area. • Always verify information at each step of the prescription-filling process. • The label should always be compared with the original prescription by at least two people.
Tips for Pharmacists	• Check prescriptions in a timely manner. • Initial all checked prescriptions. • Visually check the product in the bottle. • Cross-reference prescription information with other validating sources. • Encourage documentation of all medication use, including over-the-counter (OTC) medications and diet supplements. • Document all clarifications on orders. • Maintain open lines of communication with patients, health-care providers, and caregivers.
Tips for Technicians	• Use the triple-check system (as discussed in Chapter 6). • Regularly review work habits, and actively look for actions to take that would improve safe and accurate prescription filling. • Verify information with the patient or caregiver when the prescription is received into the pharmacy and when the filled prescription is sent out of the pharmacy. • Observe, listen, and report pertinent information that may affect the safety or effectiveness of drug therapy to the pharmacist. • Keep your work area free of clutter.

Physiological Causes of Medication Errors   Remembering that each patient has a unique response to medication can best highlight the importance of medication safety. Each person is genetically unique, and the speed at which a person can remove medications from the body varies tremendously. For instance, G6PD (glucose-6-phosphate dehydrogenase) is an enzyme that helps to remove medications from the body. A lack of G6PD is the most common human enzyme deficiency in the world. A patient with this enzyme deficiency, taking a medication that depends upon this enzyme to be removed from the body, could come to serious harm or even death. Even if this particular problem is caught and corrected before harm occurs, it would still be considered a medication error.

Social Causes of Medication Errors   Patients in the outpatient setting can also contribute to medication errors through incorrect administration. As a result, the medication does not work well, does not work at all, or may cause harm. Social causes of medication errors include failure to follow medication therapy instructions because of cost, noncompliance, failure to take therapy as the physician instructs, or misunderstanding instructions (perhaps because of language barriers). Patients can contribute to medication errors by doing the following:

- forgetting to take a dose or doses
- taking too many doses
- dosing at the wrong time
- not getting a prescription filled or refilled in a timely manner
- not following directions on dose administration
- terminating the drug regimen too soon

Such social causes may result in an adverse drug reaction, or a subtherapeutic or toxic dose. For example, over 50% of patients on necessary long-term medication are no longer taking their medication after 1 year. Any of these circumstances could result in lasting harm or in death, depending on the drug or the disease being treated. In any event, all of these social circumstances would be considered a medication error.

Categories of Medication Errors

An exact listing of medication errors is difficult to create, because the possible causes of a medication error can often be too numerous to count. However, categorizing errors into types or groups often aids in the identification and prevention of possible causes. Classic examples of medication errors are grouped into five major categories and are listed below.

- An **omission error** occurs when a dose is not given. An omission occurs when the next dose is due, but the previous dose was not administered.
- A **wrong dose error** occurs when a dose is either above or below the correct dose by more than 5%.
- An **extra dose error** occurs when a patient receives more doses than were prescribed by the physician.
- A **wrong dose form error** occurs when any dose form or formulation is given to the patient that is not the accepted interpretation of the physician order. Examples include a drug given by mouth for a drug ordered as an intramuscular (IM) injection, a capsule formulation dispensed instead of a tablet, or an immediate-release drug dispensed instead of a controlled-release drug.
- A **wrong time error** occurs when any drug is given 30 minutes or more before or after it was prescribed, up to the time of the next dose. This is a common error in the hospital and nursing home. This does not include prn (i.e., as needed) orders.

Another way of categorizing medication errors is to define them by what causes the failure of the desired result. The purpose of defining errors in this way is to clearly identify what the error was, where the error took place, and through closer examination to determine a specific cause (i.e., the *why*). Medication errors can be categorized within three basic definitions of failure:

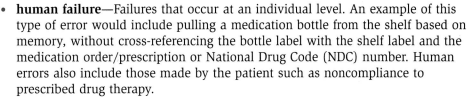

- **human failure**—Failures that occur at an individual level. An example of this type of error would include pulling a medication bottle from the shelf based on memory, without cross-referencing the bottle label with the shelf label and the medication order/prescription or National Drug Code (NDC) number. Human errors also include those made by the patient such as noncompliance to prescribed drug therapy.
- **technical failure**—Failures that result from location or equipment. An example of this type of failure would include the incorrect reconstitution of a medication because of a malfunction of a sterile-water dispenser *or* failure to properly operate automated equipment.
- **organizational failure**—Failures because of organizational rules, policies, or procedures. An example of this type of failure would include a policy or rule requiring preparing or admixing parenteral drugs such as cancer chemotherapy in an inappropriate setting.

Root Cause Analysis of Medication Errors

Root cause analysis is a logical and systematic process used to help identify what, how, and why something happened in order to prevent recurrence. Using some of the basic principles of root cause analysis, any person can examine his or her own work flow to determine the opportunities for potential error, determine what type of failure the potential error may fall into, and create a list of specific potential causes. Identifying specific potential causes allows a person to take specific actions to prevent the potential error and, as a result, improve patient safety. The actions taken improve the quality of work being done and therefore improve patient outcomes.

A medication error by handlers and preparers of medications has many causes. Three of the most common causes include the following:
- An **assumption error** occurs when an essential piece of information cannot be verified; therefore an assumption is made. An example of an assumption error that a pharmacy technician might make would be misreading an abbreviation on a prescription.
- A **selection error** occurs when two or more options exist, and the wrong option is chosen. An example of a selection error that a pharmacy technician might make would be mistakenly using a look-alike or sound-alike drug instead of the prescribed drug.
- A **capture error** occurs when focus on a task is diverted elsewhere and therefore the distraction *captures the person's attention*, preventing the person from detecting the error or causing an error to be made. An example of a capture error might be taking a phone call in the middle of filling a prescription order and, as a result, dispensing the wrong number of tablets (i.e., the correct number was forgotten and not double-checked at the conclusion of the phone call).

In relation to capture errors it is important to look at your own work habits to determine when and where in the prescription-filling process it is safe to allow focus on a task to be diverted. In other words, when completing a medication-related task, is there a place in the process when stopping and answering the telephone is *not* appropriate? When would it be appropriate to allow for such an interruption? Knowing *when* and *when not* to allow interruptions is vitally important in maintaining individual safety practices.

PRESCRIPTION-FILLING PROCESS IN COMMUNITY AND HOSPITAL PHARMACY PRACTICE

Safety Note

Each person who participates in the filling process has the opportunity to catch and correct a medication error.

A thorough review for potential causes of medication error in work practices begins with outlining work tasks in a step-by-step manner. Figure 12.1 is an example of a step-by-step prescription-filling process for community and hospital pharmacy practice settings. For the most part the filling process in both settings is identical; however, in the hospital setting medications pass through an extra set of hands—the nurse's—before reaching the patient. This extra set of hands provides both an extra opportunity to prevent medication errors, as well as an additional source of potential medication errors.

Once work practices are broken into individual steps, each step should be reviewed to determine what information is necessary to complete the step and what resources can be used to verify the information. In addition, consideration should be given to the possible errors that might result if information is missed or verification is not performed.

Therefore thinking of each step in three parts is helpful:

- information that needs to be obtained or checked
- resources that can be used to verify information
- potential medication errors that would result from a failure to obtain or check the necessary information using the appropriate resources

Step 1: Receive Prescription and Review Patient Profile

Table 12.2 lists the information needed and the resources used to avoid potential errors in the first step of the prescription-filling process.

Figure 12.1

Prescription-Filling Process
Although each step in this process can be a source of medication error, it can also be a place where the pharmacy personnel can correct a medication error.

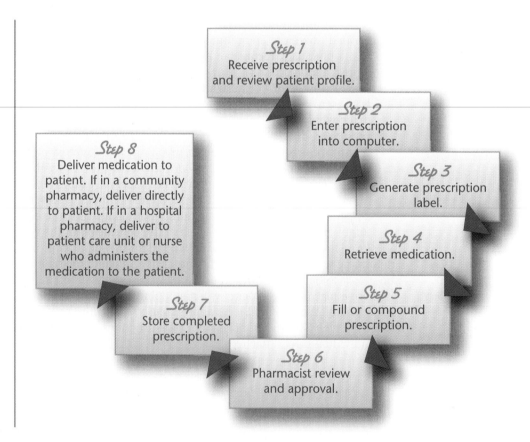

Step 1
Receive prescription and review patient profile.

Step 2
Enter prescription into computer.

Step 3
Generate prescription label.

Step 4
Retrieve medication.

Step 5
Fill or compound prescription.

Step 6
Pharmacist review and approval.

Step 7
Store completed prescription.

Step 8
Deliver medication to patient. If in a community pharmacy, deliver directly to patient. If in a hospital pharmacy, deliver to patient care unit or nurse who administers the medication to the patient.

Table 12.2 Step 1: Receive Prescription and Review Patient Profile

Information to Check	Resources to Verify Information	Potential Errors Resulting from Failure to Check/Verify Information
Legibility: Can the prescription be clearly read?	physician, patient, an independent reviewer such as pharmacist or nurse	prescription misread
Prescriber Information: Is the prescription valid? Did the prescriber sign the prescription? For narcotic prescriptions, is the prescriber's Drug Enforcement Administration (DEA) number listed? Is the prescription dated? Are the prescriber's name, address, and phone number printed on the prescription?	physician, pharmacist, nurse	out-of-date (i.e., invalid) prescription filled; fraudulent prescription filled; patient receives medication not intended for him or her
Patient Information: Is all necessary information included? Is this prescription for this patient? Are the patient's name, date of birth, address, phone number, and allergies provided? Does the information match the profile?	physician, patient, immediate family member, patient profile, pharmacist, nurse	incorrect patient selected; source of harm to the patient not able to be identified; contraindicated drug dispensed
Medication Information: Is all necessary information included? Are drug name, dose, dose form, route of administration, refills, directions for use, and dosing schedule included? Is the prescription dated?	patient, physician, family member, patient profile	wrong medication dispensed; wrong form/formulation dispensed; wrong dose dispensed; patient administers incorrectly; out-of-date (i.e., invalid) prescription filled
Drug Screening: Does the prescribed medication interact with other conditions or medications listed on the profile?	patient, physician, family member, patient profile, interaction screening program, insurance provider electronic messages, drug information resources (e.g., books, call centers, package inserts, patient information handouts)	contraindicated drug dispensed; drug-drug or drug-disease interaction takes place

Before a new prescription begins the prescription-filling process, an initial check of all key pieces of information is vital. A thorough review substantially reduces the chances that an unidentified error will continue through the filling process.

The first and most basic prescription review begins by deciding whether or not all the information is clear and legible. Can you read and understand it? Any unclear information should be clarified before any further action is taken.

Before considering the details of the information contained in a prescription, determining whether the prescription is, in fact, a valid and legal prescription is important. The requirements for a valid prescription may vary from state to state, and every technician should be familiar with the requirements of the state in which he or she practices. Does the prescription contain all the information necessary to be valid? For example, a prescription is valid for up to 1 year (less in some cases) from the date of its writing. Validity cannot be determined if the prescription is not dated. If not determined to be valid, then the prescription should not be filled.

A prescription contains three basic types of information: (1) physician information, (2) patient information, and (3) medication information. Physician information should be sufficient to determine whether a licensed and qualified prescriber wrote the prescription. Generally, the physician's contact information should be included. No prescription or medication order is valid without the signature of the prescriber. In the community setting, prescriptions lacking a presriber signature are not fillable (verbal prescriptions are an exception to this rule). Any verbal prescription order should include all the information necessary to verify that the caller is in fact a valid prescriber or his or her designated agent. In hospital settings, a physician signature is still required to validate a prescription; however, orders given verbally are generally honored, provided a signature is received within 24 hours.

Patient information should include enough detail to ensure that unique individuals can be pinpointed. Full names, addresses, dates of birth, and phone numbers give multiple points to cross-reference and separate patients that might otherwise have very similar information (e.g., patients with same first and last names). Date of birth and allergies should always be included, because this information helps to confirm the appropriateness of the medication information.

Medication information should include the drug name, strength, dose, dose form, route of administration, refills or length of therapy, directions for use, and dosing schedule. The absence of any one of these pieces of information opens the way for medication errors, such as dispensing of the wrong medication, wrong form or formulation, wrong dose or strength, or filling of an invalid prescription. Prescribing errors include poor handwriting, using nonstandard abbreviations, confusing look-alike and sound-alike drug names (see Appendix E), and using "as directed" instructions (which does not allow a pharmacist to verify normal recommended dose scheduling and reinforce correct dosing regimen to patients). A leading zero should precede a decimal point (e.g., 0.3). A zero should never follow a decimal (e.g., 3.0), because a tenfold error occurs if the decimal point is not detected.

Opportunities for medication errors increase as the number of medications a patient may take increases. This is a common occurrence with many older patients. For every prescription, a review of the profile should include a check for existing allergies and multiple drug therapy. A medication review should be performed to check for drug interactions or duplication of therapy.

Step 2: Enter Prescription into Computer

Table 12.3 lists the information needed and the resources used to avoid potential errors in the second step of the prescription-filling process.

Data entry into the computer system is simply the act of moving several important pieces of information from the prescription to the computer. The ability to perform this function accurately can make the difference between a patient receiving a correct and appropriate medication or a prescription that could cause the patient serious harm or death. With so much at stake, concentration and focus on how information is entered is very important. As each piece of information is entered, the prescription should be compared with choices from the computer menu. Check the brand and generic names and their spelling to determine whether the prescription and computer agree. Special attention should be paid to doses, formulations, concentration, and the increments of measure. Prescriptions that contain unapproved error-causing abbreviations should be confirmed with the prescriber (see Appendix A).

Does the form or formulation match the route of administration? Be aware that certain concentrations or formulations of a given medication may be associated with a particular route of administration. A common example of the potential for mismatching of form or formulation to route of administration is Depo-Medrol and

Table 12.3   Step 2: Enter Prescription into Computer

Information to Check	Resources to Verify Information	Potential Errors Resulting from Failure to Check/Verify Information
Are data choices from the computer menu and those on the prescription the same?		look-alike or sound-alike drug selection error made
Does the spelling on the prescription match the drug selection options?	cross-check brand/generic names for identical spelling	look-alike or sound-alike drug selection error made
Do the increments of measure on the drug selection options match the prescription? (e.g., gram versus milligram versus microgram)	cross-check measure prescribed with drug choices listed	patient given incorrect dose
For the dose selected, do available strengths or concentrations match? Does the dose or concentration have leading or trailing zeros? Does it require a decimal?	cross-check dose written with available strengths or concentrations on selection menu; cross-check doses or concentrations that use decimals, leading or trailing zeros	patient given incorrect dose
Do available forms match route selected?	match route to formulation choices (e.g., via injection to intravenous [IV] or intramuscular [IM] drugs; via oral route to capsule/tablet/liquid/lozenge)	inappropriate form or formulation selected

Web Link

Check the Institute for Safe Medication Practices Web site at **www.ismp.org** for dangerous abbreviations or dose designations.

Solu-Medrol. Both are injectables and have similar doses, depending on the clinical situation. However, Depo-Medrol is for intramuscular (IM) administration only and is a cloudy suspension when reconstituted. Solu-Medrol is for intravenous (IV) administration and is a clear solution. A serious and potentially fatal medication error could occur if a suspension were inadvertently administered by the IV route.

Once information entry has taken place, each data element of the completed entry should be compared with the same data elements on the original prescription, before the entry process is finalized.

Step 3: Generate Prescription Label

Safety Note

Confirm that information entered into the computer matches the original prescription.

Table 12.4 lists the information needed and the resources used to avoid potential errors in the third step of the prescription-filling process.

Use of technology presents its own unique opportunities for error. In most circumstances, errors caused by technology depend on the user; however, inherent technology malfunctions and program "glitches" do happen. Therefore good safety practices should include a check for the accuracy of any technology (e.g., computers, scales, pumps, dispensers) in the prescription-filling process. Cross-check the label output from the computer with the original prescription to make sure that a typing error or inherent program malfunction did not alter the information. Is the correct patient name on the label? Are the drug, dose, concentration, and route information identical to the original prescription?

Table 12.4   Step 3: Generate Prescription Label

Information to Check	Resources to Verify Information	Potential Errors Resulting from Failure to Check/Verify Information
Has the patient information been cross-checked?	compare label generated with original prescription	wrong patient, medication, or dose selected
Are the label and original prescription identical?	compare label generated with original prescription	wrong patient, medication, or dose selected
Are the leading or trailing zeros and unapproved abbreviations correct?	check with pharmacist or prescriber	incorrect dose selected
Do all the data elements match the original prescription (e.g., patient information, medication information, physician information)?	use additional information generated on label reference for verification (e.g., brand/generic names, National Drug Code [NDC], manufacturer name, addresses, phone numbers, age, date of birth)	inappropriate form or formulation selected wrong patient, medication, or dose selected

Step 4: Retrieve Medication

Table 12.5 lists the information needed and the resources used to avoid potential errors in the fourth step of the prescription-filling process.

Products can contribute to errors with look-alike labels, similarities in brand or generic names, and similar pill shapes or colors. Use NDC numbers, drug names, and other information available on manufacturers' labels or patient information handouts to verify selection of the correct product. Use both the original prescription and the generated label when selecting a manufacturer's drug product from the storage shelf. For example, Adderall and Inderal are similar brand names of medication, but a cross-reference of generic names reveals two very different names—*amphetamine salts* and *propranolol*.

Table 12.5   Step 4: Retrieve Medication

Information to Check	Resources to Verify Information	Potential Errors Resulting from Failure to Check/Verify Information
Has the available information on the manufacturer's label been used to verify the medication selection?		
Do the brand and generic name on the label match the product container?	original prescription, shelf- or bin-labeling systems, manufacturer names, NDC numbers, brand/generic name; pictographic medication verification references or computer programs	medication selection error made
Do the dose strength and form on the label match the product container?	original prescription, shelf- or bin-labeling systems, manufacturer names, NDC numbers, brand/generic name; pictographic medication verification references or computer programs	incorrect dose, form, or formulation selected
Do the National Drug Code (NDC) and manufacturer name match those listed on the label?	bin-labeling systems, NDC numbers; pictographic medication verification references or computer programs	incorrect dose, form, or formulation selected

Wherever possible use NDC numbers as a cross-check option, because each NDC number is specific to a particular form and specific strength for each medication (discussed in Chapter 3). Therefore the NDC numbers of two forms of a medication, even at the same strength, would not match (nor would two different strengths of the same form of the same medication).

Accidental substitution of one drug or pharmaceutical ingredient for another is one of the most serious events that can occur in pharmacy practice. Differences in potency or toxicity and not receiving the drug prescribed for treatment or prevention present significant risk of harm or possible death; therefore extreme care must be taken not to substitute drugs that have similar names. Appendix E includes a list compiled by the Institute for Safe Medication Practices (ISMP) containing drug names that are near homonyms (i.e., words that sound alike) or homographs (i.e., words that are similar in spelling). The appendix includes tips designed by ISMP for preventing dispensing errors.

In one infamous case, *Toppi vs. Scarf, 1971,* a pharmacist accidentally dispensed Nardil, an antidepressant, instead of Norinyl, a contraceptive. The woman who received the wrong drug gave birth to a child, and the Michigan Court of Appeals held the pharmacist liable not only for the medical expenses incurred in the woman's pregnancy but also for the costs of raising the child.

Some pharmacy practices possess a computer-based "pill identification" program and use a shelf-labeling system to organize inventory. Such identification programs allow the pharmacist or technician to visually verify the medication dispensed with a picture of the medication. These sources of information should be used to verify selection of the correct medication.

Step 5: Fill or Compound Prescription

Safety Note

When compounding, do not allow interruptions and prepare products one at a time.

Table 12.6 lists the information needed and the resources used to avoid potential errors in the fifth step of the prescription-filling process.

Calculation and substitution errors are frequent sources of pharmacy-related medication errors. A technician should write out the calculation and have a second person check the answer. Great care should be taken when reading labels and preparing compounded products. Using more than one container of product, preparing more than one product at a time, distractions, and interruptions can all

Table 12.6   Step 5: Fill or Compound Prescription

Information to Check	Resources to Verify Information	Potential Errors Resulting from Failure to Check/Verify Information
Have the amount to be dispensed and the increment of measure (e.g., gram, milligram, microgram) been reviewed?	amount dispensed (count twice), original prescription	incorrect quantity or incorrect dose dispensed
Does the prescription require a calculation or measurement conversion?	write out calculation and conversions; ask another person to review calculation	incorrect dose dispensed
If using equipment, has the equipment been calibrated recently?	equipment (check calibration), pharmacist, patient information handout, package insert	incorrect dose dispensed
Does the medication dispensed require warning or caution labels?	pharmacist, patient information handout, package insert	administration error made by patient

contribute to medication errors. Do not allow interruptions or distractions during filling or compounding. If you must stop before filling is complete, then be sure to start over from the beginning.

In addition, all equipment should be maintained, cleaned, and calibrated on a regular basis. This principle is not limited to sophisticated equipment alone. The simple act of cleaning counting trays and spatulas on a regular basis is an important part of medication safety. Consider the potential for serious harm to a patient if the residue or dust from an allergy-causing medication contaminates the patient's prescription. For example, penicillins or sulfa-containing medications should be counted on "dedicated" counting trays because of the high prevalence of penicillin and sulfa allergy in the general population. Cleaning the counting tray with isopropyl alcohol after each of these drugs is dispensed is also recommended.

Caution and warning labels applied to a prescription container are intended to serve as reminders to patients about the most critical aspects of drug handling or administration. In most pharmacy settings with computerized systems, the caution and warning labels are generated with the label and coordinate with the more detailed patient information handouts. These labels serve as a continuous reminder of the most crucial aspects of proper medication administration and should always be included with prescription labeling. Before affixing the auxiliary labels to the prescription vial, ask the pharmacist which ones are priority. Often up to six labels will be printed or needed but only three may fit on the vial. Be sure to ask what the policy is at your practice site.

Step 6: Review and Approve Prescription

Table 12.7 lists the information needed and the resources used to avoid potential errors in the sixth step of the prescription-filling process. (Note: The pharmacist must be the one to review and approve the prescription in the sixth step.)

The pharmacist is legally responsible for verifying the accuracy and appropriateness of any prescription that is filled, but, it is not practical for pharmacists to verify each step in the filling process. Rather, a pharmacist verifies the quality and integrity of the *end product*. Thus providing all available resources that are useful to ensure

Table 12.7   Step 6: Pharmacist Review and Approval

Information to Check	Resources to Verify Information	Potential Errors Resulting from Failure to Check/Verify Information
Did the pharmacist review the prepared medication?	original prescription, stock medication bottle or vial, calculations	
Can the pharmacist verify the validity of the prescription with the finished product and the information you provide?	original prescription	invalid or out-of-date prescription filled
Can the pharmacist verify the patient information with the finished product and the information provided?	original prescription, patient profile, patient, physician or nurse	wrong patient given medication
Can the pharmacist verify the correctness of the prepared prescription based on the medication information provided?	physical look of prepared medication; calculations and conversions (provide them), original manufacturer's container, pictographic medication verification, programs, package insert	medication selection error made; incorrect dose, form, or formulation selected; incorrect medication administered

accurate verification is vital to patient safety. The easiest way to determine what information and resources are important to the verifying pharmacist is to ask whether the information provided with the medication filled allows the pharmacist to *retrace* the technician's steps in filling the prescription. Can the pharmacist determine whether the prescription is valid, the patient information is accurate, and the medication was correctly prepared from the information provided with the finished product? One useful exercise to help you become aware of what is needed by a pharmacist is to practice checking another's work. Trade finished products with another technician, if possible. Try to check each other's work. Can you retrace the steps taken to fill the prescription? Can you validate all the key pieces of information? Undertaking this exercise on a regular basis will help to highlight "bad habits" or short cuts that may open the way for medication errors to occur.

Safety Note

The pharmacist must always check the technician's work.

Step 7: Store Completed Prescription

Table 12.8 lists the information needed and the resources used to avoid potential errors in the seventh step of the prescription-filling process.

Ensuring the integrity of medication is an important part of medication safety. Many medications are sensitive to light, humidity, or temperature. A failure to properly store medications may result in loss of drug potency or effect. In some cases improper storage of a drug may result in a degraded product that causes serious harm. The following examples illustrate this type of problem:

- Freezing of certain insulins results in changes in the formulation and absorption by the body. Once thawed and administered, the result is a drug that may show a different effect.
- Nitroglycerin is a product used for angina (i.e., heart pain). Nitroglycerin molecules adhere to plastics; therefore sublingual tablets and other nitroglycerin products must be stored in original glass containers under airtight conditions. Failure to maintain proper storage results in loss of drug effect.
- Overheating of fentanyl patches alters how the drug is released from the patch, resulting in a possible overdose.[2]

Simple measures like well-organized and clearly labeled storage systems help to keep a patient's medications together and separate from those of other patients. Orderly storage decreases the chances that a patient would receive a prescription intended for someone else or would not receive a medication because it was given to

Table 12.8   Step 7: Store Completed Prescription

Information to Check	Resources to Verify Information	Potential Errors Resulting from Failure to Check/Verify Information
Are storage conditions appropriate for the medication (e.g., humidity, temperature, light exposure)?	package insert	medication becomes degraded
Are each patient's medications adequately separated?	physical review of medications placed in bags, boxes, or bins	patient receives medication not intended for him or her; patient fails to receive medication (i.e., omission)
Are storage areas kept neat and orderly?	use of organization systems (e.g., bins, boxes, bags, alphabetizing, consolidation)	patient receives medication not intended for him or her; patient fails to receive medication (i.e., omission)

[2] *Pharmacist Letter* 21 (2005): 210806.

another patient. Both scenarios are medication errors, and depending on the drug in question, each presents the potential to cause serious harm or death if the error goes undetected.

Step 8: Deliver Medication to Patient

Table 12.9 lists the information needed and the resources used to avoid potential errors in the eighth step of the prescription-filling process. In a community pharmacy setting, the medication ultimately will be received by the patient (or a designated representative) directly, whereas in the hospital the medication is received by the nurse. In either case the opportunity exists to verify the prescription information against the knowledge and expectations of the patient or the caregiver. In situations in which the patient directly receives the medication, confirm the patient's name, the medication he or she expects to receive, and the patient's knowledge of proper use. Comparing the completed prescription against the information provided by the patient allows for a final opportunity to capture potential errors that were unrecognized in the filling process, as well as potential errors resulting from gaps or misunderstandings in the patient's knowledge. In this way, errors such as receipt of medications into the wrong hands or missing medications (i.e., omission of therapy) as well as drug, dose form, and administration errors are captured. Asking basic questions of the patient such as, "Do you know what your medicine is for and how to use it?" or calling to the patient's attention the auxiliary warning and caution labels on the medication bottle may uncover unexpected drug interactions or side effects, or a patient in need of counseling to enhance his or her understanding of correct administration.

In some community pharmacies a "show-and-tell" technique is employed to prevent medication errors and provide patient education. When the patient comes to the pharmacy to pick up the prescription, the pharmacy technician or pharmacist opens the vial and shows the drug product to the patient. This added step not only

Table 12.9   Step 8: Deliver Medication to Patient

Information to Check	Resources to Verify Information	Potential Errors Resulting from Failure to Check/Verify Information
Will the look of the pill be new to the patient or caregiver?	prescription label, patient, patient education handouts, patient profile	administration error made; patient noncompliant with medication instructions
Is the patient receiving medications intended for him or her?	patient, caregiver, original prescription, patient profile, bar code identification system	patient receives medication not intended for him or her; patient fails to receive medication (i.e., omission)
Does the patient or caregiver understand the instructions for use?	pharmacist, patient education handouts, drug information resources	administration error made; patient noncompliant with medication instructions; drug interactions, adverse reactions, degradation of medication occurs because of improper handling or storage
Does the patient or caregiver know what to expect?	pharmacist, patient education handouts, drug information resources	side effects and adverse reactions occur, clinical effect not achieved
Are all the medications prescribed for the patient included?	consolidation of medications into one bag, bin, or box; use of organization systems (e.g., bins, boxes, bags, alphabetizing, consolidation)	patient fails to receive medication (i.e., omission), therapy not completed

Safety Note

Pharmacy technicians cannot instruct patients. If a technician suspects that a patient requires instruction, then the technician should alert the pharmacist.

helps the patient identify the drug he or she will be taking, but also provides an extra opportunity for the technician or pharmacist to check that the correct drug product was put into the vial. If the patient notices that a refilled drug looks different than a previously filled drug, the patient has a chance to point this out and have this discrepancy verified. Medication errors can be caught before they ultimately reach the patient in this final check system.

In hospital settings, the medication passes through an extra set of hands (usually a nurse). Adding the caregiver to the pharmacy practice provides an additional person to confirm the accuracy and appropriateness of the medication; however, the addition of a new step in the process creates a new opportunity for a medication error to take place. The task of medication delivery to the nursing station is mainly filled by technicians; therefore the technician is in the best position to search for potential errors. Take the time to notify the nurse that a newly prescribed medication has been delivered to the floor. This opens the door of communication to ask whether the nurse knows about the medication. Ask whether the medications delivered were all that they were expecting. If unit dose medication carts are returned to the pharmacy with unused regularly scheduled medication, then the pharmacist or pharmacy technician should follow up with the nurse to determine if an error of omission occurred.

In the treatment of certain diseases such as cancer, multiple drug therapy combinations, including investigational medications, are prescribed together because they work in concert to treat the disease. If a particular drug is missing from the drug therapy combination, then treatment is incomplete. In addition, many of these drugs are extremely toxic. Any dose error could be fatal; therefore an opportunity to communicate with the nurse or physician when these medications are delivered to the treatment area is also an opportunity to verify that doses prepared are in fact correct.

Like any omission, incomplete therapy is also a medication error. Without the cooperative efforts of pharmacy technicians to ensure safe medication use, a patient's well-being is not safeguarded, and the best health outcome is not achieved.

MEDICATION ERROR PREVENTION

Learning to prevent medication errors means carefully examining potential points of failure and using available resources to verify information that is given or decisions that are made. Keeping in mind that the most common error in dispensing and administration is drug identification, a pharmacy technician becomes a very valuable asset in ensuring drug safety because the pharmacy technician "owns" a substantial portion of the prescription-filling process. A pharmacy technician is often the person who first examines a prescription when it is submitted for filling, and is just as likely to be the last person to handle a medication before it reaches the patient.

Safety Note

Incorrect drug identification is the most common error in dispensing or administration.

Consequently the pharmacy technician often has the most opportunities to prevent a medication error. In addition, pharmacy technicians are also in a position to identify potential sources of error beyond prescription dispensing, because they are the ones who may interact with a patient or nurse when a prescription comes in or goes out of the pharmacy.

Many medication errors also occur during prescribing and administration. Prescriptions often pass first through the hands of a pharmacy technician once they are received from a physician or patient. Prescribers are responsible for ensuring the "five Rs" or five rights (Figure 12.2). In other words, they must ensure that the drug prescribed is the right drug for the right patient, at the right strength, given by the right route, and administered at the right time. Pharmacy practice overlays the physician responsibilities and thereby facilitates patient safety and error prevention by processes that verify the following:

- The correct patient is being given the medications, and other associated medications are correct.
- The correct drug is dispensed.
- The correct dose is prepared, whether for a child or adult, to maintain a correct body concentration or blood level.
- The correct route of administration is indicated.
- The appropriate dose form is prepared (e.g., a tablet would not be dispensed for administration by nasogastric [NG] tube, and antibiotic capsules would not be appropriate for administration to an infant).
- The correct administration times and the correct conditions for administration (e.g., medications that must be taken with or without food) are indicated.

Patient Education

Importantly, patients and caregivers must have the basic knowledge needed to administer, handle, and support safe medication use. Pharmacy technicians can encourage patients to ask questions, relay complete medical and allergy history, and carefully check medications (both prescription and over-the-counter [OTC]) for information as to when they should be taken. The pharmacy technician should be actively involved in monitoring for potential errors. Although pharmacy technicians cannot instruct patients, they can encourage patients to become informed about their conditions and to ask the pharmacist basic questions about the prescribed medications. Patients should understand 10 key pieces of information about every medication taken:

1. what the brand and generic names are
2. what the medication looks like
3. why they are taking the medication, and how long they will have to take it
4. how much to take, how often, and the best time or circumstances to take a medication
5. what to do if they miss a dose
6. what medications or foods interact with what they are taking
7. whether the medication prescribed is in addition to or replaces medication currently taken

Figure 12.2

Five Rs for Patient Drug Administration

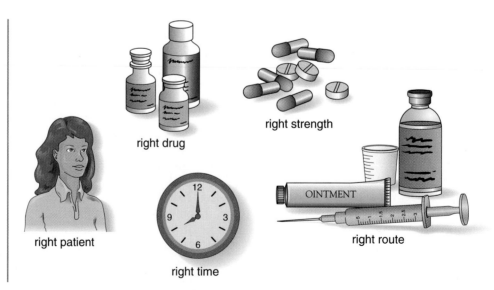

right drug

right strength

right patient

right time

right route

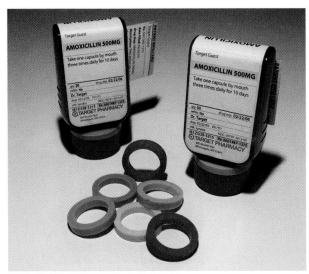

The Target ClearRx packaging is designed to help patients manage their medications by providing information in a clear and easy-to-read format.

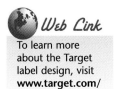

Web Link

To learn more about the Target label design, visit **www.target.com/pharmacy**

8. what common side effects can be expected and what to do when encountered
9. what special precautions should be taken for each particular drug therapy
10. where and how to store the medication

By encouraging patients to ask questions and helping them to connect with the pharmacist or appropriate healthcare provider, you will assist patients in becoming more informed and empower them to be advocates for their own safety and health.

Innovations to Promote Safety

The physical pharmacy work setting can have a major contribution to the overall safety of any work environment. Adequate space and clean, well-lit conditions are just some of the basics. Table 12.10 outlines work environment practices a pharmacy can create to promote safety and reduce errors.

Many examples exist of efforts made to minimize the possibility of medication errors. A most recent example in community pharmacy practice is the effort of Target Pharmacies to visually redesign the packaging of dispensed medications to help patients safely take their medication. The design uses colored rings to help patients identify medications intended for them, as opposed to those intended for other family members. In addition, the new design provides a clear, easy-to-read label for patient administration instructions and cautions that includes a pullout patient information card or printout.

Moving from a paper-based system to an integrated computerized filling system is an easy and very common example of how hospitals improve efficiency and allow resources to be redirected to increase patient safety and improve quality of patient care. An example of this type of change and safety improvement occurred at Medcenter One Health Systems in Bismarck, ND. Originally the hospital operated a paper-based medication administration system. With this system, the hospital reported about 305 medication administration errors, and estimated an additional 50% went unreported. Pharmacists spent 90% of their time on order entry and distribution. It has long been shown that when a pharmacist is actively involved in medication decisions, safety and outcomes for patients are substantially improved.[3]

Table 12.10 Work Environment Practices to Promote Safety

- Automate and bar-code all fill procedures.
- Maintain a clean, organized, and orderly work area.
- Provide adequate storage areas with clear drug labels on the shelves.
- Encourage prescribers to use common terminology and only safe abbreviations.
- Provide adequate computer applications and hardware.

[3] Personal communication, Dr. Marc Perlman, McKesson Provider Technologies.

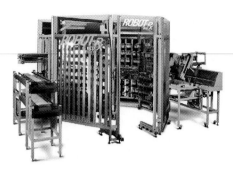

Robot-based medication dispensing increases efficiency and speed of medication delivery without compromising safety. The robot uses bar codes to validate drug selection, significantly reducing the chances of drug selection errors.

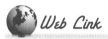

Web Link

Learn more about McKesson's technologies at **www.mckesson.com**

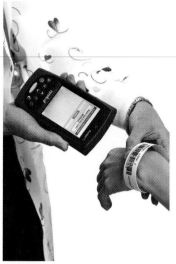

Bar coding technologies enhance medication administration safety by creating a standardized way to validate the five rights: right patient, right drug, right strength, right time, and right route.

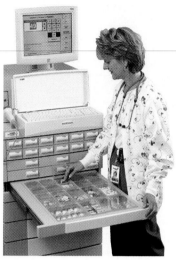

Automated dispensing cabinets like this one are maintained primarily by technician staff and provide a safe and efficient means to deliver medications to patients.

The hospital converted its paper-based system to an electronic medication administration system (Admin-Rx), which used a computer-based bar code validation program that worked together with automated dispensing cabinets (AccuDose-Rx) and robotic filling systems (ROBOT-Rx). These technologic advances empowered the pharmacy technician staff to become more productive and, as a result, pharmacists were freed to become more involved in patient care. In the end, medication-dispensing errors dropped from 11% to almost zero.

MEDICATION ERROR AND ADVERSE DRUG REACTION REPORTING SYSTEMS

If it is true that what is not known cannot be fixed, then the first step in prevention of medication errors is collection of information. Fear of punishment is always a concern when any error arises; as a result, people may decide not to report an error at all, leaving the door open for the same error to occur again and again. For this reason, anonymous or *no-fault* systems of reporting have been established. The focus of no-fault reporting is on fixing the problem and not fixing the blame.

State Boards of Pharmacy

Many efforts have been made to create a safe and comfortable atmosphere for individuals to report medication errors. Currently more than 20 states have mandatory error-reporting systems, but most state officials admit medical errors are still under-reported, mostly because of fear of punishment and liability. States like Florida, Texas, and California have worked to reduce the fear of reporting by passing new regulations that allow pharmacists to document errors and error-prone systems without worry of punishment as long as steps are taken to eliminate weaknesses that might allow such errors to continue. Most boards of pharmacy will not punish pharmacists for errors as long as there was a good faith effort to fill correctly. In addition, legislatures have proposed new laws that will protect error reports from subpoena. These error reports must be separate from medical records, because all medical records can be subpoenaed, including prescription records.

The task of error reporting is best performed by the authority in charge; however, pharmacy technicians are an integral part of the error identification, documentation, and prevention process. An understanding of the *what, when, where,* and *why* of error reporting is important for pharmacy technicians just like pharmacists. Keep in mind that the final and most important piece of medication error reporting is the delicate task of informing the patient that a medication error has taken place. This is commonly the task of the pharmacist. The circumstances leading to the error should be explained completely and honestly. Patients should understand the nature of the error, what if any effects the error will have, and how he or she can become actively involved in preventing errors in the future. Generally speaking, people are more likely to forgive an honest error but rarely will accept a hiding of the truth.

Joint Commission on Accreditation of Healthcare Organizations

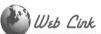

Web Link

Learn more about the Joint Commission International Center for Patient Safety at **www.jcipatient safety.org**

Organizations also contribute to error-reporting efforts by creating a centralized point through which all members may channel information safely. A well-established example is the Sentinel Event Policy created by the Joint Commission on Accreditation of Healthcare Organizations (JCAHO) in 1996. A **sentinel event** is an unexpected occurrence involving death, serious physical or psychologic injury, or the potential for occurrences to happen. When a sentinel event is reported, the organization (i.e., hospital, pharmacy, managed-care company) is expected to analyze the cause of the error (i.e., perform a root cause analysis), take action to correct the cause, monitor the changes made, and determine whether the cause of the error is eliminated. Accreditation of hospitals is dependent on demonstrating an effective medical and medication error–reporting system.

United States Pharmacopeia

Web Link

Learn about the Medication Errors Reporting Program and MEDMARX at **www.usp.org/ patientsafety**

Many professional organizations support patient safety efforts by gathering medical error information and using the data to create tools to support professionals in specific settings or situations. The United States Pharmacopeia (USP) supports two types of reporting systems for the collection of medical errors and adverse drug reactions. The first is the Medication Errors Reporting Program, designed to allow healthcare professionals to report medication errors directly. The second is an Internet-based program for use by hospitals and health systems known as **MEDMARX**. MEDMARX allows institutions to document, analyze, track, and trend adverse events specific to the institution. Both error-reporting programs support research into medication-related adverse events and then use the information to develop medication-specific patient safety initiatives.

Federal Drug Administration

The government body responsible for approving the safety of medications and medical devices, the Food and Drug Administration (FDA), also collects adverse event reports for medications and medical devices through a program known as **MedWatch**. The FDA uses this information to track unrecognized problems or issues that were not apparent when the medication or medical device was approved. The recognition of a problem or potential for error does not mean the product will be removed from the marketplace. Many times, improving of prescribing information, education of healthcare professionals or the public, or perhaps a simple name change may be all that is necessary to reduce or eliminate a safety risk. The FDA provides an adverse event reporting form for documenting (Figure 12.3).

Institute for Safe Medication Practices

The Institute for Safe Medication Practices (ISMP) is a nonprofit healthcare agency whose membership is primarily comprised of physicians, pharmacists, and nurses. The mission statement of this organization is "to understand the causes of medication errors and to provide time-critical error reduction strategies to the healthcare community, policy makers and the public."

Figure 12.3
MedWatch Adverse Event Reporting Form

U.S. Department of Health and Human Services

MEDWATCH

The FDA Safety Information and Adverse Event Reporting Program

For VOLUNTARY reporting of adverse events and product problems

Page ___ of ___

Form Approved: OMB No. 0910-0291 Expires: 04/30/03
See OMB statement on reverse

FDA Use Only

Triage unit sequence #

PLEASE TYPE OR USE BLACK INK

A. Patient information

1. Patient identifier — In confidence
2. Age at time of event: or Date of birth:
3. Sex — ☐ female ☐ male
4. Weight — ___ lbs or ___ kgs

B. Adverse event or product problem

1. ☐ Adverse event and/or ☐ Product problem (e.g., defects/malfunctions)
2. Outcomes attributed to adverse event (check all that apply)
   - ☐ death ______ (mo/day/yr)
   - ☐ life-threatening
   - ☐ hospitalization - initial or prolonged
   - ☐ disability
   - ☐ congenital anomaly
   - ☐ required intervention to prevent permanent impairment/damage
   - ☐ other: ______
3. Date of event (mo/day/yr)
4. Date of this report (mo/day/yr)
5. Describe event or problem
6. Relevant tests/laboratory data, including dates
7. Other relevant history, including preexisting medical conditions (e.g., allergies, race, pregnancy, smoking and alcohol use, hepatic/renal dysfunction, etc.)

C. Suspect medication(s)

1. Name (give labeled strength & mfr/labeler, if known) #1 #2
2. Dose, frequency & route used #1 #2
3. Therapy dates (if unknown, give duration) from/to (or best estimate) #1 #2
4. Diagnosis for use (indication) #1 #2
5. Event abated after use stopped or dose reduced
   #1 ☐yes ☐no ☐doesn't apply
   #2 ☐yes ☐no ☐doesn't apply
6. Lot # (if known) #1 #2
7. Exp. date (if known) #1 #2
8. Event reappeared after reintroduction
   #1 ☐yes ☐no ☐doesn't apply
   #2 ☐yes ☐no ☐doesn't apply
9. NDC # (for product problems only) - -
10. Concomitant medical products and therapy dates (exclude treatment of event)

D. Suspect medical device

1. Brand name
2. Type of device
3. Manufacturer name & address
4. Operator of device
   - ☐ health professional
   - ☐ lay user/patient
   - ☐ other: ______
5. Expiration date (mo/day/yr)
6. model # ______ catalog # ______ serial # ______ lot # ______ other # ______
7. If implanted, give date (mo/day/yr)
8. If explanted, give date (mo/day/yr)
9. Device available for evaluation? (Do not send to FDA)
   ☐ yes ☐ no ☐ returned to manufacturer on ______ (mo/day/yr)
10. Concomitant medical products and therapy dates (exclude treatment of event)

E. Reporter (see confidentiality section on back)

1. Name & address — phone #
2. Health professional? ☐ yes ☐ no
3. Occupation
4. Also reported to
   - ☐ manufacturer
   - ☐ user facility
   - ☐ distributor
5. If you do NOT want your identity disclosed to the manufacturer, place an " X " in this box. ☐

FDA

Mail to: MEDWATCH
5600 Fishers Lane
Rockville, MD 20852-9787

or FAX to:
1-800-FDA-0178

FDA Form 3500

Submission of a report does not constitute an admission that medical personnel or the product caused or contributed to the event.

Web Link

Get an adverse event reporting form at **www.fda.gov/medwatch/getforms.htm**

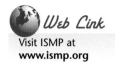
Web Link

Visit ISMP at
www.ismp.org

ISMP in concert with the USP provides a confidential national voluntary program called MERP (Medication Errors Reporting Program). According to the program, medication errors include (1) wrong drug, strength, or dose; (2) confusion over look-alike and sound-alike drugs; (3) incorrect route of drug administration; (4) calculation or preparation errors; (5) misuse of medical equipment; and (6) errors in prescribing, transcribing, dispensing, or monitoring medications. Reports can be completed on-line.

ISMP has sponsored national forums on medication errors, recommended the addition of labeling or special hazard warnings on potentially toxic drugs, encouraged revisions of potentially dangerous prescription writing practices, and first promoted the now common practice of using the leading zero. ISMP is active in disseminating information to healthcare professionals and consumers such as e-mail newsletters, journal articles, and videotape training exercises. This organization has both FDA safety alerts and ISMP hazard alerts posted on its Web site.

Chapter Terms

assumption error error that occurs when an essential piece of information cannot be verified and is guessed or presumed

capture error error that occurs when focus on a task is diverted elsewhere, and therefore the error goes undetected

extra dose error error in which more doses are received by a patient than were prescribed by the physician

human failure error generated by failure that occurs at an individual level

medical error any circumstance, action, inaction, or decision related to healthcare that contributes to an unintended health result

medication errors medical errors in which the source of error or harm includes a medication

MEDMARX Internet-based program for use by hospitals and healthcare systems for documenting, tracking, and trending medication errors

MedWatch FDA reporting system for adverse events resulting from medications and medical devices

omission error error in which a prescribed dose is not given

organizational failure errors generated by failure because of organizational rules, policies, or procedures

root cause analysis logical and systematic process used to help identify what, how, and why something happened to prevent recurrence

selection error error that occurs when two or more options exist and the wrong option is chosen

sentinel event unexpected occurrence involving death or serious physical or psychologic injury or the potential for occurrences to happen

technical failure error generated by failure because of location or equipment

wrong dose error error in which the dose is either above or below the correct dose by more than 5%

wrong dose form error error in which the dose form or formulation is not the accepted interpretation of the physician order

wrong time error medication error in which any drug is given 30 minutes or more before or after it was prescribed, up to the time of the next dose, not including as needed orders

Chapter Summary

- Pharmacy technicians play a crucial role in the prevention of medication errors.
- Knowing the potential causes and categories of medication errors is the first step toward preventing them from happening.
- Specific practices, careful work habits, and a clean work environment promote patient safety and decrease illness and injury caused by medication errors.
- Medication errors caused by patients have physical and social causes.
- Once errors are identified, corrective measures should be put in place and permanent elimination of the source of error should be the goal.
- Ensuring the integrity of medication is an important part of medication safety.
- Although pharmacy technicians cannot instruct patients concerning their medications, they can encourage them to ask questions of the pharmacist.
- Helping patients to become more informed will empower them to be advocates for their own safety and health.
- Several medication error reporting systems exist. Pharmacy personnel should be familiar with these sources and utilize them to confidentially report errors so that they do not occur again.

Chapter Review

Knowledge Inventory

Choose the best answer from those provided.

1. For every 250 prescriptions dispensed in a community pharmacy, how many will contain a medication error of some type?
   a. none
   b. 1
   c. 4
   d. 25

2. Which example is *not* a patient-caused medication error?
   a. The patient takes an antibiotic with meals when instructions say to take it on an empty stomach.
   b. The patient forgot an antibiotic dose yesterday, so he or she takes an extra dose today.
   c. The patient did not receive a sufficient quantity of antibiotic suspension from the pharmacy.
   d. The patient takes antibiotics left over from the last time he or she was sick.

3. A wrong dose error occurs when a dose is either above or below the correct dose by more than
   a. 1%.
   b. 3%.
   c. 5%.
   d. 8%.

4. A patient applied a heating pad to an area where he or she also applied a fentanyl patch, causing the patch to release all of the medication at once, resulting in an overdose. This is an example of
   a. a wrong dose error where the cause of failure is technical.
   b. a wrong dose form error where the cause of failure is human or patient-related.
   c. All of the above
   d. None of the above

5. Filling a prescription with Toprol when the drug requested was Toprol XL is an example of which type of error?
   a. assumption error
   b. selection error
   c. capture error
   d. None of the above

6. When receiving a new prescription, which of the following should a technician avoid doing?
    a. verify all drug information with the pharmacist, appropriate drug references, and/or the prescriber when handwriting is difficult to read;
    b. use a trailing zero when the dose written is for a whole number
    c. cross-check patient information on the written prescription with the patient
    d. verify that the patient has not experienced any new drug allergies and that all profile information is current and correct

7. Which of the following sources of information is useful to verify that the correct medication has been selected from the shelf to fill the prescription order?
    a. generic and/or brand names on drug container
    b. NDC number
    c. drug name on original prescription
    d. All of the above

8. Where can the patient find information regarding the most crucial aspects of administration and proper storage and handling of a medication?
    a. on the patient information handout
    b. on the original prescription
    c. on the auxiliary warning and caution labels
    d. by asking the pharmacist

9. At a minimum, patients and caregivers should understand 10 key pieces of information about their prescription. Which of the following pieces of information is *not* included in those 10 key pieces of information?
    a. the name of their medication
    b. best times to pick up the prescription
    c. where to store the medicine
    d. pill shape and color
    e. the names of all other medications

10. A sentinel event is
    a. an unexpected occurrence involving death or serious physical or psychologic injury or the potential for the occurrence to happen.
    b. an unexpected outcome as the result of a drug reaction or side effect.
    c. a computer program that looks out for medication errors in a hospital pharmacy.
    d. None of the above

Pharmacy in Practice

1. At a minimum, patients and caregivers should understand 10 key pieces of information about their prescription. Name five of those key pieces of information.

2. Table 12.1 outlines seven activities pharmacists can do to reduce errors. Choose one, and briefly describe how a pharmacy technician can support a pharmacist engaged in these activities to improve patient safety.

3. Using Appendix E, locate at least two pairs of drug names that are spelled similarly. Write a brief commentary on the differences between the drugs in each pair and what might happen if they were accidentally switched in the pharmacy and given to the patient. Would this mixup be life threatening?

Improving Communication Skills

1. Many times a patient may have a question but may hesitate to ask the nurse, pharmacist, or physician, because he or she is "so busy." Anytime a patient hesitates to ask a question or better understand his or her own condition, a chance to improve the patient's health or avoid an adverse event is lost. What could you do or say as a pharmacy technician to help the customer make the connection to the needed information?

2. Using Appendix E, locate at least two pairs of drug names that are sound-alike names when spoken out loud. Say them to a classmate across the room to see how easily they can be mistaken for each other. Repeat the exercise with other drug names and other students.

Internet Research

1. Choose a state and visit that state's board of pharmacy Web site. Review the state regulations, and identify the information that must be present on a prescription to be "valid" in that state.

2. Visit www.fda.gov/medwatch/index.html and prepare a summary of what is new in the last 2 weeks. How is a MedWatch report made? What information is contained in a MedWatch report?

3. Visit the Target "ClearRx" Web site at www.target.com/pharmacy and click "See what's new." Watch the video. What changes were made to improve Target medication vials? Discuss how these changes might improve patient safety.

Human Relations and Communications

Learning Objectives

- Explain the role of the pharmacy technician as a member of the customer care team in a pharmacy.
- State the primary rule of retail merchandising, and explain its corollaries.
- Provide guidelines for proper use of the telephone in a pharmacy.
- Explain the appropriate responses to rude behavior on the part of others in a workplace situation.
- Identify the importance of verbal and nonverbal communication skills.
- Define discrimination and harassment, and explain the proper procedures for dealing with these issues.
- Discuss the importance of protecting patient privacy in the pharmacy.
- Identify and discuss the important areas of the Health Insurance Portability and Accountability Act regulations.

In addition to being an important part of the healthcare system, the community pharmacy is also a place of business, and the technician must be sensitive to customer service responsibilities similar to those appropriate in any retail setting. A customer service approach is important in the hospital setting as well, especially when providing support and information to other healthcare providers. Examples of providing first-rate customer service are provided for both retail and hospital pharmacy settings. In all pharmacy practice settings, maintaining patient confidentiality and following federal legislation protecting patient privacy are crucially important.

PERSONAL SERVICE IN THE CONTEMPORARY PHARMACY

Since the Millis Report in 1975 and the Hepler-Strand Report of 1990, the pharmacy profession has undergone an extensive self-analysis and re-evaluation of its duties and goals (see Chapter 1). The upshot of this re-examination of the profession has been an increased emphasis on clinical pharmacy, or the provision of more information and counseling regarding medications. It is now almost universally recognized that the pharmacist is far more than a dispenser of drugs. The pharmacist has the following equally important duties:

- Identify any known allergies, drug interactions, or other contraindications for a given prescription.
- Make certain that a given medication will not be harmful to a patient given that patient's medical and prescription history.
- Ensure that a patient understands what medication he or she is taking, why he or she is taking it, how it should be taken, and when it should be taken.
- Triage self-limited illnesses and recommend appropriate over-the-counter (OTC) or diet supplements to the patient.

Just as the pharmacist increasingly plays a clinical role, so the pharmacy technician increasingly is expected to be much more than simply a cash register operator, a stock person, and an all-around pharmacy "gofer." Today the technician is viewed as an important part of the customer service team within the pharmacy.

In the 1960s and 1970s, at the height of the era of mass merchandising, customers grew used to large, impersonal supermarkets, department stores, and pharmacy superstores, with their numbered rows of merchandise and automated, bar-coded checkout stations. In the 1980s, retail merchandisers began to realize that the mass-merchandising model adopted in the 1960s was terribly flawed. Customers missed the days of personal service (i.e., attending to the individual customer's needs) associated with the small, independent, neighborhood pharmacy of the past, where everyone affectionately called the pharmacist "Doc."

For this reason, many of the large department store chains reorganized their operations to create separate small operational entities, known as *boutiques*, within their larger stores. They also began extensive training programs to improve the quality of customer service. In pharmacy, as well, a new and welcome emphasis on personal service has returned.

One mass marketing research firm conducted an experiment involving bank tellers. In the experiment, one group of tellers was instructed to lightly touch customers on the hand or wrist at some point during each teller transaction. A second control group was instructed to carry out transactions as usual, without this "personal touch." Exit surveys of customer satisfaction were then conducted, with dramatic results. Although largely unaware that they had been touched during their teller transactions, those customers who had been touched reported a 40% higher satisfaction rate with the overall quality of service of their banks. The lesson to be learned from this research is not that one should make a habit of touching customers; indeed, touching should probably be avoided in most cases. However, a little personal attention goes a long way. A courteous tone of voice, a smile, eye contact, a listening ear, and a bit of assistance finding merchandise or holding a door can go a long way toward making customers think of the pharmacy in which you work as a pleasant place in which to do business.

Attitude and Appearance

Attitude is the overall emotional stance a worker adopts toward his or her job duties, customers, employer, and coworkers. **Appearance** is the overall look an employee has on the job, including dress and grooming. Pharmacy technicians often conduct their jobs unobtrusively (i.e., behind the scenes), stocking items in the pharmacy area, retrieving stock for compounding operations, maintaining records, filling bottles, and cleaning. Even if the immediate task is not customer-oriented, the technician should remember the primary rule of retail merchandising:

> *At all times you are representing your company to the patient or customer. Remember that in a pharmacy you are, in a legal sense, an agent of your employer and entering into a contract to provide care to the patient. Your employer must "answer" for all of your actions.*

This rule has a number of corollaries, and these are presented in the following sections.

Appear Professional Customers hope for the highest degree of cleanliness and professionalism from their pharmacy. After all, they are entrusting their health or the health of their loved ones to the operation for which you work. A pharmacy employee with unkempt hair or a uniform smock thrown over a pair of jeans makes a bad impression. The customer may not directly register these facts and yet goes away with a vague impression that the pharmacy is not a professional operation. You should wear

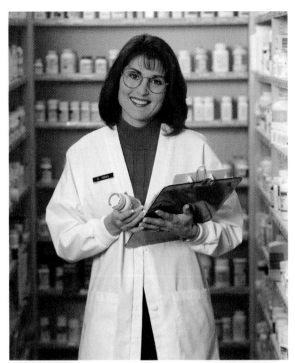
A pharmacy technician should always be well groomed, neat, and professional looking while working in the pharmacy.

a clean lab coat and nametag at all times. This sets the desired professional atmosphere and immediately identifies you as an employee of the pharmacy. However, the technician must follow the dress code of the pharmacy. The dress code may be crisp and professional or more relaxed and casual.

Respond to Customers Modern community pharmacies are often large, complex places. When customers enter, the first thing they often do is stand in the middle of the floor, looking around for the part of the store where the product they seek is to be found. A good pharmacy employee thus continually scans the area around him or her, looking for customers who are lost, confused, or need help. In the hospital setting, your customer may be a physician, a nurse, or another hospital worker who needs your help.

A pharmacy technician must be observant of customer needs. Often a customer will be reluctant to ask for help to avoid imposing on the technician or pharmacist's time. It is important to **triage** customer needs in everyday practice, by sorting requests or needs and ranking them by the priority of their needs. This triage is sometimes as simple as responding to customer requests in order of their arrival at the pharmacy. In the community pharmacy, many things may be happening at once: you are cashiering a sale, the phone is ringing, a customer is waiting for help in the over-the-counter (OTC) aisle, and you have five patients waiting to pick up their prescriptions. Try to acknowledge the customers by a simple statement, such as, "I will be right with you." Then when attending to their needs you might say something like, "Thank you for waiting." Keeping your eye on the customer and meeting his or her needs applies to any retail operation. However, in other situations, such as a stat order in the hospital pharmacy, the order of requests needs to be ignored in response to a more urgent medical situation.

Know Your Pharmacy Few things are as frustrating to a customer as asking for help and getting an insufficient or inaccurate response. Often a customer is uncertain about what he or she is looking for or whom to ask for help. Once you spot that uncertain look, ask courteously, "May I help you?" Then, after the customer's response, you may have to ask some clarifying questions. If, for example, the customer is looking for aspirin, then he or she may need to know not only where OTC analgesic products are stocked in the store but also where to locate a specific analgesic (e.g., baby aspirin, aspirin for a migraine, liquid form for children, an enteric-coated form for persons whose stomachs cannot tolerate conventional analgesic dose forms). If possible, escort the customer to the place where the merchandise is located, and help him or her to find it.

In other cases the customer may want to know whether to take aspirin or another OTC analgesic like ibuprofen; he or she may ask whether it is acceptable to take ibuprofen with blood pressure medication. The pharmacy technician can triage or sort out different requests by the customer. Those involving product location, availability, or price can be handled by the technician. In any case involving professional judgment, you may say to the customer, "That is a good question; let me have you speak with the pharmacist."

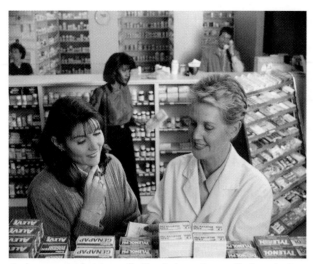
A pharmacy technician will often help customers find products in the retail pharmacy.

Smile and Make Eye Contact The goodwill you communicate will come back to you. Making a personal connection with the customer is very important. Learning and greeting patients by name is very important in community pharmacy. Patients are far more likely to return to a pharmacy where they have received personal attention than to one where they have not. Some pharmacists have learned sign language so that they can communicate with patients who are hearing impaired without the need of an interpreter or the chance of misreading lips.

Eye contact is especially important to older patients and patients who may be deaf or hard of hearing. A person who is hard of hearing learns to informally "read lips" to supplement the voice that he or she hears. If you speak with your head turned away, then the person may hear you but not be able to fully interpret what you have said. Remembering to make eye contact will ensure you are looking directly at the person. In addition, older generations of Americans often associate eye contact with honesty, sincerity, and respect.

Use Common Courtesies In every interaction with a customer, use courteous words and phrases. Begin and end interactions, even the briefest ones, with ceremonial courtesies such as, "Good afternoon" and "Have a nice day." "Please" and "Thank you" should become a part of your regular vocabulary. In between, practice courteous speech, as demonstrated in these examples:

> Poor: What do you want?
> Better: May I help you?
> Poor: It's over there.
> Better: That's in aisle three. Follow me, and I'll show you.
> Poor: It's $8.39.
> Better: That will be $8.39 please.
> Poor: Next?
> Better: May I help whoever is next? or Hello, Mr. Ray. Are you here to pick up a refill?

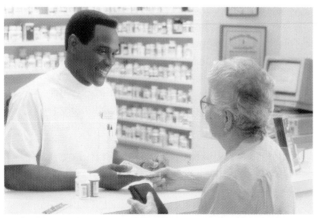
A pharmacy technician should maintain good eye contact and pleasant attitude while talking, with the patient.

Be Sensitive to Cultural and Language Differences Often pharmacies are located in areas catering to a diverse customer base. If you cannot understand a customer because of a language difference, then do not speak louder or in an exaggeratedly slow and punctuated manner. Simply enunciate your words and avoid using slang terms or abbreviations, because the person may not be familiar with them. Apologize courteously for your language deficiency if necessary, and find another store employee who can communicate in the customer's native tongue. If a translator is not available, then the pharmacist may have available some simple counseling sheets that use

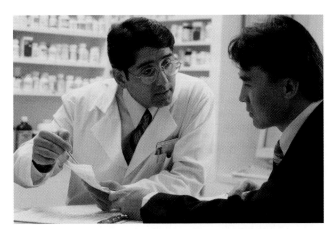
Pharmacy technicians will need to be able to assist customers from other cultural groups.

drawings, diagrams, and clocks made especially for this purpose. Some computer software programs print patient information in different languages.

Cultural differences should also be taken into account. If the pharmacy where you are employed has a large group of patients from a particular culture, then you should make an effort to become familiar with that culture's diet, health habits, beliefs, and courtesies. Knowing more about the culture will help you to provide higher-quality service and will show customers that you care about them.

Follow Policies and Procedures Many pharmacies, especially within large retail chains, have a **policy and procedure manual** covering a wide range of activities including technician responsibilities in customer care. A policy and procedure manual outlines all activities in the pharmacy; the larger the pharmacy and the more complex the organization, the more important it is for each employee to follow departmental guidelines.

Make sure you are thoroughly familiar with these guidelines and abide by them in your routine interactions. Deviations from these written procedures could have adverse consequences in a legal case in which a medication error occurred. Individual pharmacists also have preferences about how prescriptions are prepared and dispensed under their guidance; although not written, these guidelines will be learned and followed as you are trained in a particular pharmacy.

Do Not Dispense Medical or Pharmaceutical Advice Remember that you are not trained or licensed to advise customers with regard to medications and their use. Use common sense to determine whether a given query from a customer exceeds the bounds of common knowledge. As a rule of thumb you should refer to a pharmacist any questions involving the proper administration, uses, or effects of a medication, whether prescription, OTC, or diet supplement, as well as any questions that require a professional "opinion or judgment."

Do not be afraid of admitting your lack of expertise. Customers will appreciate that you are concerned enough to make sure they receive accurate information. When a question deals with the effects or administration of a medication, ask the customer to wait for a moment while you get someone who can provide a professional answer to the question. In some instances technicians may provide medication-related information when providing refills and when directed to do so by a pharmacist.

Of course, a technician should use common sense with regard to providing customers with information. In the case of OTC medications, sometimes customers simply need basic information that is readily available on the OTC packaging. For example, a customer might ask what an analgesic is, when an enteric-coated analgesic is appropriate, which alternative brands are available, and other routine questions that can be safely answered without referring the customer to the pharmacist.

Customers will also arrive at the pharmacy and speak or inquire about physicians, specialists, and other healthcare professionals. General information may be given, but opinions on the competence of a particular physician or healthcare provider should not be given out by anyone in the pharmacy. You should at all times avoid making disparaging comments about other healthcare providers. If such comments are made, and the person's professional reputation is questioned, then the person may sue you for slander.

Safety Note
Do not provide medical advice. Direct such questions to the pharmacist.

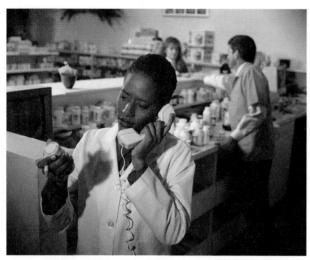
Pharmacy technicians need to be able to communicate effectively over the phone, to both customers and healthcare professionals.

Telephone Courtesies

Customers and healthcare professionals often contact pharmacies by telephone. The following are some guidelines for using the telephone properly:

- When you answer the phone, identify yourself and the pharmacy, as follows: "Good morning. This is Ball Ground Pharmacy. My name is Tracy. How may I help you?"
- Always begin and end the conversation with a conventional courtesy, such as "Good morning" and "Thank you for calling." Stay alert to what the caller is saying and use a natural, conversational voice. You should be friendly but not too familiar with the caller. When speaking to patients who are hard of hearing, speak clearly, pronounce each word distinctly, and be prepared to repeat yourself.
- If the caller is calling in a new prescription, you may need to turn over the phone to a licensed pharmacist. In most states technicians are not allowed by law to take prescriptions over the telephone. However, you should learn the regulations for the state in which you are employed.
- If the caller has questions about the administration or effects of a medication or about a medical condition, adverse reaction, or drug interaction, place the customer on hold and refer the call to a licensed pharmacist.
- Make sure that any information you provide is accurate. Giving incorrect directions to a customer in need of a prescription can be a life-threatening mistake.
- Depending on the regulations in your state and the procedures of your pharmacy, you may be authorized to handle prescription transfers or to provide information related to prescription refills. Follow the procedures outlined by your supervising pharmacist.
- If a customer is calling about a medical emergency or a prescription error, then refer the call to your supervising pharmacist.

Interprofessionalism

In the course of their duties, pharmacy technicians encounter, personally or on the telephone, many other professionals and paraprofessionals, including pharmacists, physicians, nurses, administrators, store managers, sales representatives, insurance personnel, and other technicians. Healthcare is a demanding industry, often requiring long hours and involving stressful, emergency situations. As a result, practitioners in the industry often suffer from fatigue and stress. Sometimes this stress

Pharmacy technicians should always approach the supervisory pharmacist with respect.

shows itself in unintentionally rude behavior. Rarely, it may present as abuse of alcohol or prescription drugs.

Busy healthcare professionals sometimes, unfortunately, speak to subordinates in an inappropriate and nonprofessional manner. Remember that the degree to which you maintain your courtesy and respect, even in the face of rudeness, is a measure of your professionalism. Return rudeness with kindness, and you will often find that, immediately or over time, the quality of your interactions will improve. If you answer the telephone and someone barks a command at you, then demonstrate your professionalism by attending to the content of the message and not to its tone.

Always refer to physicians, chiropractors, osteopathic professionals, and dentists using the title "Doctor." In the presence of patients refer to the pharmacist as "Doctor" if he or she has achieved a Doctor of Pharmacy degree. Some states have designated all pharmacists as "doctors" in recognition of their professional experience. Refer to other supervisors using appropriate courtesy titles such as "Sir," "Madam," or "Ma'am." When the technician refers to the pharmacist as "Doctor," this raises the level of customer respect not only for the pharmacist but also for the technician, who is the doctor's assistant. A degree of formality is always in order until you are requested to use more informal modes of address in day-to-day operations.

OTHER ASPECTS OF PROFESSIONALISM

Other aspects of professionalism include appropriate behavior, verbal and nonverbal communication, and conflict resolution.

Professional Behavior

Healthcare professionals of all levels are expected to abide by both written laws and ethical guidelines. **Decorum** means proper or polite behavior or that which is in good taste in the pharmacy workplace. Arguing with your supervisor in public would be an example of inappropriate decorum. Another set of unwritten rules to be followed is often referred to as **etiquette**. Etiquette is difficult to describe and is often recognized most easily when it is not being followed. For example, being disrespectful to a physician would be an obvious violation of etiquette.

Respect should be shown to all who work in a healthcare facility, because each person has an important job to do that contributes to the overall healthcare provided to the patient. However, additional respect should be shown to those with a high level of medical training and those responsible for managing the facility where you are employed. Personal relationships with coworkers or pharmacists are also discouraged in most practice settings.

Personal telephone calls and visits should be made only during breaks. Telling ethnic or off-color jokes and making disparaging comments about others is not acceptable. When in doubt as to what the expected behavior is in a situation, it is best to be quiet, watch, learn from someone else in the pharmacy that is a suitable model, and perform your assigned task.

A more experienced pharmacy technician may act as a mentor for a new technician.

Verbal and Nonverbal Communication

Communicating effectively takes practice. Once you have the knowledge and vocabulary needed to function effectively in the pharmacy, you will acquire verbal communication skills with time. Model yourself after someone whom you admire, but keep in mind that some of your coworkers have a different role and thus different communication needs and styles. Verbal communication skills take practice, and pronouncing medical terms and drug names is one hurdle that you can overcome with study. Listening and asking a coworker to pronounce words for you are the best ways to learn. Repeat difficult words to yourself several times. You may also find it helpful to keep a pocket-sized reference on drug names handy and make notes in it regarding pronunciation and usage.

A pharmacy technician needs good verbal communication skills in the receipt of prescriptions and also when assisting the patient for an OTC medication. The technician performs a valuable service by gathering information and relaying this information to the pharmacist. Asking **open-ended questions** to the patient such as, "Please describe your headache pain for me" is more preferable. **Closed questions** are asked in a yes-or-no format such as, "Do you have a headache?" or "Have you tried aspirin?" An open-ended question allows the patient to share more information about his or her illness and is more helpful to the pharmacist in recommending the best treatment.

Nonverbal communication is easy to understand, and one needs only to pay attention to the other party to interpret what is being conveyed. From the time we are small children we learn how to interpret nonverbal communication. Facial expression, eye contact, body position, and tone of voice are all methods of communicating without using words. Mannerisms and gestures often indicate agreement or disagreement. The mood of the other party can often be determined through nonverbal communication. Although each individual is unique and may exhibit unusual habits with certain moods, many generalizations can be made regarding nonverbal communication. Simple observation and listening can be a very effective way to supplement the verbal portion of what you are hearing.

The following examples demonstrate nonverbal communication in the pharmacy.

Poor: Talking to a patient while filling a prescription or answering the phone.

Better: Ask the patient to wait a moment, complete filling the prescription or place the telephone caller on hold (or have another staff member take the call), and go down to the front counter or private counseling area and talk to the patient. Determine if you can help the patient or direct the patient to speak with the pharmacist if necessary.

Poor: Showing surprise through open-mouth facial expressions when a patient shares a diagnosis with you (e.g. HIV, gonorrhea, syphilis, or depression).

Better: Be nonjudgmental with minimal facial expressions and try to assist the patient with the information or products he or she needs. Be empathetic and show genuine concern. Remember all patient medical information is confidential and protected by law.

Poor: Talking to a patient about an OTC recommendation with arms crossed some distance from the patient.

Better: Move closer to the patient, ask open-ended questions, listen carefully, and be aware of both your body movements and those of the patient. Crossed-arms often convey some barrier to communication, such as you are too busy to help the patient.

Safety Note

All patient medical information is confidential and protected by law.

The flip side of verbal communication is, of course, listening. Listening to the words and the voice that you are hearing is important. You should maintain eye contact with the person speaking and send the speaker nonverbal signals to indicate that you are genuinely interested in what he or she is saying. Learn to tolerate your own silence. Ask questions to clarify issues and repeat portions of the conversation to confirm that you have correctly heard what was said. Always use a nonjudgmental expression and tone of voice. Never let the patient feel that he or she is imposing or that your time is more valuable than the patient's.

Discrimination and Harassment

As with any job, you should bear in mind that **discrimination** (i.e., preferential treatment or mistreatment) and **harassment** (i.e., mistreatment, sexual or otherwise) are not only unethical but also against the law. Generally speaking, a romantic or sexual involvement with coworkers, and especially with coworkers in supervisory or subordinate positions, is inadvisable.

If you find yourself the object of discrimination or harassment, then first try to resolve the issue with the person or persons involved. Do your best to maintain your composure and to express your discomfort calmly and rationally. If discrimination or harassment persists, then you may need to discuss the matter with a supervisor. If unsuccessful, make inquiries regarding the discrimination and harassment laws and procedures in your state as a last resort.

The law requires all businesses, pharmacies included, to post information related to workplace discrimination and harassment. Bear in mind that in the past, sexual harassment was defined as unwanted physical contact or as the act of making sexual conduct a condition for advancement, preferential treatment, or other work-related outcomes. Recently, however, the Supreme Court redefined sexual harassment more generally as the creation of an unpleasant or uncomfortable work environment through sexual action, innuendo, or related means. Therefore know that you do not have to put up with off-color jokes if you do not wish to hear them, and be aware that you must not contribute in any way to creating an environment that is uncomfortable for your coworkers. One person's innocent remark, made in a spirit of fun, can be another person's grounds for a legal action.

Disputes involving duties, hours, pay, and other matters are common occurrences in occupations of all kinds. Try to resolve work-related disputes through rational, calm, private discussion with the parties involved. If you are seeking a raise in pay, then prepare for the meeting by outlining your accomplishments; most pharmacies invest a significant amount of time in training a pharmacy technician and would not want to lose such a valuable employee. Most large pharmacies, including chain stores and hospital pharmacies, will have personnel policy manuals detailing procedures for resolving disputes.

PATIENT CONFIDENTIALITY

In our electronic age all health professionals must understand the importance of maintaining patient confidentiality. If a patient cannot trust the pharmacist or pharmacy technician with medical information, then both trust and a good customer may be lost. A pharmacy technician may be discussing sensitive medical issues with a patient in the course of trying to help identify or locate a product in the pharmacy. A patient may request a private conversation with a pharmacist to discuss a medical issue. Finally, this section will discuss the effect of some of the Health Insurance

Portability and Accountability Act (HIPAA) regulations on pharmacy. Maintaining patient confidentiality must remain a very high priority for the pharmacy technician.

Respect the Customer's Privacy

Pharmacies sell many products related to private bodily functions and conditions (e.g., condoms and other contraceptives, feminine hygiene and menstrual products, suppositories, hemorrhoid remedies, enemas, adult diapers, catheters, bed pans, scabicides). Often customers find asking about such products embarrassing and have to get up the nerve to request assistance. If you find discussing such matters embarrassing, then you will need to overcome your reservations quickly.

As a pharmacy employee, you are part of the healthcare profession and must adopt a helpful, no-nonsense, professional attitude toward the body and its functions. Responding to an inquiry about such a product with promptness, courtesy, respect, and a certain degree of nonchalance often relieves your customer's embarrassment and demonstrates your professionalism. Speak in a clear voice but not so loudly that other customers or employees will be privy to your private exchange with the customer.

In addition, often a patient's illness can be determined by his or her medication history. A patient receiving antiviral prescriptions for human immunodeficiency virus (HIV), or antibiotics for gonorrhea, or antidepressants for depression, or chemotherapy for cancer requires the same amount of privacy as in a physician's office. This information cannot even be shared with a family member without the expressed written permission of the patient. You would not want information on your health to be made public. Violations of confidentiality of medical information can have serious legal ramifications (see following section) and can potentially cost you your job and career as a technician.

A patient has the right to expect medical information will be kept confidential. Pharmacies will have policy statements that define patient privacy rights and how patient information will be used and protected by the pharmacy. These policy statements should be explained to all new pharmacy customers at the time that they first visit the pharmacy. Pharmacies also ask customers to sign an information sheet that

Figure 13.1

New Customer Information Form

Pharmacy New Customer Information
Confidential

Name: _____

Date of Birth: _____

Address: _____

City: _____ State: _____ ZIP code: _____

Phone Numbers

Home: _____ Work: _____ Cell: _____

Drug Allergies: _____

Food Allergies: _____

I declare all of the above information to be accurate to the best of my knowledge. The signature below also gives this pharmacy permission to contact my physician and/or healthcare provider regarding my care. I also certify that this pharmacy has informed me of its privacy policy.

Signature: _____ Date: _____

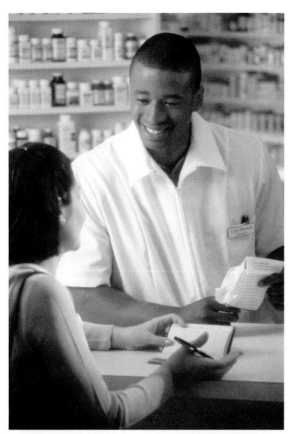

The pharmacy technician should make every effort to make the customer comfortable. This includes maintaining customer privacy by appropriately bagging medications and other purchases.

gives important information about the patient and also ensures that the patient has been informed of the pharmacy's privacy policy. Figure 13.1 is an example of this information form.

Privacy should be maintained as you update customer information. If, for example, you are stationed at the pharmacy window and need information for the customer's patient profile, then let the customer know why you need the information. Tell the customer, for example, "I need some information for your prescription profile so that we can better serve you. May I ask you a few questions? Thank you. What is your full name and address?" You may also need to verify insurance information; most customers are accustomed to presenting a card or proof of insurance regularly at the physician's office and will not be upset once the procedure is explained.

When a patient is picking up a prescription, confirm his or her identity and what he or she is picking up. Keep your tone of voice low so as not to broadcast to nearby customers what the patient is receiving. Many pharmacies now have a private counseling area for prescription pickup, where the patient can have a higher degree of privacy.

Health Insurance Portability and Accountability Act

Privacy of the patient's medical record and information regarding medical conditions and prescriptions is also an important legal issue. Both state and federal law govern patient confidentiality. Generally where conflict exists, the law that is the most stringent is the one that should be followed. It would be worthwhile for the pharmacy technician to know the laws in the state where he or she is practicing; if the technician moves to another state, then the regulations and laws may change. Many states have specific laws protecting patients with HIV or acquired immunodeficiency syndrome (AIDS).

As was introduced in Chapter 2, the Health Insurance Portability and Accountability Act (HIPAA) is a comprehensive federal law passed in 1996. All healthcare facilities (including pharmacies in all practice settings) that access, store, maintain, or transmit patient identifiable medical information must comply with these regulations. Failure to do so can result in severe civil and criminal penalties. Although HIPAA covers many areas, the following are those that are related to security and patient confidentiality.

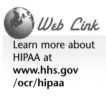

Web Link

Learn more about HIPAA at **www.hhs.gov /ocr/hipaa**

Privacy and Security As discussed earlier in this chapter, maintaining the privacy and security of health information is extremely important. Who should have access to what information internally or outside the pharmacy? A good example would be a high school teenager receiving birth control pills from the family planning clinic; that information cannot be shared with her parents or anyone else without her permission.

How can unnecessary access to patient health information be limited, especially in large organizations such as hospitals, chain pharmacies, research sponsors, or insurance providers? In the course of diagnosing or treating the patient, the physician and pharmacist may exchange information without restriction or expressed written permission of the patient. However, if a retail pharmacist wanted a copy of a recent hospital discharge summary, or a copy of the patient's most recent laboratory results, then written permission by the patient may need to be obtained. Most pharmacies will try to have written documentation that patients have read and understood the store policy.

Other examples of situations in which some but not all health information is shared are investigational drug studies and communications between a patient's insurance provider and his or her employer. How much information about the patient does the sponsor (often a pharmaceutical company) of an investigational drug study need to know? In nearly all cases, studies must be designed so that patients cannot be identified. An insurance company processing a prescription reimbursement has the right to know which drug and dose were dispensed, but it may not be necessary to share that information with the patient's employer. In the past there were occasional instances where an insurance company shared medical information with an employer, resulting in employee job termination. No such information is shared with the employer under HIPAA today.

Each pharmacy can develop its own mechanism to implement, communicate, audit, and document compliance with HIPAA regulations. Depending on the size of the pharmacy (i.e., independent, chain, hospital), formal training programs with annual refresher courses may be used. A prerecorded educational program may be an alternative. Each pharmacy should have a set of policy and procedures in its manual to cover the HIPAA regulations. A breach of confidentiality is often a sufficient reason for immediate termination, so it behooves the technician to know and understand the policy. To protect the pharmacy's interests, patients may be asked to document that they have read and understood the pharmacy's privacy statement called a *notice of privacy practices*.

Patient Identifiers A common term used in HIPAA is **protected health information (PHI)**. Personal health information must be protected from unauthorized use and access. Obviously a physician, nurse, pharmacist, and pharmacy technician have access to medical information to serve the needs of the patient. A pharmacy technician, for example, may be able to determine a medical diagnosis from the medications that are dispensed in the pharmacy (e.g., a patient receiving combination antiretroviral therapy most likely has an HIV infection). All health professionals are bound by law and ethics not to disclose this information outside of the workplace.

To be in compliance, any information that can identify the patient must be removed or concealed from view. **Patient identifiers** are defined as any information that could identify the patient. Examples of patient identifiers are listed in Table 13.1.

In the pharmacy, shredding all patient-related information rather than simply discarding it in the trash is common practice. Even used prescription vials with patient-labeled information must be discarded appropriately (i.e., *black out* the patient name with a marking pen, or peel the label from the vial and discard). Investigational drug studies collate medical data such that PHI remain confidential. As a technician, be extra vigilant and sensitive to maintaining patient confidentiality. In addition, you must be sure to understand the policy and procedures of your pharmacy. If you see potential violations, bring them to the attention of your pharmacist supervisor.

Table 13.1   Patient Identifiers

name
address and ZIP code
relatives
employer
date of birth
telephone number or fax number
e-mail address
social security number
medical record number
health plan identification number
account number
vehicle identification
certificate or license number
uniform resource locater (URL) or Internet protocol (IP) address
fingerprint or voiceprint
photo

Electronic Data Transactions   HIPAA sets standards for the electronic submission of patient medical information and provides safeguards to protect the confidentiality of patient information. Access to some medical information (or fields of information) may be restricted to certain healthcare professionals. Frequent password renaming and resets are another way to limit access. The Internet is usually not a completely secure place to transmit electronic information; therefore you should avoid sending e-mails containing patient information or identifiers (see Table 13.1) on the subject line.

The electronic transmission of medical and insurance information improves the revenue of a community pharmacy (more prescriptions can be dispensed, more rapid reimbursement, fewer claims rejections), contains cost (fewer personnel needed for billing claims), and provides better patient care (more time to review patient profile and counsel patient). The efficiencies of transmitting medical information electronically must be balanced against the need to maintain patient confidentiality.

Many examples exist of electronic transmission of data in the pharmacy. Almost every third-party insurance transaction involves the electronic submission of data with immediate on-line adjudication (as discussed in Chapter 7). A fax request for refill authorization to the physician's office is a common practice. Electronic prescriptions from handheld personal digital assistants (PDAs) may replace written prescriptions in the near future.

Chapter Terms

appearance physical look an employee has on the job, including dress and grooming

attitude disposition a worker adopts toward his or her job duties, customers, employer, and coworkers

closed questions questions that require a yes or no answer

decorum behavior that is in good taste

discrimination preferential treatment or mistreatment

etiquette unwritten rules of behavior

harassment mistreatment, sexual or otherwise

nonverbal communication communication without words through facial expression, body contact, body position, and tone of voice

open-ended questions questions that require a descriptive answer, not yes or no

patient identifiers any demographic information that can identify the patient such as name, address, phone number, social security number, or medical identification number

policy and procedure manual book that outlines activities in the pharmacy, defines the roles of individuals, and lists guidelines

protected health information (PHI) medical information that is protected by HIPAA such as medical diagnoses, medication profiles, and results of laboratory tests

triage ranking of patients for treatment or customer care by the priority of their needs

Chapter Summary

- Community pharmacies are returning to the concept of the small, customer-oriented neighborhood pharmacy of the past.
- Increased emphasis on personal service (i.e., attention to the needs of individual customers) requires the technician to consider carefully all interactions with pharmacy customers.
- Customer orientation involves dressing and grooming oneself neatly, maintaining a constant lookout for customers in need of assistance, knowing the layout of the store and the location of its merchandise, smiling and using courteous language, providing explanations as necessary to customers, being sensitive to language differences, following established policies and procedures, and referring requests for medical or pharmaceutical advice to competent professionals.
- Common courtesy should be used in all telephone communications and conversations with both patients and healthcare professionals.
- A request for information about adverse effects and drug interactions should always be referred to a supervising pharmacist.
- A no-tolerance policy exists with regard to discrimination and harassment in the pharmacy workplace.
- A pharmacy technician must be sensitive to maintaining patient privacy, confidentiality of medical information, and compliance with all state and federal HIPAA regulations.

Chapter Review

Knowledge Inventory

Choose the best answer from those provided.

1. In the 1980s, retail merchandisers began to rethink their previous
    a. personal service-merchandising model.
    b. mass-merchandising model.
    c. customer service model.
    d. retail service model.

2. The emotional stance that a worker adopts toward his or her job duties is called
    a. tone.
    b. mood.
    c. attitude.
    d. appearance.

3. Which of the following is the primary rule of retail merchandising?
    a. Always dress and groom yourself neatly.
    b. Respect the customer's privacy.
    c. Explain necessary interactions to the customer.
    d. At all times you are representing your company to the customer.

4. Decorum means
    a. proper or polite behavior, or behavior that is in good taste.
    b. dissatisfaction with services provided.
    c. lack of understanding of the options available.
    d. ability to negotiate for goods and services.

5. A pharmacy technician should never
    a. waste time walking a customer across the store to show him or her the location of an item on the shelves.
    b. dispense advice regarding the use of a medication.
    c. attempt to speak to a customer in the customer's native language.
    d. take a written prescription from a customer.

6. When asking a customer for information for the patient profile, the pharmacy technician should explain
    a. how and when the prescription should be administered.
    b. why the pharmacy needs this information.
    c. the parts of the label of the prescription.
    d. the differences between the payment policies of various third-party insurance providers.

7. Preferential treatment or mistreatment based on race, gender, age, or other criteria is known as
    a. harassment.
    b. discrimination.
    c. innuendo.
    d. decorum.

8. When answering a drugstore telephone, a person should identify himself or herself and the name of the
    a. supervising pharmacist.
    b. pharmacy.
    c. customer.
    d. prescribing physician.

9. An underage teen is on a birth control pill. All of the following can review this medical information at the pharmacy *except* the
    a. parent.
    b. physician.
    c. pharmacist.
    d. teen.

10. HIPAA involves all the following *except*
    a. medication profile.
    b. medical diagnoses.
    c. insurance provider.
    d. laboratory results.

Pharmacy in Practice

1. Working in a small group, recall your own experiences visiting drugstores or pharmacies. Make a list of problems you have encountered in pharmacies (e.g., slow service, lack of a comfortable place in which to wait while a prescription was being filled, difficulty in finding an item). As a group, brainstorm some ways to solve such problems and to improve customer service.

2. Imagine you are a drugstore manager who operates a 24-hour pharmacy in a big-city, urban neighborhood with the following demographics:
    10% Vietnamese-speaking customers
    26% Spanish-speaking customers
    16% Korean-speaking customers
    32% English-speaking customers
    16% customers who speak other languages (e.g., Thai, Laotian, Hmong, Russian, Latvian, Polish)

    With other students, brainstorm a list of steps you might need to take to meet the needs of the customers whom you serve.

3. With other students in a small group, brainstorm a list of positive experiences you have had in retail merchandising establishments of all kinds. Using this list, draw up a list of recommendations for making a customer's experience in a pharmacy retail establishment a positive one.

Improving Communication Skills

1. As a class, identify four students to play the following roles: a customer, a physician, a pharmacy technician, and a supervising pharmacist. Have them act out some typical telephone calls to the pharmacy, including a customer calling to find out when a prescription will be ready, a physician calling in a prescription, a customer asking medical advice, a customer asking for signs of an overdose, and a customer with a complaint. After each call critique what was said and done by the technician taking the telephone call.

2. Conduct the following role-play activities with other students: (1) a male who is obviously embarrassed asks a female technician for information on condoms; (2) a female who is embarrassed asks a male technician for information on feminine hygiene products. Perform other scenarios with other products until each student has played a role. After each scenario is played out, critique the technician's response. Discuss the kinds of problems that can arise in such situations and how they might be avoided.

3. Tone of voice can communicate many different types of feelings. Consider how you would say the following sentences out loud to communicate the feeling in parentheses.
   a. I love my job.   (Nobody else may love it, but I do.)
   b. I love my job.   (I more than like my job—I love it.)
   c. I love my job.   (I may not like anything else, but I love my job.)
   d. I love my job.   (I don't like my boss, but I like my job.)
   e. I love my job.   (You have got to be kidding!)

   Try repeating the sentence using your own feelings, and see if your classmates can interpret your true feelings about your job. Ask yourself if you know how you sound.

4. The culture of the United States is changing constantly and becoming more diversified. Patients are often influenced by a wide variety of factors in their culture, religion, and community. Explain in writing why it is important for a pharmacist and the pharmacy employees to get to know individual patients, their families, and their cultural beliefs. Include three examples or case illustrations in your explanation.

Internet Research

1. Visit the Keirsey Web site at www.keirsey.com, register (free), and take the Temperament Sorter II self-evaluation test.
   a. What type person are you?
   b. Were the descriptions of your personality type accurate?
   c. How will knowing your own type and the type of your coworkers assist your communication skills?
   d. Which personality types do you communicate with easily, and which are more difficult for you?

2. Do an Internet search to identify the laws of your state relating to patient confidentiality of medical information and how they affect community pharmacy practice. How do they differ from HIPAA? Are they more or less stringent than HIPAA?

Your Future in Pharmacy Practice

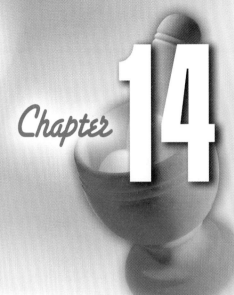

Chapter 14

Learning Objectives

- Describe the format and content of the Pharmacy Technician Certification Examination.
- Explain the criteria for recertification for pharmacy technicians.
- Discuss the major principles of the Code of Ethics of the American Association of Pharmacy Technicians.
- Identify a variety of strategies for successful adaptation to the work environment.
- Make a plan for a successful job search.
- Write a résumé and a cover letter.
- Prepare for and successfully complete an interview.
- Discuss some trends for the future of the pharmacy profession and their impact on pharmacy technicians.

The past 30 years have seen dramatic changes in the pharmacy profession, especially as the role of the technician expands and becomes integral to practice. Exciting changes are afoot, including a movement toward national certification and more formalized training and education of pharmacy technicians. Increasingly, technicians are finding more opportunities for placement in new roles and responsibilities. This chapter presents useful information on these trends and provides skills to prepare you for becoming a pharmacy technician.

INCREASING YOUR EMPLOYABILITY

As you have learned in previous chapters, the pharmacy technician career field continues to undergo dramatic changes. Throughout the country, pharmacy technicians are gaining recognition for the vital role they play in providing a wide range of pharmaceutical services in various employment settings. The occupational outlook for the pharmacy paraprofessional is quite bright. In many parts of the country, technicians are now receiving official recognition from state boards of pharmacy and are usually required to register with the state. Registration means that individuals working in a pharmacy as a technician must submit information on where they live and work to the state board of pharmacy. This process allows state boards to track technician employment, especially when drug diversion or illegal activity is suspected.

At least half of states recognize national certification (Figure 14.1). Some, like Texas, require certification to work as a technician in that state. Others recognize it through their state regulations in some way. For instance, Colorado pharmacies may use a higher technician-to-pharmacist ratio if at least one technician is certified. Whether required by the state or not, both hospitals and community pharmacies are increasingly calling for technicians to become certified by taking the national Pharmacy Technician Certification Examination (PTCE). Often certification is a requirement for

Figure 14.1

States Recognizing Pharmacy Technician Certification

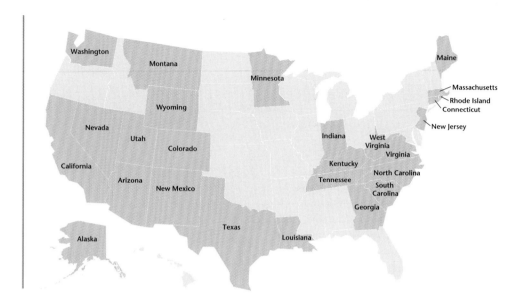

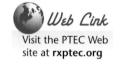

Web Link

Visit the PTEC Web site at **rxptec.org**

initial employment. With other employers, incentives are in place for technicians to become certified once employed.

Some states are also beginning to recognize the value of formal technician education. For instance, South Carolina now requires completion of an accredited technician education program in addition to PTCB certification and 1000 hours of work experience to be a certified pharmacy technician. Some people and organizations within the profession, including the Pharmacy Technician Educators Council (PTEC), are calling for the development of a 2-year associate degree standard for technician training. With these new requirements, technicians are given greater responsibilities—even allowed to check the work of other technicians in some settings.

All of these developments point to an increase in the presence, responsibilities, and status of the technician within the pharmacy community. As a result, today's employers expect more (and deliver more) to their technician employees. This section provides some useful information to help you to meet these increased demands and to place your best foot forward as you enter the field.

Professionalism and the Technician

Just as pharmacists are required to obtain **credentials** such as graduating from an accredited pharmacy school, sitting for a licensure examination, and perhaps completing a residency, pharmacy technicians are increasingly asked to seek credentials. Credentials are defined simply as *documented evidence of qualifications*. This documentation of their qualifications is moving the role of technicians forward in the profession of pharmacy. Now, being a pharmacy technician is not simply having a job in a pharmacy; rather, it is a chosen career path recognized as a **paraprofessional**.

As a paraprofessional in healthcare, technicians have specific expectations for job performance. Technicians are part of the pharmacy profession, and professionals are expected to do the following:

- be qualified to perform the duties required
- use their specific knowledge and skills to perform the duties required
- adhere to a code of ethical conduct

These expectations are held for all health professionals, elevating their job responsibilities beyond that of a mere employee. Patients come to trust healthcare professionals and paraprofessionals. This trust obligates pharmacy technicians to serve the public good and benefit the lives of patients.

Although type and length of technician education and training still vary widely, only one credential for technicians is recognized nationally—**Certified Pharmacy Technician (CPhT).** This credential is quickly becoming preferred or even required for employment in many areas.

Certification and the National Certification Examination

In January of 1995, the American Pharmacists Association (APhA)—along with the American Society of Health-System Pharmacists (ASHP), the Illinois Council of Health-System Pharmacists (ICHP), and the Michigan Pharmacists Association (MPA)—created the Pharmacy Technician Certification Board (PTCB). The mission of the PTCB is to establish and maintain criteria for certification and recertification of pharmacy technicians on a national basis. A nonprofit testing company, the Professional Examination Service (PES), administers the **Pharmacy Technician Certification Examination (PTCE)**, which candidates must pass to become certified and receive the title of CPhT. Although not universal, employers are increasingly encouraging certification. Sometimes certification is required for newly hired technicians. Other employers are often willing to pay for the training pharmacy technicians must take in preparation for the certification examination and may even pay the examination fee. Of course, technicians often receive higher pay once they are certified. According to the PTCB, over 200,000 technicians have become certified since its inception.

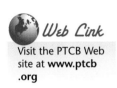

Web Link

Visit the PTCB Web site at **www.ptcb .org**

The PTCE is a multiple-choice examination containing a total of 140 questions (125 questions are graded and 15 questions are sample questions being tested for possible use in graded portions of future tests). The questions are organized into three sections, each of which is weighted differently. Anyone who does not have a felony conviction, has graduated from high school, has a general equivalency diploma (GED), or has obtained the foreign equivalent may sit for the examination. The goal of the PTCE is to verify the candidate's knowledge and skill base for activities performed by pharmacy technicians under the supervising pharmacist. It is comprehensive in its scope in that no specific pharmacy setting or specialty is emphasized. Skills and knowledge from both the community and institutional settings are required to pass this examination. No previous education, training, or work experience is required before taking the examination, but such work will assist a candidate in preparing for it. Table 14.1 details the content of the examination as specified by the PTCB. (State laws and regulations and job center policies and procedures may also specifically define the functions and responsibilities of pharmacy technicians.) These activities are characterized under three broad function areas:

1. assisting the pharmacist in serving patients (66% of examination)—covers topics such as prescription interpretation, patient profile maintenance, prescription filling and processing, compounding, calculations, and customer service
2. maintaining medication and inventory control systems (22% of examination)—covers topics such as ordering pharmaceuticals and devices, maintaining records and drug stock, repackaging, and quality control measures
3. participating in the administration and management of pharmacy practice (12% of examination)—covers topics such as working with third-party payers, operating computer and automated dispensing technology, and maintaining federal laws and practice standards

Candidates for certification are given 3 hours to complete the examination. The blueprint for the examination is listed in Table 14.1; check the PTCB Web site for modifications. Points are not deducted for incorrect answers on the examination, so it pays to answer every question. Candidates must receive a score of 650 or higher to pass and receive certification. So far, the PTCB reports that 80% of those who have taken the examination have passed. More specifically, anywhere from 77 to 82% of examination takers pass it each year. A technician may retake the examination as many times as is necessary to achieve a passing score. However, an application fee applies each time one takes the examination.

Candidates should bring with them to the examination photo identification; a silent, handheld, nonprogrammable, battery-operated calculator; and a supply of No. 2 pencils with erasers. No reference materials, books, papers, or other materials may be taken into the examination room. The PTCB recommends that persons taking the examination be familiar with the material in "any of the basic pharmacy technician training manuals."

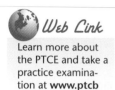

Web Link

Learn more about the PTCE and take a practice examination at **www.ptcb.org**

Table 14.1   The Contents of the Pharmacy Technician Certification Examination

I. *Assisting the Pharmacist in Serving Patients*

1. Receive prescription or medication order(s) from patient/patient's representative, prescriber, or other healthcare professional:
   - Accept new prescription or medication order from patient/patient's representative, prescriber, or other healthcare professional.
   - Accept new prescription or medication order electronically (e.g., by telephone, fax, or computer).
   - Accept refill request from patient/patient's representative, prescriber, or other healthcare professional.
   - Accept refill request electronically (e.g., by telephone, fax, or computer).
   - Contact prescriber/originator for clarification of prescription or medication order refill.

2. At the direction of the pharmacist, assist in obtaining from the patient/patient's representative such information as diagnosis or desired therapeutic outcome, medication use, allergies, adverse reactions, medical history and other relevant patient information, physical disability, and reimbursement mechanisms.

3. At the direction of the pharmacist, assist in obtaining from prescriber, other healthcare professionals, and/or the medical record such information as diagnosis or desired therapeutic outcome, medication use, allergies, adverse reactions, medical history and other relevant patient information, physical disability, and reimbursement mechanisms.

4. At the direction of the pharmacist, collect data (e.g., blood pressure, glucose) to assist the pharmacist in monitoring patient outcomes.

5. Assess prescription or medication order for completeness (e.g., patient's name and address), accuracy (e.g., consistency with products available), authenticity, legality, and reimbursement eligibility.

6. Update the medical record/patient profile with such information as medication history, allergies, medication duplication, as well as drug-disease, drug-drug, drug-laboratory, and drug-food interactions.

7. Process a prescription or medication order:
   - Enter prescription or medication order information onto patient profile.

- Select the product(s) for a generically written prescription or medication order.
- Select the product(s) for a brand name prescription or medication order (consulting established formulary as appropriate).
- Obtain medications or devices from inventory.
- Measure, count, or calculate finished dose forms for dispensing.
- Record preparation of prescription or medication, including any special requirements, for controlled substances.
- Package finished dose forms (e.g., blister pack, vial).
- Affix label(s) and auxiliary label(s) to container(s).
- Assemble patient information materials.
- Check for accuracy during processing of the prescription or medication order (e.g., matching National Drug Code [NDC] number).
- Verify the measurements, preparation, and/or packaging of medications produced by other technicians.
- Prepare prescription or medication order for final check by pharmacist.

8. Compound a prescription or medication order:
   - Assemble equipment and/or supplies necessary for compounding the prescription or medication order.
   - Calibrate equipment (e.g., scale or balance, total parenteral administration [TPN] compounder) needed to compound the prescription or medication order.
   - Perform calculations required for usual dose determinations and preparation of compounded intravenous (IV) admixtures.
   - Compound medications (e.g., ointments, reconstituted antibiotic suspensions) for dispensing according to prescription formula or instructions.
   - Compound medications in anticipation of prescription or medication orders (e.g., bulk compounding for a specific patient).
   - Prepare sterile products (e.g., TPNs, piggybacks).
   - Prepare chemotherapy.
   - Record preparation and/or ingredients of medications (e.g., lot number, control number, expiration date).

continues

Table 14.1   The Contents of the Pharmacy Technician Certification Examination—Continued

9. Provision of medication to patient/patient's representative:
   - Store medication before distribution.
   - Provide medication to patient/patient's representative.
   - Place medication in dispensing system (e.g., unit dose cart, robotics).
   - Deliver medication to patient-care unit.
   - Record distribution of prescription medication.
   - Record distribution of controlled substances.
   - Record distribution of investigational drugs.
10. Determine charges and obtain reimbursement for services.
11. Communicate with third-party payers to determine or verify coverage and obtain prior authorizations.
12. Provide supplemental information (e.g., patient package leaflets, computer-generated information, videos) as requested/required.
13. Ask patient whether counseling by pharmacist is desired.
14. Perform drug administration functions under appropriate supervision (e.g., perform drug/IV rounds, anticipate refill of drugs/IVs).
15. Assist the pharmacist in monitoring patient laboratory values (e.g., blood pressure, cholesterol values).

II. Maintaining Medication and Inventory Control Systems

1. Identify pharmaceuticals, durable medical equipment, devices, and supplies to be ordered (e.g., want book).
2. Place orders for pharmaceuticals, durable medical equipment, devices, and supplies (including investigational and hazardous products and devices), and expedite emergency orders in compliance with legal, regulatory, professional, and manufacturers' requirements.
3. Receive goods and verify against specifications on original purchase orders.
4. Place pharmaceuticals, durable medical equipment, devices, and supplies (including hazardous materials and investigational products) in inventory under proper storage conditions.
5. Perform nonpatient-specific distribution of pharmaceuticals, durable medical equipment, devices, and supplies (e.g., crash carts, nursing station stock, automated dispensing systems).
6. Remove from inventory expired/discontinued/slow-moving pharmaceuticals, durable medical equipment, devices, and supplies.
7. Remove from inventory recalled pharmaceuticals, durable medical equipment, devices, and supplies.
8. Communicate changes in product availability (e.g., formulary changes, recalls) to pharmacy staff, patient/patient's representative, physicians, and other healthcare professionals.
9. Implement and monitor policies and procedures to deter theft and/or drug diversion.
10. Maintain a record of controlled substances received, stored, and removed from inventory.
11. Perform required inventories and maintain associated records.

12. Maintain record-keeping systems for repackaging, bulk compounding, recalls, and returns of pharmaceuticals, durable medical equipment, devices, and supplies.
13. Compound medications in anticipation of prescription/medication orders (e.g., bulk compounding).
14. Perform quality assurance (QA) tests on compounded medications (e.g., for bacterial growth; for sodium, potassium, dextrose levels; for radioactivity).
15. Repackage finished dose forms for dispensing.
16. Participate in QA programs related to products and/or supplies (e.g., formulary revision, nursing unit audits, performance evaluations of wholesalers).
17. Communicate with representatives of pharmaceutical and equipment suppliers.

III. Participating in the Administration and Management of Pharmacy Practice

1. Coordinate written, electronic, and oral communications throughout the practice setting (e.g., route phone calls, faxes, verbal and written refill authorizations), and disseminate policy changes.
2. Update and maintain information (e.g., insurance information, patient demographics, provider information, reference material).
3. Collect productivity information (e.g., the number of prescriptions filled, fill times, money collected, rejected claim status).
4. Participate in quality improvement activities (e.g., medication error reports, customer satisfaction surveys, delivery audits, internal audits of processes).
5. Generate QA reports.
6. Implement and monitor the practice setting for compliance with federal, state, and local laws, regulations, and professional standards (e.g., materials safety data sheet [MSDS], eyewash centers, Joint Commission on Accreditation of Healthcare Organizations [JCAHO] standards).
7. Implement and monitor policies and procedures for sanitation management, handling of hazardous waste (e.g., needles), and infection control (e.g., protective clothing, laminar flow hood, other equipment cleaning).
8. Perform and record routine sanitation, maintenance, and calibration of equipment (e.g., automated dispensing equipment, balances, robotics, refrigerator temperatures).
9. Maintain and use manual or computer-based information systems to perform job-related activities (e.g., update prices, generate reports and labels, perform utilization tracking/inventory).
10. Maintain software for automated dispensing technology, including point-of-care drug dispensing cabinets.
11. Perform billing and accounting functions (e.g., personal charge accounts, third-party rejections, third-party reconciliation, census maintenance, prior authorization).
12. Communicate with third-party payers to determine or verify coverage.
13. Conduct staff training.
14. Aid in establishing, implementing, and monitoring policies and procedures.

Source: Pharmacy Technician Certification Board (PTCB), www.ptcb.org/exam/content.asp (accessed October 11, 2005). Used with permission.

Recertification

Recertification is required by the PTCB every 2 years. To be recertified, one must earn a total of 20 hours credit in pharmacy-related continuing education, with at least one of these hours being in pharmacy law. Certified technicians receive notification of the need for recertification approximately 60 days before their certification lapses. Pharmacy-related continuing education can be found in professional organization meetings and Web sites, employers, and professional journals.

Hierarchy of Technician Positions

Because of expanded recognition of technician credentials, a hierarchy of pharmacy technician job descriptions has evolved especially in institutional settings. Although specific job descriptions will vary between organizations, many institutions now have different levels of technician responsibilities. If certification is not required for an entry-level technician, then it is usually required for higher levels. Often, corresponding job titles will be something like Technician I and II or Entry-Level Technician and Technician Specialist. The difference in responsibility grows and expands as one moves up the company ladder. For higher levels, added job responsibilities beyond basic competence for an entry-level technician may include the following:
- prioritization of work
- demonstrated initiative and ability to work independently
- trouble shooting and critical thinking
- supervision of others
- staff training responsibilities
- advanced communication skills (e.g., writing, word processing)
- advanced computer application skills
- advanced calculations
- billing and documentation procedures
- inventory ordering and purchasing

In some cases intravenous (IV) preparation duties may be reserved for higher-level technicians because of new regulations and standards implemented by JCAHO and the United States Pharmacopeia (i.e., USP Chapter 797).

Professional Organizations

Being part of a profession means taking an active role in advancing the profession. As a paraprofessional in pharmacy, technicians have an obligation to make their views heard in the local, state, and national forums that discuss issues facing their field. The future of the technician role is in the hands of those within the profession. This self-governance, something that is increasing for technicians, is one characteristic of a **professional**. As the status and role of pharmacy technicians increase, it is important for those within the profession to get involved in decisions and movements affecting it.

Ways to get involved vary widely. Some examples include:
- volunteering to serve on a committee of your local, state, or national pharmacy organization (most of which have technician representation)
- running for office in your local chapter of the National Pharmacy Technician Association (NPTA) or American Association of Pharmacy Technicians (AAPT)
- participating in your state's annual pharmacy legislative day activities
- attending a national pharmacy technician conference

Report what you learn to your employer and fellow technicians at work. Learning about issues facing technicians and taking ownership in the decisions made to advance their roles will give technicians control over their own destinies.

Some issues that face technicians currently are standardization of technician training or education, expansion of technician responsibilities to assist with the projected

Web Link

Visit the resources provided in the Pharmacy Library of this book's Internet Resource Center (IRC) at **www.emcp .com** for a listing and description of professional organizations in which technicians can become active.

shortages in pharmacy workforces, and implementation of state requirements for national certification. Locate your local technician organizations, and inquire about how you can participate in decisions affecting the future practice of pharmacy.

ETHICS IN PHARMACY PRACTICE

Ethics is the study of standards of conduct and moral judgment that outlines rightness or wrongness of human conduct and character. Ethics is a process for reflection and analysis of behavior when the proper course of action is unclear. It is the basis on which we make judgments. In addition, it is the system or code of conduct of a particular person, group, or profession. It is not necessarily part of one's religious beliefs, because even an atheist can have a sense of right and wrong conduct. However, religion often has an influence on one's personal ethics.

The most important benefit of studying ethics is to internalize a framework or set of guidelines based on high professional standards that will guide our decision making and actions. It is important to be aware of situations one may find himself or herself in while working in healthcare and to examine and discuss how one may react and behave when faced with those situations. Determining what the ethical choice is in such situations ahead of time can avoid the paralyzing quandary one may face when confronted with questionable circumstances.

All of us face hundreds of situations when our moral beliefs seem unfounded, uninformed, and anything but a foundation on which to base a moral decision. Through ethical study, an individual may be able to make decisions using a moral compass and to understand and respect the viewpoints of others. Pharmacy technicians, working side by side with pharmacists, must recognize and adopt the accepted ethical standards of pharmacy practice.

Not all behaviors in pharmacy practice are done solely because of the law. Moral obligations exist that are not legal obligations and vice versa. Using the best priced medication within choices of generics, true disclosures of prescription wait times, and providing accurate information on out-of-stock situations are examples of these obligations. Laws governing the practice of pharmacy do not always dictate what the proper behavior is in every situation encountered in pharmacy. For example, some debate has arisen over prescribed emergency contraceptives. Although these prescriptions may be entirely valid and legal, some pharmacists reserve the right to refuse to dispense such medication because they consider it morally or ethically unsound. The correct way to address such situations is not always outlined in laws and regulations.

Ethical codes are based on the belief that a relationship of trust exists between a professional (i.e., the pharmacist) and client (i.e., the patient). Two reasons for this exist. First, professional service is not standardized; it is unique and personal. These essential qualities cannot be specified in a contract or purchased. Second, the patient often hardly knows what to ask for, let alone how it can be provided. Therefore the patient is vulnerable to the services provided by the pharmacist.

Employees categorized as *professional* are held to high standards of conduct. To be considered professionals, they must meet selected criteria. First, professionals hold a specialized body of knowledge, which enables the practitioner to perform a highly useful social function. A pharmacist is considered a professional not because he or she can type or dispense medications but because of his or her knowledge about drugs and how to help patients make the best use of medicine.

A second characteristic of a professional is that the individual has a set of attitudes that influence his or her professional behavior. The basic attitude is an unselfish concern for the welfare of others, called *altruism*.

Finally, a third characteristic of a professional is social sanction. More than licensing, social sanction also creates trust between society (i.e., patients) and professionals (i.e., pharmacists). Social sanction rewards the professional with status, income, and power.

Code of Ethics Statements

Codes of ethics statements regarding professional behavior are often written as formal documents and supported by professional organizations. These statements provide language to aid in the decision-making process when ethical dilemmas present themselves in pharmacy practice. Tables 14.2 and 14.3 present codes of ethics for pharmacy technicians and pharmacists, respectively.

Dilemmas and Questions Facing Healthcare Professionals

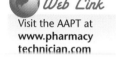
Web Link
Visit the AAPT at
www.pharmacy technician.com

Ethics can help a pharmacy professional to determine how best to handle an ethical dilemma. An **ethical dilemma** is a situation that calls for a judgment between two or more solutions, not all of which are necessarily wrong.

Deciding what action to take when faced with an ethical dilemma in the pharmacy requires consideration of the circumstances, choosing an action, and justifying the action. To do this, you should ask certain questions:

Table 14.2 Code of Ethics for Pharmacy Technicians

Preamble

Pharmacy technicians are healthcare professionals who assist pharmacists in providing the best possible care for patients. The principles of this code, which apply to pharmacy technicians working in all settings, are based on the application and support of the moral obligations that guide all in the pharmacy profession in relationships with patients, healthcare professionals, and society.

Principles

1. A pharmacy technician's first consideration is to ensure the health and safety of the patient and to use knowledge and skills most capably in serving others.

2. A pharmacy technician supports and promotes honesty and integrity in the profession, which includes a duty to observe the law, maintain the highest moral and ethical conduct at all times, and uphold the ethical principles of the profession.

3. A pharmacy technician assists and supports the pharmacist in the safe, efficacious, and cost-effective distribution of health services and healthcare resources.

4. A pharmacy technician respects and values the abilities of pharmacists, colleagues, and other healthcare professionals.

5. A pharmacy technician maintains competency in practice and continually enhances professional knowledge and expertise.

6. A pharmacy technician respects and supports the patient's individuality, dignity, and confidentiality.

7. A pharmacy technician respects the confidentiality of a patient's records and discloses pertinent information only with proper authorization.

8. A pharmacy technician never assists in the dispensing, promoting, or distributing of medications or medical devices that are not of good quality or do not meet the standards required by law.

9. A pharmacy technician does not engage in any activity that will discredit the profession and will expose, without fear or favor, illegal or unethical conduct in the profession.

10. A pharmacy technician associates and engages in the support of organizations that promote the profession of pharmacy through the use and enhancement of pharmacy technicians.

Source: Copyright by the American Association of Pharmacy Technicians (AAPT). Reprinted with permission.

- What is the dilemma?
- What pharmaceutical alternatives apply?
- What is the best alternative, and can it be justified on moral grounds?

Pharmacy technicians must recognize and accept the ethical standards of pharmacy practice and apply them when working side by side with pharmacists. They must also understand decision-making processes and become personally involved in

Table 14.3   Code of Ethics for Pharmacists

Preamble

Pharmacists are health professionals who assist individuals in making the best use of medications. This Code, prepared and supported by pharmacists, is intended to state publicly the principles that form the fundamental basis of the roles and responsibilities of pharmacists. These principles, based on moral obligations and virtues, are established to guide pharmacists in relationships with patients, health professionals, and society.

Principles

  I. *A pharmacist respects the covenantal relationship between the patient and pharmacist.*

   Considering the patient-pharmacist relationship as a covenant means that a pharmacist has moral obligations in response to the gift of trust received from society. In return for this gift, a pharmacist promises to help individuals achieve optimum benefit from their medications, to be committed to their welfare, and to maintain their trust.

  II. *A pharmacist promotes the good of every patient in a caring, compassionate, and confidential manner.*

   A pharmacist places concern for the well-being of the patient at the center of professional practice. In doing so, a pharmacist considers needs stated by the patient, as well as those defined by health science. A pharmacist is dedicated to protecting the dignity of the patient. With a caring attitude and a compassionate spirit, a pharmacist focuses on serving the patient in a private and confidential manner.

  III. *A pharmacist respects the autonomy and dignity of each patient.*

   A pharmacist promotes the right of self-determination and recognizes individual self-worth by encouraging patients to participate in decisions about their health. A pharmacist communicates with patients in terms that are understandable. In all cases, a pharmacist respects personal and cultural differences among patients.

  IV. *A pharmacist acts with honesty and integrity in professional relationships.*

   A pharmacist has a duty to tell the truth and to act with conviction of conscience. A pharmacist avoids discriminatory practices, behavior or work conditions that impair professional judgment, and actions that compromise dedication to the best interests of patients.

  V. *A pharmacist maintains professional competence.*

   A pharmacist has a duty to maintain knowledge and abilities as new medications, devices, and technologies become available and as health information advances.

  VI. *A pharmacist respects the values and abilities of colleagues and other health professionals.*

   When appropriate, a pharmacist asks for the consultation of colleagues or other health professionals or refers the patient. A pharmacist acknowledges that colleagues and other health professionals may differ in the beliefs and values they apply to the care of the patient.

  VII. *A pharmacist serves individual, community, and societal needs.*

   The primary obligation of a pharmacist is to individual patients. However, the obligations of a pharmacist may at times extend beyond the individual to the community and society. In these situations, the pharmacist recognizes the responsibilities that accompany these obligations and acts accordingly.

  VIII. *A pharmacist seeks justice in the distribution of health resources.*

   When health resources are allocated, a pharmacist is fair and equitable, balancing the needs of patients and society.

Source: Copyright by the American Pharmacists Association (APhA) and adopted October 27, 1994. Reprinted with permission.

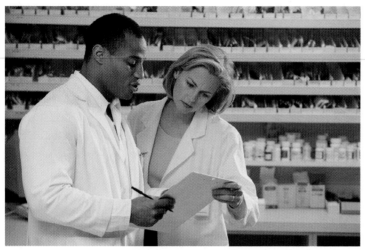
A pharmacy technician will often discuss issues with the pharmacist, such as whether to fill a questionable Schedule II prescription.

obtaining facts relevant to a dilemma, evaluating the alternatives, and determining the correct solutions.

As modern pharmacy practice continues to evolve, new questions will arise that challenge pharmacy personnel in new decision-making deliberations. Advances in medical health, pharmaceutical delivery systems, and new medication development will change how pharmacists and pharmacy technicians conduct their daily work. The answers to such ethical practice questions deserve both individual and profession-wide debate. As with any politically, professionally, and emotionally charged topic, a variety of opinions will surface. The pharmacy technician must learn to respect differences without prejudice when those differences occur in a work team or with a patient.

ADJUSTING TO THE WORK ENVIRONMENT

If you have not worked before or if your work experience has been sporadic, then getting used to your job as a technician might seem like getting used to life in a foreign country. You will have to adjust to a new "work culture," to different behaviors, to unfamiliar customs, and even to a new "language," the technical jargon of the profession. The following list provides some advice for making your adjustment to the job a comfortable one:

- attitude—Do not give in to the temptation to behave in ways that are elitist or superior. Remember you are part of a healthcare team, and cooperation is extremely important.
- reliability—Healthcare, like teaching, is one of those industries in which standards for reliability are very high. One simply cannot, for example, show up late for work or take days off arbitrarily without good reason. Unreliable employees in the healthcare industry do not keep their jobs for long. Therefore make sure that your employer can always depend on you to arrive at work on time. Staying late does not make up for a tardy arrival. Remember that tardiness can play havoc with other people's work schedules and work loads. Finish your grooming and eating before you enter your work area.
- accuracy and responsibility—In a pharmacy, one rarely has the leeway to be partially correct. As discussed in Chapter 12, an error, even a small one, can have dire consequences for a patient or customer, as well as for the pharmacy. Develop work habits to ensure accuracy, and expect to be held responsible for what you do on the job. Work steadily and methodically. Keep your attention on the task at hand, and always double-check everything you do.
- relating to your supervisor—Always show your supervisor a reasonable degree of deference and respect. Ask your supervisor how he or she prefers to be addressed. Be respectful of your supervisor's experience and knowledge. If tensions arise between you and your supervisor, then take positive steps to lessen them. Remember that your supervisor has power over your raises, promotions, benefits, and references for future employment. When you disagree with him or her, it is best to discuss these differences in private.

- personality—It may come as some surprise to you, but personality is one of the greatest predictors of job success. Be positive, cooperative, self-confident, and enthusiastic.
- performance—Demonstrate that you can get things done and that you put the job first. Employers expect you to devote your full attention to your responsibilities for the entire length of your shift. Rushing through a task because it is close to the end of your shift places patient care at risk. Maintaining attentiveness and accuracy is always important even if it is close to quitting time.
- questioning—Sometimes people are afraid to ask questions because doing so might make them appear less intelligent or less knowledgeable. Nothing could be further from the truth. When you do not know how something should be done, always ask.
- dress—Follow the dress code of the company or institution for which you work.
- receptivity—Listen to the advice of others who have been on the job longer. Accept criticism gracefully. If you make a mistake, then "own up" to it. If you are criticized unfairly, then adopt a nondefensive tone of voice and explain your view of the matter calmly and rationally. This behavior is part of performing with integrity, an important part of being a professional.
- etiquette—Every workplace has its unique culture. Especially at first, pay close attention to the details of that culture. Pick up on the habits of interaction and communication practiced by other employees, and model the best of these.
- alliances—In all organizations, two kinds of power systems exist: (1) formal, or organizational ones, and (2) informal ones, based upon alliances. Cultivate alliances on the job, but make sure that you are not seen as part of a clique. Even as a new employee, you will begin to build power through making alliances. If a problem or an opportunity arises, then you will probably hear about it first through your allies on the job. If a change in the workplace affects you, then advance notice may give you the time to plan a strategic response.
- reputation—Many people assume that if they work hard and are loyal, they will be rewarded. This is often but not necessarily always true. Management personnel may be so involved with their own concerns that you remain little more than a face in the crowd. Being pleasant to others will help you to be noticed, as will making helpful or useful suggestions. Do not keep your professional qualifications a secret. Join professional organizations. Serve on committees within the institution. When you have won an award or achieved some other success, see that your name is publicized in, for example, institutional newsletters, community newspapers, or the newsletters of professional organizations. Give presentations at professional meetings, civic groups, churches, or synagogues. Write articles for publication in professional publications. In short, avoid hiding your light under a bushel.
- luck—Most of the big lucky breaks in life come through knowing the right people at the right time. So, by cultivating alliances, you can, more than you might expect, control your luck.
- crisis—When a crisis occurs, do not overreact. Take time, if you can, to think and then act, and do not keep the crisis a secret from your supervisor.

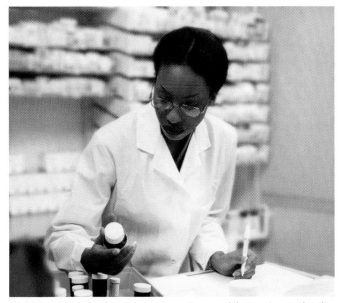

Maintaining medication inventory requires careful attention to detail and accurate documentation.

- learning—Pharmacy is a rapidly changing field. Accept the idea of continuing education as a way of life. You need not take formal course work every year (unless you are doing so to maintain your certification), but do make a point to read and to attend professional meetings to learn about the latest trends. Think of the job-related learning that you do as a regular "information workout," as necessary to your employment fitness as aerobic workouts are to your physical fitness.
- expertise—How can you become a person who makes things happen? Become highly knowledgeable about a specialty within your field. Become the most expert technician that you can become in that area; then move on and master another area. Soon, others will be asking your advice, and your reputation will build.
- reflectiveness about your career—There will never be a time in your career to coast and relax. Good career chances can come your way at any time in life, so make a regular habit of taking the time to think about your career and where you are headed. Planning lends structure and substance to your career management.

JOB SEARCH

Before you can implement the excellent strategies introduced in the preceding section, you must, of course, find the right job. Many people find the prospect of job hunting overwhelming. Avoid such negative thinking. Instead, think of the job hunt as an adventure, a period of exploration that can lead to exciting new possibilities. Taking the following steps can make the job search successful.

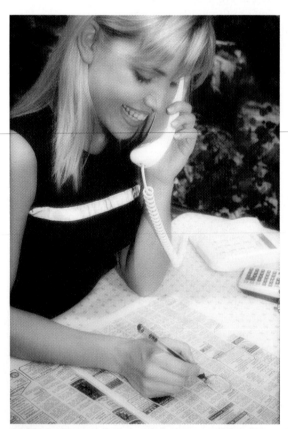

Taking the job search process one step at a time can help you successfully find a position as a pharmacy technician.

Clarify Your Career Goals

It will be very difficult to find a job if you are not sure what you are looking for. Do you want to work in a community pharmacy? Do you want to work in a hospital, a long-term care facility, or a home infusion pharmacy? If you have uncertainties about the setting in which you wish to work, then arrange to interview some people who work in these settings. In addition, do some thinking about what you want out of the job. Are you interested in jobs with opportunities for advancement in retail management? Are you more interested in customer care or prescription dispensing? Do you want to master the preparation of parenterals, compounding, ordering and inventory, billing, or maintenance of a drug information library? Think about what you want to do; then look for jobs that suit your ambitions. Many schools have career counselors who can help you to answer such questions. Make an appointment to visit and talk to one of these individuals.

Write a Good Résumé

Make use of some of the excellent résumé-writing software now available, or contact a résumé-writing service. A résumé is a brief written summary of what you have to offer an employer. It is a sales tool, and

Table 14.4   The Parts of a Résumé

Heading	Give your full name, address, and telephone number. Remember to include your ZIP code in the address, area code in the phone number, and your e-mail address if you have one a potential employer can use to contact you.
Employment Objective	This is the first thing an employer wants to know. The objective should briefly describe the position you are seeking and some of the abilities you would bring to the job. Identify the requirements of the position you are applying for; then tailor the employment objective to match those requirements.
Education	Give your college, city, state, degree, major, date of graduation, and additional course work related to the job, to the profession, or to business in general. State your cumulative grade point average (GPA) if it helps to sell you (3.0 or higher).
Experience	In reverse chronological order, list your work experience, including on-campus and off-campus work. Do not include jobs that would be unimpressive to your employer. Be sure to include cooperative education experience. For each job, indicate your position, employer's name, the location of the employment, the dates employed, and a brief description of your duties. Always list any advancements, promotions, or supervisory responsibilities. Include any certifications, registrations, or licensures on your résumé.
Skills	If you do not have a lot of relevant work experience, then include a skills section that details the skills that you can use on the job. Doing so is a way of saying, "I'm really capable. I just haven't had much opportunity to show it yet."
Related Activities	Include any activities that show leadership, teamwork, or good communication skills. Include any club or organizational memberships, as well as professional or community activities that help to sell your skills. Simple hobbies and pastimes are not recommended for inclusion because they may seem trivial.
References	State that these are *available on request.*

the product you are selling is yourself. A résumé is an opportunity to present your work experience, your skills, and your education to an employer. Table 14.4 outlines the general topics to be included in a chronological résumé.

Make sure that your résumé follows a consistent, standard format, like the one shown in Figure 14.2. Limit it to a single page. Type it, or print it on a high-quality printer, using high-quality 8½- × 11-inch paper. Many special résumé papers are available from stationery and office supply shops. However, ordinary opaque white paper is acceptable. Although outlandish colors and textures may seem unique and serve to set you apart, they are usually viewed as unprofessional. Remaining conservative when selecting stationery is best to ensure that your résumé conveys a professional image.

Be sure to check your résumé very carefully for errors in spelling, grammar, usage, punctuation, capitalization, and form. No one wants to hire a sloppy technician. Once your résumé is complete, you should always have another person read through it and check for errors in spelling, grammar, and vocabulary, because it is easy to overlook such things.

Establish a Network

Tell everyone you know that you are looking for a job. Identify faculty, acquaintances, friends, and relatives who can assist you in your job search. Identify persons within employers' organizations who can give you insight into their needs. If you complete any rotations or internships as part of your schooling, then ask your supervisors and

Figure 14.2

Sample Résumé

BRENDA COLLINS
1700 Beltline Blvd.
My Town, CO 29169
(345) 555-3245

Objective: Position as pharmacy technician that makes use of my training in dispensing and compounding medications, ordering and inventory, patient profiling, third-party billing, and other essential functions

Education	Diploma in Health Science—Pharmacy	August 20XX–May 20XX
	My Town Technical College in My Town, CO	
	Program Accredited by American Society of Health-System Pharmacists (ASHP)	
	Dean's List	
Certification	(awaiting results)	July 20XX
	National Pharmacy Technician Certification Exam	
Skills	Converting units of measure	
	Setting up ratios and proportions for proper performance of pharmacy calculations	
	Preparing aseptic intravenous (IV) solutions	
	Proper interpretation of prescriptions and physician's orders	
	Proper interpretation and updating of prescription records	
	Attention to clerical detail	
	Operation of pharmacy computer systems and software	
	Preparation of compounded prescription products	
Employment	Clerk	January 20XX to present
	Arborland Pharmacy in Erewhon, CO	
	Duties included customer service, operating cash register, and stocking inventory.	
	Sales Associate	September 20XX–January 20XX
	Mother's Sporting Goods in My Town, CO	
	Duties included customer service and operating a cash register.	

References available on request.

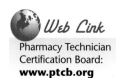

Pharmacy Technician Certification Board: **www.ptcb.org**

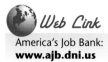

America's Job Bank: **www.ajb.dni.us**

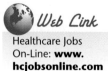

Healthcare Jobs On-Line: **www. hcjobsonline.com**

coworkers about anticipated openings. If you perform well as a student-in-training, then you will be viewed as a good potential employee. Even previous graduates of your educational program can provide valuable information about hiring practices. Join professional associations, attend meetings, and network with colleagues and potential employers.

Identify and Research Potential Employers

Your school may have a career placement office. Use the services of that office. Check the classified ads in newspapers. Go to a career library and look up employers in directories. Look up potential employers in telephone directories. Make use of career opportunities posted on Web sites and job search Web sites; many local hospitals also have a Web site that is used to post job vacancies.

Write a Strong Cover Letter

The cover letter, or letter of application, is the first communication that you send to an employer. It is generally sent in response to a job advertisement or posting or before a cold call to a potential employer. Your résumé should accompany the cover letter. Both the cover letter and the résumé should be typed or printed on the same kind of paper, and both should be placed in a matching business envelope addressed by means of typing or printing on an inkjet or laser printer. The letter should be single-spaced, using a block or modified block style. In the block style, all items in the letter begin at the left margin. In the modified block style, the sender's address, the complimentary close, and the signature are left aligned from the center of the paper, and all other parts of the letter begin at the left margin.

The cover letter should highlight your qualifications and call attention to your résumé. Remember that a sloppy cover letter will detract from even the most professional résumé. As with your résumé, proofread the cover letter carefully for errors in spelling, grammar, usage, punctuation, capitalization, and form. Address the letter, when possible, to a particular person, by name and by title, and make sure to identify the position for which you are applying. Sometimes it takes extra investigation to find out these details, but it shows initiative and professionalism if the letter is addressed to the specific person (with his or her correct degree and title) doing the hiring. A letter addressed *to whom it may concern* will not get the same reception as one addressed to the actual pharmacist manager in charge of hiring. Realize also that pharmacists may have different degrees—Registered Pharmacist (RPh), Bachelor of Science in Pharmacy (BS Pharm), or Doctor of Pharmacy (PharmD). If necessary, call the employer to get the correct spelling of the recipient's name. Do not make assumptions. No one likes to receive correspondence with his or her name spelled incorrectly. Use the format shown in Table 14.5 for your letter. Figure 14.3 shows a sample cover letter.

Prepare for the Interview

Review your research on the employer and role-play an interview situation. Get plenty of sleep, and eat well on the day before and the day of the interview. Find out

Table 14.5   Suggested Format for Cover Letters

First Paragraph	In your initial paragraph, state why you are writing, what specific position or type of work you are seeking, and how you learned of the opening (e.g., from the placement office, the news media, a friend). If you learned of the opening through networking, then be sure to mention who told you about the position. It may help to get the employer's attention.
Second Paragraph	Explain why you are interested in the position, the organization, or the organization's products and services. Again, this may take some investigation but shows desire and thoroughness. State how your academic background makes you a qualified candidate for the position. If you have had some practical experience, then point out your specific achievements.
Third Paragraph	Refer the reader to the enclosed résumé—a summary of your qualifications, training, and experience. If specific items on your résumé require a special explanation, tactfully and positively point them out; you can include work experience from outside of pharmacy, but be sure that it relates to skills you will use as a technician.
Fourth Paragraph	Indicate your desire for a personal interview and your flexibility as to the time and place. Repeat your telephone number, as well as the best times to reach you in the letter. If you use e-mail as a preferred method of communication, then let the employer know that. Close your letter with a statement or question to encourage a response, or take the initiative by indicating a day and date on which you will contact the employer to set up a convenient time for a personal meeting.

Figure 14.3

Sample Cover Letter in Block Style

February 1, 20XX

James Green, PharmD
Pharmacy Manager
Main Street Community Pharmacy
1500 Main Street
My Town, CO 29201

Dear Dr. Green:

I learned of Main Street Community Pharmacy's need for a pharmacy technician through the Placement Office at My Town Technical College. I was pleased to learn of an opening for a technician at the very pharmacy that my family has frequented for years.

I believe that my education and experience would be an asset to Main Street Community Pharmacy. In May, I graduated from My Town Technical College's pharmacy technician training program, and I just took the National Pharmacy Technician Certification Examination. I would welcome the opportunity to apply what I have learned to a career with your pharmacy. I bring to the job a number of assets, including a 3.4 grade point average, commitment to continuing development of my skills as a technician, a willingness to work hard, and a desire to be of service.

As you can see from my enclosed résumé, I already have some experience in pharmacy as a clerk. I am a responsible person, concerned with accuracy and accountability, and someone whom you can depend upon to carry out the technician's duties reliably. Although not in pharmacy directly, I also have plenty of experience dealing with customers in my position as a sales associate. Working with the public is something I am quite comfortable with and enjoy greatly.

I would appreciate an opportunity to discuss the position with you. I will call next week to inquire about a meeting. Thank you for considering my application.

Sincerely,

Brenda Collins
1700 Beltline Blvd.
My Town, CO 29169

Enc.: résumé

everything that you can about the company or institution before you go for an interview. Better yet, do this work before you write the cover letter that you send with your résumé. Knowing details about a potential employer can help you to assess whether the employer is right for you and can win points in your cover letter or interview.

During the interview, follow the guidelines provided in Table 14.6 and be prepared to answer the questions in Table 14.7. Rehearse answers to these questions before the interview. Doing so out loud can help you identify the wording choices you want to use and help to avoid mixing up words in the actual interview. When coming up with answers to such questions, bear in mind the employer's point of view. Try to

Table 14.6 Guidelines for Job Interviews

1. Find out the exact place and time of the interview.
2. Know the full name of the company, the address, the interviewer's full name, and the correct pronunciation of the interviewer's name. Call the employer, if necessary, to get this information.
3. Know something about the company's operations.
4. Be courteous to the receptionist, if one exists, and to other employees. Any person with whom you meet or speak may be in a position to influence your employment.
5. Bring to the interview your résumé and the names, addresses, and telephone numbers of people who can provide references.
6. Arrive 10 to 15 minutes before the scheduled time for the interview.
7. Wear clothing and shoes appropriate to the job.
8. Greet the interviewer and call him or her by name. Introduce yourself at once. Shake hands only if the interviewer offers to do so. Remain standing until invited to sit down.
9. Be confident, polite, poised, and enthusiastic.
10. Look the interviewer in the eye.
11. Speak clearly, loudly enough to be understood. Be positive and concise in your comments. Do not exaggerate, but remember that an interview is not an occasion for modesty.
12. Focus on your strengths. Be prepared to enumerate these, using specific examples as evidence to support the claims you make about yourself.
13. Do not hesitate to ask about the specific duties associated with the job. Show keen interest as the interviewer tells you about these.
14. Avoid bringing up salary requirements until the employer broaches the subject.
15. Do not chew gum or smoke.
16. Do not criticize former employers, coworkers, working conditions.
17. At the close of the interview, thank the interviewer for his or her time and for the opportunity to learn about the company.

Table 14.7 Interview Questions

1. Why did you apply for a job with this company?
2. What part of the job interests you most and why?
3. What do you know about this company?
4. What are your qualifications?
5. What did you like the most and the least about your work experience? (Note: Explaining what you liked least should be done in as positive a manner as possible. For example, you might say that you wish that the job had provided more opportunity for learning about this or that and then explain, further, that you made up the deficiency by study on your own. Such an answer indicates your desire to learn and grow and does not cast your former employer in an unduly negative light.)
6. Why did you leave your previous job? (Again, avoid negative responses. Find a positive reason for leaving, such as returning to school or pursuing an opportunity.)
7. What would you like to be doing in 5 years? How much money would you like to be making? (Keep your answer reasonable, and show that you have ambitions consistent with the employer's needs.)
8. What are your weak points? (Again, say something positive, such as, "I am an extremely conscientious person. Sometimes I worry too much about whether I have done something absolutely correctly, but that can also be a positive trait.")
9. Why do you think you are qualified for this position?
10. Would you mind working on the weekends or overtime? How do you feel about traveling?
11. Do you prefer working with others or by yourself? Do you prefer a quiet or a noisy environment?
12. If you could have any job you wanted, then what would you choose and why?
13. Tell me a little about yourself.
14. What are your hobbies and interests?
15. Why did you attend [the college that you attended]?
16. Why did you choose this field of study?
17. What courses did you like best? What courses did you like least? (Again, couch your responses to both questions in positive ways.)
18. What have you learned from your mistakes?
19. What motivates you to put forth your greatest efforts?
20. Do you plan to continue your education?

imagine what you would want if you were the employer, and take the initiative during the interview to explain to the employer how you can meet those needs.

Some interviewers will pose hypothetical situations and ask for your response, or they may ask you to describe a past experience and how you handled it. These types of questions require you to think on your feet and talk about your problem-solving skills. At the least, be ready to describe a situation or two from your past where you have had to deal with a difficult coworker or member of the public. Choose a situation where you are pleased with how you responded, and describe the measures you took to improve the end result. Interviewers should not ask you questions about your religion, marital status, or if you have or plan to have children. You are not obligated to answer questions like these.

After the interview, follow up with a note thanking the interviewer for seeing you and (within an appropriate time) a telephone call. Be persistent but not pushy.

TRENDS IN PHARMACY PRACTICE

One of the wonderful things about a career in pharmacy is that the profession changes continually. Consider how different the average community pharmacy of today is from the druggist's shop at the turn of the century, in which premanufactured medicines were novelties and rows of bottled tonics and elixirs vied for customers' attention with open barrels of hard candies. Doubtless the profession will change as much or more in the next 30 years as it did in the past 100 years, and that is a lot of change. The following are but a few of the exciting developments that lie in store.

Workforce Issues

As the volume of prescriptions rises and our reliance on drug therapy increases, the need for qualified personnel in the pharmacy profession continues to grow. The number of prescriptions filled was expected to be 3.27 billion in 2005, and some estimate this volume will double over the next 5 to 15 years. Consequently, the need for pharmacists to handle this increased work load is expected to double as well. By 2020, up to 400,000 pharmacists may be needed to handle the increased prescription volume. The number of pharmacists, however, is expected to increase only 30% (from less than 200,000 to 260,000) over that same period. Therefore the need for well-trained, qualified technicians will be critically needed to bridge the gap between the volume of work to be done and the available personnel to do it.

As the pace of work in pharmacies around the country increases, the demands on pharmacists for more direct patient care, drug therapy assessment, and cognitive duties also expand. Pharmacists are increasingly called out of the pharmacy to handle patient care situations and consultations with prescribers. Technicians must step in to manage the workflow and prescription-processing system to keep up with these new demands on the pharmacists' time.

New Medicines and New Drug Development Technologies

Every day, new medicines come to market, many involving new drug development technologies such as genetic engineering. To work in pharmacy is to be at the front lines when new medications are introduced to combat acquired immunodeficiency syndrome (AIDS), cancer, heart disease, cystic fibrosis, and other challenging diseases.

New Dose Forms and Drug Delivery Mechanisms

New dose forms and drug delivery mechanisms are not introduced as often as new drugs, but here, as well, the pace of innovation is increasing rapidly. The past few years have seen the introduction of such innovations as ocular inserts, liposomes, and monoclonal antibodies. We are not far away from combining wearable intravenous (IV) infusion pumps with continuous sensory meters creating in effect an "artificial pancreas." What the future holds is anyone's guess, but the one certainty is that new dose forms and delivery mechanisms will continue to emerge.

Robotics

Robotic machinery is already used in many institutional settings for unit dose repackaging procedures. It is being installed in the community pharmacy setting with greater frequency. Robotics will likely play a larger role in the future pharmacy, providing, for example, automated compounding, filling, labeling, and record keeping in a single device.

Continued Growth in Clinical Applications

The pharmaceutical care movement continues to grow. In the future, more and more of the pharmacy professional's time and energies will be given to educational and counseling functions. For instance, more pharmacies offer specialty diabetes and asthma education and management services. Technicians could find themselves working more one-on-one with patients to choose a glucose meter and learn to use it.

Increased Emphasis on Home Healthcare

The home healthcare industry is one of the most rapidly growing of all industries in the developed world. The reasons behind this growth include reduced cost, improvements in technology that make home care more practical, and the preference of individuals for remaining at home rather than in institutions. The growth of the home care industry shows no signs of abating; therefore in the future, more pharmacists and technicians will find themselves servicing this industry.

Increased Emphasis on Managed Care

Managed care has been applying rational and fiscal conservation to the healthcare system since the early 1990s. The increased emphasis on primary and preventive care with attention to cost-effective medical services that managed care introduced has in effect revolutionized our healthcare system. As such, the practice of pharmacy has felt the squeeze. Pharmacy is increasingly called upon to provide the most appropriate drug therapy at the lowest cost possible. Technicians will find new opportunities available in support roles with pharmacists who work closely with programs and efforts to encourage smart but inexpensive drug use. The nature of this work may differ greatly in its day-to-day, hands-on time with drug products. Increased communication, writing, and computer application skills will be necessary for technicians specializing in managed care settings.

Increased Technician Responsibility and Specialization

Some states are already experimenting with allowing trained technicians to check the work of other technicians. Other states allow the pharmacy technician to accept new prescriptions from a doctor's office. Expect, in the future, for technicians to be given ever more responsibility and for more and more technicians to become specialized in particular areas of service.

Increased Geriatric Applications

As the population of the United States ages, the importance of geriatric pharmacy will increase. The aging of the population will place great financial burdens on the healthcare system as a whole and on pharmacy in particular, leading inevitably to political decisions that will affect the functions of the pharmacist and the technician.

In addition, as Medicare Part D is implemented, more older patients will have some coverage for prescription costs where they did not before. Although this is good news, the program is complex and can be confusing to a population that already finds navigating the healthcare system difficult. Personnel in the pharmacy will need to assist older patients to get information about their rights and to help them understand what level of coverage they have for prescription drugs.

Increased Healthcare and Drug Costs

As we spend more on healthcare in the United States, employers that offer health insurance as a benefit are paying more and experiencing greater drains on their bottom lines. As they ask employees to share in the financial burden of these increased costs, patients themselves are becoming more sensitive to the costs of healthcare and prescription drugs. Pharmacies will need to work with patients to identify cost-effective and affordable options for drug therapy.

Chapter Terms

Certified Pharmacy Technician (CPhT) pharmacy technician who has passed the PTCE

credentials documented evidence of qualifications

ethical dilemma situation that calls for a judgment between two or more solutions, not all of which are necessarily wrong

ethics study of standards of conduct and moral judgment that outlines the rightness or wrongness of human conduct or character

paraprofessional trained person who assists a professional person

Pharmacy Technician Certification Examination (PTCE) examination developed by the Pharmacy Technician Certification Board (PTCB) that technicians must pass to be certified and receive the title of CPhT

professional someone with recognized expertise in a field where expectations are that they use their knowledge and skills to benefit others and to operate with some autonomy in an ethical manner

recertification periodic updating of certification

Chapter Summary

- The occupational outlook for the pharmacy technician is very promising. Increasingly, states are requiring national certification and possibly formal education.
- Certification is offered through the Pharmacy Technician Certification Board (PTCB).
- Technicians will have increasing opportunities for job advancement as requirements for certification and training increase.
- Preparing to work in an institutional or community-based pharmacy requires serious thought about one's attitude, reliability, accuracy, sense of responsibility, personal appearance, organizational skills, and ability to relate to others.
- Writing a comprehensive, attractive résumé and cover letter is an important part of a carefully planned job search.
- Preparing for a job interview is integral to obtaining a desirable technician position.
- New trends in healthcare, drug costs, and the nature of pharmacy work will affect the role of technicians.

Chapter Review

Knowledge Inventory

Choose the best answer from those provided.

1. The organization that certifies pharmacy technicians is the
   a. Pharmacy Technician Certification Board (PTCB).
   b. Committee for the Certification of Pharmacy Technicians.
   c. Pharmacy Technician Review Council.
   d. American Society of Pharmacy Technicians.

2. The Pharmacy Technician Certification Examination (PTCE) is
   a. an essay examination.
   b. a multiple-choice examination.
   c. a true-or-false examination.
   d. All of the above

3. When taking the PTCE, the candidate is allowed to bring into the room
   a. two reference works of his or her choosing.
   b. scrap paper on which to do calculations.
   c. a calculator.
   d. one pharmacy technician training manual.

4. A majority of the PTCE tests candidates on
   a. assisting the pharmacist in serving patients.
   b. medication and inventory control systems.
   c. administration of pharmacy operations.
   d. insurance billing

5. Once a technician becomes certified (i.e., a CPhT), he or she can get recertified every 2 years by obtaining how many continuing education credits/hours?
   a. 2
   b. 15
   c. 20
   d. 60

6. Which of the following is true in regard to the code of ethics for pharmacy technicians?
   a. The basis for the code of ethics is built entirely upon laws and regulations governing pharmacy practice.
   b. Technicians have a duty to maintain competence and continually enhance their knowledge of practice.
   c. A technician's first consideration is to engage in the support of organizations that promote the profession of pharmacy and the role of technicians.
   d. All of the above

7. A standard résumé does *not* list
   a. the job objective.
   b. employment history.
   c. name, address, and telephone number of the applicant.
   d. names, addresses, and telephone numbers of references.

8. A candidate without a great deal of work experience can compensate for this deficiency by emphasizing the
   a. employment history section of the résumé.
   b. references section of the résumé.
   c. job objective section of the résumé.
   d. skills section of the résumé.

9. The cover letter sent with a résumé should highlight one's
   a. qualifications.
   b. personality.
   c. network of connections.
   d. need for the job.

10. The increased emphasis and needs of the geriatric population will affect pharmacy technicians most specifically in which of the following ways?
    a. Increased computer application skills will be necessary for technicians to deal with the demands of this particular patient population.
    b. Robotics will play a larger role in the pharmacy, and technicians will have to work more closely with them to serve this population.
    c. Technicians will have to become familiar with Medicare Part D to assist these patients in gaining needed information about this drug coverage program.
    d. Technicians must step in to manage prescription-processing systems, because pharmacists are increasingly called upon to provide greater clinical services.

Pharmacy in Practice

1. Using reference texts and the Internet, compile a list of three potential employers of pharmacy technicians in each of the following areas: community pharmacy, hospital pharmacy, long-term care, and home infusion. Each list should include the name of the employer, the address, the telephone number, and a contact person. Collect the lists prepared by students in the class to make a master list.

2. Choose one potential employer of pharmacy technicians, and research to find more information about the employer. Write a brief report providing information that might be of interest to a potential employee of this pharmacy or institution. Write a résumé and cover letter that you might use to apply for a job as a pharmacy technician.

3. Consider the following ethical dilemma facing pharmacy personnel: A pharmacist's religious beliefs preclude him or her from dispensing an emergency contraceptive prescription. Write a brief report on how this applies to the technician working under the supervision of this pharmacist. What would you do in such a situation if presented with a prescription for emergency contraception?

Improving Communication Skills

1. Practice role playing an interview situation with other students in your class. Use the interview questions supplied in this chapter. Develop or update your résumé. Share your résumé with another student. Ask that student to critique and identify your strengths from your résumé.

2. Debate with another student whether border states should encourage drug importation from outside the United States (e.g., from Canada).

Internet Research

1. Visit the Web site of the Pharmacy Technician Certification Board (PTCB) at www.ptcb.org and compile a checklist of tasks to be done to apply for the examination.

2. Write an e-mail to the PTCB and order information on the PTCE.

3. Search the Web for the American Association of Pharmacy Technicians (AAPT). Some areas have a local chapter with a Web site. Locate the contact person's name, the next meeting dates, and times.

4. Search the Internet for news on which states allow "right-to-die" or physician-assisted suicide prescriptions. Report on what procedures must be taken to fill such a prescription in the pharmacy. What ethical dilemma might pharmacy personnel encounter in a state where such prescriptions are legal?

5. The ethical implications of the Human Genome Project are very serious and involve the pharmacy directly. Physicians may someday be able to instantly diagnose a disease based on the patient's genetic makeup. In addition, drug therapies may be designed specifically for a patient based on his or her genetic makeup. Physicians, pharmacists, and many members of the healthcare team will need to access a patient's genetic information. Consider some of the ethical implications of this project, and prepare for a class discussion by listing some of the considerations involved and your opinion regarding this issue.

Common Pharmacy Practice Abbreviations

Appendix **A**

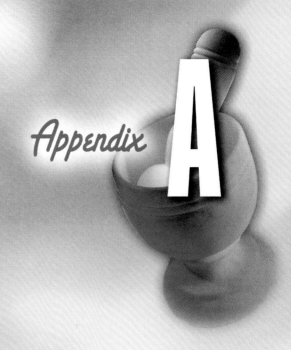

Healthcare professionals have developed their own shorthand for many aspects of patient care, and it is reflected in the abbreviations used in prescription directions.

Many of the abbreviations used in prescriptions are derived from the initials of Latin or Greek phrases. Others come from medical terminology in English, and some even combine terms from multiple languages. Tables A.1–A.7 list some of the most common abbreviations used in pharmacy practice. These should be committed to memory.

Some prescribers may write abbreviations using capital letters or periods. However, periods should not be used with metric units or medical abbreviations as they can be a source of medication errors.

When abbreviations are standardized (to have only one meaning) and are clearly written or printed, they are useful because they save space and time. Abbreviations can cause problems, however, if they are misinterpreted. Sometimes, this occurs when the same set of letters can have two different meanings. For example, the abbreviation "IVP" means "IV Push" or "administer by injection into the vein from a syringe" when used on a hospital prescription order for an intravenous medication. In another context, however, "IVP" designates "intravenous pyeolograms," an x-ray examination of the kidneys, bladder, and urinary tract.

Abbreviations are also problematic when they are not typed or written clearly. The abbreviation "q 6pm," for example, means "every evening at 6 PM," but if written hastily or printed on a fax machine low in toner, it may appear to say "q6h," meaning every 6 hours. The abbreviation "qhs" means "nightly at bedtime," but could be misread as "qhr," meaning "every hour." Some abbreviations are so error-prone that the Joint Commission on Accreditation of Healthcare Organizations (JCAHO) has declared that they are absolutely unacceptable for use in accredited institutions. These are listed in Table A.8. In addition, the symbols > and < should be avoided and written out: "greater than" and "less than".

Safety Note

Do not use periods with abbreviations.

Safety Note

Pay special attention when interpreting abbreviations on prescriptions.

Web Link

Visit **www.ismp.org** for more error-prone abbreviations.

Table A.1 Amounts

Abbreviation	Derivation	Meaning
aa	*ana*	of each
ad	*ad*	up to, so as to make
C	—	Celsius
cc	—	cubic centimeter (mL)
dtd	*datur talis dosis*	dispense such doses
F	—	Fahrenheit
g	*gramma*	gram
gr	*granum*	grain
gtt	*guttae*	drop(s)
h, hr	*hora*	hour
L	*litre*	liter
lb	*libra*	pound
m^2	—	square meter
mcg, µg		microgram
mEq	—	milliequivalent
mg	—	milligram
mg/kg	—	milligrams of drug per kilogram of body weight
mg/m^2	—	milligrams of drug per square meter of body surface area
ℳ	—	minim
mL	—	milliliter
#	*numerus*	number
qs	*quantum sufficiat*	a sufficient quantity
qsad	*quantum sufficiat ad*	a sufficient quantity to make, up to
s̄s̄	*semis*	one half
stat	*statim*	immediately
T	—	temperature
tbsp	—	tablespoonful
tsp	—	teaspoonful
unit	*unitas*	unit
w/v	—	weight-to-volume ratio
&	—	and
+	—	and

Table A.2 Bodily Functions or Conditions

Abbreviation	Meaning
BM	bowel movement
BP	blood pressure
BS	blood sugar
CA	cancer
CHF	congestive heart failure
DT	delirium tremens
GT	gastrostomy tube
HA	headache
HBP	high blood pressure
HT, HTN	hypertension
NKA	no known allergies
NKDA	no known drug allergies
N&V, N/V	nausea and vomiting
SCT	sickle-cell trait
SOB	shortness of breath
URI	upper respiratory infection
UTI	urinary tract infection
VS	vital signs
WBC	white blood cell (count)

Table A.3 Drugs and Drug References

	Abbreviation	Derivation	Meaning
Drugs	APAP	—	acetaminophen
	ASA	acetylsalicylic acid	aspirin
	HC	—	hydrocortisone
	HCTZ		hydrochlorothiazide
	LCD	liquor carbonis detergens	coal tar solution
	MS	—	morphine sulfate
	NTG	—	nitroglycerin
	PCN	—	penicillin
	SMZ/TMP	—	sulfamethoxazole/trimethoprim
	TCN	—	tetracycline
	ZnO	—	zinc oxide
References	NF		National Formulary
	PDR		Physician's Desk Reference
	USP		United States Pharmacopeia

Table A.4 Dose Forms, Solutions, and Delivery Systems

Abbreviation	Derivation	Meaning
amp	*ampulla*	ampule
aq	*aqua*	water
cap	*capsula*	capsule
D$_5$LR	—	5% dextrose in lactated Ringer's solution
D$_5$NS	—	5% dextrose in normal saline solution
DW	—	distilled water
D$_5$W	—	5% dextrose in water
D$_{10}$W	—	10% dextrose in water
ECT	—	enteric-coated tablet
elix	*elixir*	elixir
fl	*fluidus*	fluid
fl oz	—	fluid ounce
inj	*injectio*	injection
IV	*intra venosus*	intravenous
IVP	—	intravenous push
IVPB	—	intravenous piggyback
KVO	—	keep vein open
NS	—	normal saline (0.9% sodium chloride)
½NS	—	half-strength normal saline (0.45%)
MDI	—	metered dose inhaler
oint	—	ointment
O/W	—	oil-in-water
RL, R/L	—	Ringer's lactate (solution)
sol	*solutio*	solution
supp	*suppositorium*	suppository
susp	*suspensus*	suspension
SWFI	—	sterile water for injection
syr	*syrupus*	syrup
tab	*tabella*	tablet
TDS	—	transdermal delivery system
TPN	—	total parenteral nutrition
ung	*unguentum*	ointment
W/O	—	water-in-oil

Table A.5 Time and Time of Administration

Abbreviation	Derivation	Meaning
ā	*ante*	before
ac	*ante cibum*	before meals
ad lib	*ad libitum*	at pleasure, freely
am	*ante meridiam*	morning, before noon
ATC	—	around the clock
bid	*bis in die*	twice a day
h, hr	*hora*	hour
hs	*hora somni*	at bedtime
noct	*nocte*	at night
p	*post*	after
pc	*post cibum*	after meals
pm	*post meridiem*	evening, after noon
post-op	—	postoperative
pp	*postprandial*	after meals
prn	*pro re nata*	as needed
q	*quaque*	each, every
qh	*quaque hora*	every hour
q3h	*quaque 3 hora*	every three hours
qid	*quater in die*	four times a day
tid	*ter in die*	three times a day
tiw	—	three times a week
wk	—	week

Table A.6 Sites of Administration/Parts of the Body

Abbreviation	Derivation	Meaning
ad	*auris dextra*	right ear
as	*auris sinistra*	left ear
au	*auris uterque*	each ear
BSA	—	body surface area
GI	—	gastrointestinal
GU	—	genitourinary
IA	—	intra-arterial
ID	—	intradermal
IM	—	intramuscular
IT	—	intrathecal
npo	*non per os*	nothing by mouth
od	*oculus dexter*	right eye
os	*oculus sinister*	left eye
ou	*oculus uterque*	each eye
per	—	by or through
po	*per os*	by mouth
R	*rectum*	by rectum, rectal
SL	*sub lingua*	sublingual
top	*topikos*	topical
vag	—	vaginally

Table A.7 Pharmacy and Provider Instructions

Abbreviation	Derivation	Meaning
c̄	*cum*	with
comp	*compositus*	compound
DAW		dispense as written
D/C	*discontinuare*	discontinue, discharge
dil	*diluere*	dilute, dissolve
disp	*dispensare*	dispense
div	*dividere*	divide
DT	—	discharge tomorrow
ECT	—	electroconvulsive therapy
m ft	*misce et fiat*	mix and make
non rep, NR	*non repetatur*	do not repeat
O_2	—	oxygen
PBO		prescribe brand only
℞	*recipe*	take
s̄	*sine*	without
sig	*signa, signetur*	write on label
sos	*si opus sit*	if there is need
TAb	—	therapeutic abortion
ut dict, ud	*ut dictum*	as directed
w/	—	with
w/o	—	without
y/o	—	years old
Δ	—	change

Table A.8 Unacceptable Abbreviations Formerly in Common Use

Unapproved Abbreviation	Intended Meaning	Misinterpretation	Correct Form to Use
μg	microgram	milligram	microgram or mcg
qd	every day	four times a day	every day
qod	every other day	daily or four times a day	every other day
SC, SQ, or sub q	subcutaneous	sublingual or 5 every	subcutaneously
U	unit	number 0 or 4	units
$MgSO_4$	magnesium sulfate	morphine sulfate	magnesium sulfate
MSO_4	morphine sulfate	magnesium sulfate	morphine sulfate

Note: Additional error-prone abbreviations are listed at www.ismp.org.

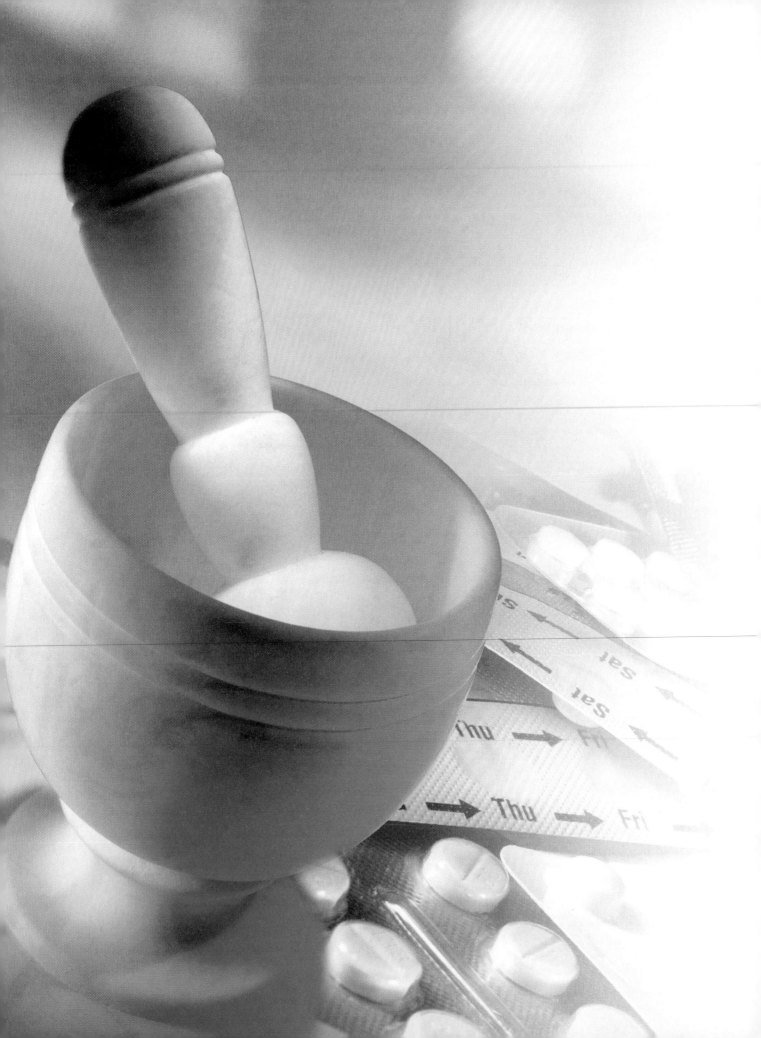

Greek and Latin Word Parts

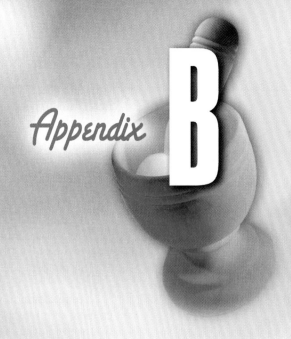

Appendix **B**

Not so long ago, a dedicated student could go a long way toward mastering the available book-learning (if not the practical knowledge) of his or her culture. Today, all that has changed. Modern education and modern information technologies have created an explosion of knowledge. One consequence of the knowledge explosion is specialization. In the seventeenth century, a single person could comprehend the whole of biological science. In the nineteenth century, that person's descendant could absorb the whole of, say, entomology, the study of insects. Today, as Harvard entomologist E. O. Wilson points out, several lifetimes is not enough time in which to learn all that is known about the behaviors of bees, wasps, termites, and other members of the single order of creatures known as *Hymenoptera*, which contains over a million known species.

To communicate precisely with other people involved in a particular field of endeavor, people find it necessary to invent new terminology, words, and phrases to describe the particular elements of their field. To communicate quickly as well as precisely, they create abbreviations and special symbols. Sometimes, the specialized words, phrases, abbreviations, and symbols used in a scientific field such as pharmacy or medicine can be intimidating. The name of a lung disease suffered by coal miners, for example, is

pneumonoultramicroscopicsilicovolcanokoniosis

and this is not even the longest of all technical words in chemistry, biology, and medicine! Do not let the foreign-sounding nature of scientific words intimidate you, however. With a little study and practice in the field of pharmacy, you will soon master most of the specialized terms and abbreviations that you need to know. Most are far shorter and far clearer than the word given above.

At the beginning of the scientific revolution, in the Renaissance, most scholars in Western Europe were deeply learned in the Greek and Latin classics, and so it is not

Web Link
Visit Medline for a list of on-line medical dictionaries at **www.nlm. nih.gov/ medlineplus/ dictionaries.html**

surprising that, when inventing new terms to describe their discoveries and observations, they borrowed bits and pieces of these ancient languages. Such coinage, based on Greek and Latin word parts, remains at the heart of scientific naming. Therefore, when you encounter in your practice as a pharmacy technician the names of procedures, parts of the body, drugs, chemicals, and so on, they will often look like this:

> **analgesic** from Greek *an*, "without," and *algos*, "pain" (def: pertaining to without pain)
>
> **sublingual** from Latin *sub*, "under, below," and *lingua*, "language, tongue" (def: under the tongue)
>
> **cardiologist** from Greek *kardia*, "heart," *-logia*, "the study of," and *ist*, "specialist" (def: person who specializes in the study of the heart)

Some common Greek and Latin word parts encountered in medical and pharmaceutical terminology are listed in the following tables. A root is a word part that forms a major internal constituent of a word. When a word root is combined with a vowel, it is referred to as a combining form. Roots are often combined with other roots and suffixes with the vowel *o*. A prefix is a word part added to the beginning of a word, and common examples are listed in Table B.1. A suffix is a word part added to the end of a word, and common examples are listed in Table B.2. Common roots and combining forms are listed in Table B.3.

Table B.1   Common Prefixes

Word Part	Meaning	Example
acu-	sharp, abrupt, sudden	acupuncture, acute
a-, ad-	towards	adsorbent, adsternal
a-, an-	without	anesthesia, apathy, anemia
ab-	from, away from	abaxial, abnormal, abscess
allo-	other, another	allopathy, AlloDerm
ana-	up to, back, again, apart	anaplastic, anabolic
ante-	before, forwards	antecubital, ante-cibum
anti-	against, opposite	antitoxin, antiseptic, antidepressant
auto-	self	autoimmune
bi-	twice, double	biceps, bisulfite
brady-	slow	bradycardia, bradytaxia
cata-	down	catabolism
circum-	around	circumoral, circumcision
con-	together	congestion, concurrent
contra-	against	contraindication
cuti-	skin	cuticle
de-	from, away from, down from	decongestant
deci-	ten	decimal
di-, dis-	two	distillation, dissect

continues

Table B.1   Common Prefixes—Continued

Word Part	Meaning	Example
dia-	through, complete	dialysis, diarrhea
dipl-, diplo-	double	diplococci, diplopia
dis-	separation	distended
dur-	hard, firm	durable
dys-	bad, abnormal	dystrophy, dyspepsia
e-, ec-, ecto-	out, from out of	ectopic
en-, endo-	into	endoarteritis, endometriosis
epi-	on, up, against, high	epidermis, epidural
eu-	well, normal, abundant	eupnea, euphoria
ex-, exo-	out, from out of	exotropia, excision
extra-	outside, beyond, in addition	extraoral, extrahepatic
hemi-	half	hemiplegia
hetero-	different	heterophilic
homo-	same	homeopathy, homogenous
hyper-	above, excessive	hyperalimentation, hypertension
hypo-	below, deficient	hypodermic, hypovolemic
im-, in-	not	impotence, inaccurate
in-	into	invasive
infra-	below, underneath	infracardiac
inter-	among, between	intercostal
intra-	within, inside, during	intravenous, intrauterine
iso-	equal, same	isomorphic, isotonic
macro-	large	macrocytic, macrophage
mal-	bad	malnutrition, malaise
mega-	large	megavitamin
megalo-	large	megalomania
meta-	change, between	metastasize, metacarpal
micro-	small	micron, microscope
mono-	one	mononucleosis, monocyte
neo-	new	antineoplastic, neonate
non-	not	nontoxic, nonsteroidal
pan-	all, across, throughout	pandemic, panacea
para-	beside, to the side of, wrong	paranasal, parasympathetic
per-	by, through, throughout	percutaneous
peri-	around	pericardium
poly-	many	polymorphonuclear, polypharmacy
post-	behind, after	postpartum, postoperative

continues

Table B.1 Common Prefixes—Continued

Word Part	Meaning	Example
pre-	before, in front	prenatal, premature infant
primi-	first	primigravida
pro-	before, in front	proptosis
pros-	besides, in addition	prosthesis
pseudo-	false	pseudoplegia
quadri-	four	quadriplegia
re-, red-	back, again	reconstitute, reduce
retro-	backwards, behind	retrovirus, retrocardiac
semi-	half	semiconscious
sub-	under, beneath	subcutaneous
super-	above, in addition, over, excessive	supersensitive
supra-	above, on upper side, excessive	suprarenal
syn-	together, with	syndrome
tachy-	rapid	tachypnea
tetra-	four	tetracycline
trans-	across, beyond, through	transocular, transfusion
tri-	three	triceps, tricyclic
ultra-	beyond, excess, more	ultrasound, ultrasensitive
uni-	one	unicellular

Table B.2 Common Suffixes

Word Part	Meaning	Example
-ac	pertaining to	cardiac
-al	pertaining to	myocardial
-algia, -algesia	pain	cephalgia, neuralgia, analgesia
-ar	pertaining to	lumbar
-ase	enzyme (makes a noun)	amylase
-ate	(makes a verb)	expectorate
-cele	herniation, prolapse	rectocele, cystocele
-cide	killer	spermicide
-centesis	surgical puncture to remove fluid	arthrocentesis, amniocentesis
-coccus	berry	staphylococcus
-clasis	break	osteoclasis
-cyte	cell	osteocyte, hepatocyte
-desis	binding, fixation	arthrodesis

continues

Table B.2 Common Suffixes—Continued

Word Part	Meaning	Example
-dipsia	thirst	polydipsia
-dynia	pain	lumbodynia, myodynia
-ectomy	removal of, cut out	appendectomy
-emesis	vomiting	hematemesis, antiemetic
-emia	condition of the blood	anemia, drepanocytemia, hypoglycemia
-genic	producing	carcinogenic, iatrogenic
-gram	a record	angiogram, myelogram
-graph	a device which records	electrocardiograph
-graphy	the process of recording	radiography
-iasis	abnormal condition	nephrolithiasis
-iatry	treatment	podiatry, psychiatry
-ism	condition, state	alcoholism
-ist	specialist	podiatrist
-itis	inflammation	colitis, rhinitis
-ium	tissue	pericardium
-ize	(makes a verb)	immunize
-lepsy	seizure	narcolepsy
-logy	study of, reasoning about	etiology, biology
-lysis	to break apart	urinalysis, hemolysis
-malacia	softening	osteomalacia
-meter	to measure	pelvimeter
-oid	resembling	ovoid, adenoid
-ol	alcohol	ethanol
-oma	tumor	melanoma
-opia	vision	myopia
-ose	carbohydrate	glucose
-ose	full of	adipose tissue
-osis	abnormal condition	halitosis, nephrosis
-path, -pathy	disease, suffering	homeopathy, cardiomyopathy
-pepsia	digestion	dyspepsia
-philia	attraction to, liking for	hydrophilia
-plasty	reshaping, repair of	rhinoplasty, tympanoplasty
-rhea	discharge, flow	diarrhea, leukorrhea
-rrha, -rrhag	discharge, flow, burst forth	hemorrhage
-sclerosis	hardening	arteriosclerosis, otosclerosis

continues

Table B.2   Common Suffixes—Continued

Word Part	Meaning	Example
-scope	device to view with one's eye	microscope, otoscope
-scopy	the process of viewing with the eye	endoscopy, ophthalmoscope
-sis	process, state of	diagnosis
-stasis	stopping, controlling, stand	hemostasis, metastasis
-stat	stop	bacteriostat, hemostat
-stomy	surgical opening	colostomy
-tomy	cut	nephrotomy
-ule	little, minute	venule
-uria	urinary condition	dysuria

Table B.3   Common Roots and Combining Forms

Word Part	Meaning	Example
acet/o	vinegar, acid, sharp	acetaldehyde
acr/o	tip, end, sharpness	acromegaly
aden/o	gland	adenoid, adenovirus
adip/o	fat	adipose, adipoma
aer/o	air	aerogel, aerosol
agon/o	contest, struggle	agonist, agony
alb/o	white	albumin, albino
alg/o	pain	analgesia, myalgia
allel/o	one another, mutual	allergen, allergic
amb/i, amph/o	both, two	amphoteric, ampicillin
ambul/o	walk	ambulatory
amni/o	membrane around the fetus	amniotic fluid, amniocentesis
amyl/o	starch	amylase, amylolysis
andr/o	male	androgen
angi/o	vessel	angiogram, angioplasty
anthrac	black	anthrax, anthracosis
aqu, aqua, aque	water	aqueous
arter/o	artery (as opposed to vein)	arterial, arteriosclerosis
arthr/o	joint	arthritis, arthralgia
asthm	shortness of breath	antiasthmatic

continues

Table B.3 Common Roots and Combining Forms—Continued

Word Part	Meaning	Example
atri	entry	atrium
aud, audit/o	hear	auditory, audiometry
aur/o	hear	aural, Auralgan
axill/o	armpit	axillary temperature
bi/o	life	biopsy, biology
blast	sprout, immature cell	erythroblastosis, osteoblast
blephar/o	eyelid	blepharoptosis
bol	throw, create	bolus, metabolism, emboli
brachi	arm	brachial artery
bronch/o	bronchus (pathway from windpipe)	bronchoscope, bronchitis
bucc/o	inside of cheek	buccal membrane
burs/o	pouchlike cavity	bursa, bursitis
calc/o	calcium	hypocalcemia
cap/o, capi	head, expansion	capillary, capitation
carb/o	carbon	carbohydrate
carcin/o	crab, cancer	carcinogen, carcinoma
cardi/o	heart	cardiology, electrocardiogram
carp/o	wrist	carpal tunnel syndrome
caus	burn	causalgia, caustic
centr/o	center	centrifuge
cephal/o	head, expansion	hydrocephalic
cerebr/o	brain	cerebrovascular accident
cervic/o	neck, cervix	cervicofacial, cervical
chem/o	chemistry	chemotherapy
chir/o	hand	chiropractic
chol/o	bile, cholesterol	cholangiogram, hypercholesterolemia
chondr/o	cartilage; grain	achondroplasia, chondroitin
chron/o	time, long	chronic, chronological
cili	eyelash, hair	cilia, penicillin
coagul/o	clot	anticoagulant
collo	glue	colloidal oatmeal
coni/o	dust	pneumoconiosis
core/o	pupil of eye	coreoplasty, coreoplegia
corp/o	body	corpuscle, corpse
crani/o	cranium, skull	craniotomy

continues

Table B.3 Common Roots and Combining Forms—Continued

Word Part	Meaning	Example
cutane/o, cuti	skin	subcutaneous, cuticle
cyan/o	blue	cyanosis, acrocyanosis
cycl/o	circle, wheel	tetracycline, tricyclic antidepressant
cyst/o	bladder, cyst	cystic fibrosis, cystitis
cyt/o	cell	cytologist
dacr/o	tear (crying)	dacryoadenitis
dactyl/o	finger	syndactylism, adactyly
demos	people	pandemic, epidemic
dent/o	tooth	dentifrice, dentalgia
derm, dermat/o	skin	epidermis, dermabrasion, dermatitis
edem, edema	excess fluid in tissues	angioedema, edematous
encephal/o	brain	electroencephalogram, encephalitis
enter/o	intestine (usually small intestines)	parenteral, enteric
erythr/o	red	erythromycin, erythrocyte
esth, esthesi/o	perception	anesthesia, paresthesia
flat	blow	antiflatulent
galact/o, lact/o	milk	galactosemia, lactorrhea
gangl	knot	ganglion
gastr/o	stomach	gastritis
gen	become, beget, produce	antigen, genetic
genesis	origin	pathogenesis, agenesis
ger/o	aged	gerontology, geriatric
gest	produce	gestation
glob	sphere, ball, round body	globule, hemoglobin
gloss/o	tongue	glossectomy, subglossal
gluc/o	sugar	glucose, Glucophage
glyc/o	sugar	glycosuria
gnos/o	state of	prognosis, diagnosis
gonad/o	reproductive organ	gonadotropin
gynec/o	female	gynecologist
hem/o	blood	hemostat, hemorrhage
hepat/o	liver	hepatitis, hepatotoxic
hidr/o	sweat	hidradenoma, hidrosis
hydr/o	water	hydrocephalus, hydrophobic
hypn/o	sleep	hypnotic
hyster/o, metr/o	uterus	hysterectomy, endometrium

continues

Table B.3 Common Roots and Combining Forms—Continued

Word Part	Meaning	Example
ichthy/o	fishy, scaly	ichthyosis
immun/o	safe, safe from	immunologist, immune
kera, kerat/o	horned, horny skin cells, cornea	keratolytic, keratin, keratoplasty
kinesi/o	motion	kinesiology, akinetic
labi/o	lip	labia, labial
lachri	tear (from the eye)	lacrimal fluid
leuk/o	white	leukemia, leukorrhea
lingu/o	tongue	sublingual
lith/o	stone	nephrolithiasis
lumb/o	lower back, loin	lumbar, lumbodynia
lymph/o	water, lymph	lymphatic system, lymphoma
mast/o	breast	mastectomy, mastitis
melan/o	black	melanoma
mening/o	membrane surrounding brain and spinal cord	meningitis, meningocele
mens	moon, month	menses, menstruation
mnem/o	memory	mnemonic
morb/o	sick	morbidity
morph/o	shape, dream	morphology, morphine
muscul/o	mouse, muscle	intramuscular, neuromuscular
myc/o	fungus	onychomycosis
myel/o	bone marrow, spinal cord	myeloid leukemia, myelogram
my/o	muscle	myocardial infarction, myalgia
myx/o, muco	slime	mucous membrane, myxedemic coma
narc/o	sleep	narcotic, narcolepsy
nas/o	nose	nasopharyngitis, nasal spray
nat/i	birth	prenatal
necr/o	dead	necrosis
nephr/o	kidney	nephritis, nephrologist
neur/o	nerve	neurotransmitter
ocul/o	eye	ocular, oculonasal
odont/o	tooth	orthodontics, odontalgia
onc/o	tumor, mass	oncology
onych/o	fingernail, toenail	onychomalacia
ophthalm/o	eye	ophthalmic, ophthalmologist
opi/o	opium	opiate

continues

Table B.3 Common Roots and Combining Forms—Continued

Word Part	Meaning	Example
optic	eye	optician
orchi, orchid/o	testes	orchiditis, orchiectomy
or/o	mouth	oral
orth/o	straight	orthodontia, orthopedics
osm/o	smell	anosmia
oste/o	bone	osteoporosis, osteopath
ot/o	ear	otic, otoscope
ox/o, oxy	oxygen	hypoxemia, anoxia
ped	child	pediatric
part	parturition, give birth	postpartum
path/o	disease, misery	pathology, nephropathy
pect/o	chest	expectorant, angina pectoris
pod, ped	foot	podiatrist, pedometer
pelvi	pelvis	pelvimetry
phag/o	eat	bacteriophage, dysphagia
pharmac/o	sorcery, poison, drug	pharmacy, pharmacokinetics
phasia	speech	aphasia
phil/o	like, love	hydrophilic, eosinophil
phleb	vein	phlebitis, phlebotomy
phon/o	voice	dysphonia, telephone
phori	carry, bear	diaphoresis
phos, phot/o	light	photosensitivity, phosphorescent
physi	nature, grow	physiological, physical therapy, epi-physeal plate
plasm, plas/o	molded, formation	neoplasm, aplastic anemia
plegi	stroke, paralysis	paraplegic, ophthalmoplegic
pleur/o	lining surrounding lungs	pleurisy, pleural effusion
pneum/o, pneumat/o	breath, air	pneumonia, pneumatic
prandial	meal	postprandial
proct/o	rectum	proctologist, Procto-Foam
psych/o	spirit, mind	antipsychotic, psychotropic
pty, ptyal/o	spit	hemoptysis
pulm/o, pulmon/o	lung	pulmonary, Pulmicort
pyr, pyr/o	fever, fire	pyrogen, antipyretic
radi/o	radiation, X-ray	radiogram
ren/o	kidney	renal, adrenal gland
retin/o	retina	retinopathy

continues

Table B.3 Common Roots and Combining Forms—Continued

Word Part	Meaning	Example
rhin/o	nose	rhinovirus, rhinitis
sarc/o	flesh	sarcoma
scler/o	hard	atherosclerosis, sclerosing agent
seb/o	fat, oil	sebum, seborrheic dermatitis
sect/o, seg	cut	section, segment, dissect
seps, sept	rot, infection	antiseptic, aseptic technique
sial	saliva	sialolith
soma	body	psychosomatic, somatropin
spasm/o	drawing tight	antispasmodic
spondyl/o	spine	spondylitis, spondylodesis
sphygm/o	heartbeat, pulse	sphygmomanometer (BP cuff)
spir/o	breathing	spirometer, inspiration
staphyl/o	cluster of grapes	staphylococcus
stern/o	breastbone	sternum
stom/o, stomy	mouth, surgical opening	stomatitis, colostomy
strept/o	wavy, twisted chain	streptomycin, streptococcus
ten/o, tend/o	stretch	tendonitis, tenosynovitis
thorac/o	chest	pneumothorax, thoracic
thromb/o	blood clot	thrombolysis, thrombosis
thyr/o	thyroid	hypothyroidism, thyroiditis
tom, tome	cut, instrument to cut	lobotomy, craniotomy
tox, toxo	poisonous	toxic, toxicology
troph, trop/o	growing, nourish, develop	atrophy, somatotropin
tympan/o	eardrum	tympanocentesis
ur/o	urine	urology
uter/o	uterus, womb	intrauterine
vas/o	blood vessel	vasodilation
ven/o, phleb/o	vein (as opposed to artery)	venule, phlebotomy
vert	turn	vertigo, divert
viscer/o	internal organs	viscera, visceromegaly
xer/o	dry	xeroderma, xerostomia

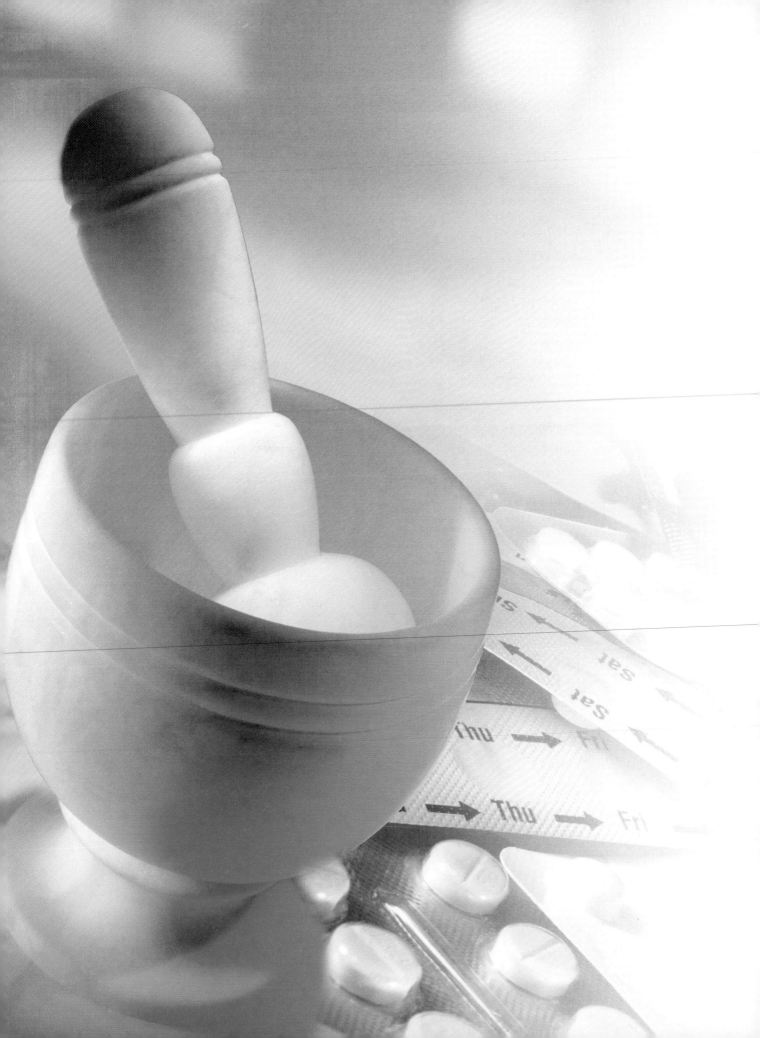

Most Commonly Prescribed Drugs

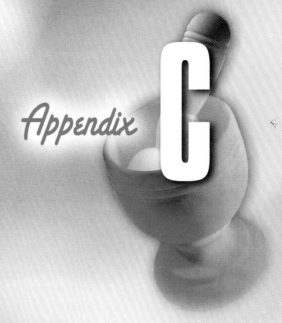

Appendix C

This table, reformatted and organized by brand name, is available on this textbook's Internet Resource Center at www.emcp.com.

Generic Name	Pronunciation	Category	Brand Name
acetaminophen-codeine	a-seat-a-MIN-oh-fen KOE-deen	analgesic	Phenaphen With Codeine, Tylenol With Codeine
albuterol	al-BYOO-ter-ole	bronchodilator	Proventil, Ventolin
alendronate	a-LEN-droe-nate	bone resorption inhibitor	Fosamax
allopurinol	al-oh-PURE-i-nole	antigout agent	Zyloprim
alprazolam	al-PRAZ-oh-lam	antianxiety agent	Xanax
amitriptyline	a-mee-TRIP-ti-leen	antidepressant	Elavil
amlodipine	am-LOE-di-peen	antihypertensive	Norvasc
amlodipine-benazepril	am-LOE-di-peen ben-AYE-ze-pril	antihypertensive	Lotrel
amoxicillin	a-mox-i-SIL-in	systemic antibacterial	Trimox
amoxicillin-clavulanate	a-mox-i-SIL-in klav-yoo-LAN-ate	systemic antibacterial	Augmentin
atenolol	a-TEN-oh-lole	antihypertensive	Tenormin
atomoxetine	AT-oh-mox-e-teen	ADHD therapy agent	Strattera
atorvastatin	a-TOR-va-sta-tin	antihyperlipidemic	Lipitor
azithromycin	az-ith-roe-MYE-sin	systemic antibacterial	Zithromax
benazepril	ben-AYE-ze-pril	antihypertensive	Lotensin
brimonidine	bri-MOE-ni-deen	antiglaucoma agent	Alphagan P
budesonide	byoo-DES-oh-nide	antiasthmatic	Pulmicort

Generic Name	Pronunciation	Category	Brand Name
bupropion	byoo-PROE-pee-on	antidepressant, smoking cessation adjunct	Wellbutrin, Zyban
calcitonin-salmon	kal-si-TOE-nin SAM-en	bone resorption inhibitor	Miacalcin
candesartan	kan-de-SAR-tan	antihypertensive	Atacand
carisoprodol	kar-eye-soe-PROE-dole	skeletal muscle relaxant	Soma
carvedilol	KAR-ve-dil-ole	antihypertensive	Coreg
cefdinir	sef-DI-neer	systemic antibacterial	Omnicef
cefprozil	sef-PROE-zil	systemic antibacterial	Cefzil
celecoxib	sel-a-KOX-ib	analgesic, antirheumatic NSAID	Celebrex
cephalexin	sef-a-LEX-in	systemic antibacterial	Keflex
cetirizine	se-TI-ra-zeen	antihistaminic, H_1 receptor	Zyrtec
cetirizine-pseudoephedrine	se-TI-ra-zeen soo-doe-e-FED-rin	antihistaminic, H_1 receptor–decongestant	Zyrtec-D
ciprofloxacin	sip-roe-FLOX-a-sin	systemic antibacterial	Cipro
citalopram	sye-TAL-oh-pram	antidepressant	Celexa
clarithromycin	kla-RITH-roe-mye-sin	systemic antibacterial, antimycobacterial	Biaxin
clonazepam	kloe-NA-ze-pam	anticonvulsant	Klonopin
clonidine	KLON-i-deen	antihypertensive	Catapres, Duraclon
clopidogrel	kloh-PID-oh-grel	antithrombotic, platelet aggregation inhibitor	Plavix
clotrimazole-betamethasone	kloe-TRIM-a-zole bay-ta-METH-a-sone	antifungal, corticosteroid	Lotrisone
conjugated estrogen	CON-ju-gate-ed ES-troe-jen	systemic estrogen, osteoporosis prophylactic, ovarian hormone therapy agent	Premarin
conjugated estrogen–medroxyprogesterone	CON-ju-gate-ed ES-troe-jen me-DROX-ee-proe-JES-te-rone	estrogen-progestin, osteoporosis prophylactic, ovarian hormone therapy agent	Premphase, Prempro
cyclobenzaprine	sye-kloe-BEN-za-preen	skeletal muscle relaxant	Flexeril
desloratadine	des-LOR-at-a-deen	antihistaminic, H_1 receptor	Clarinex
dextroamphetamine-amphetamine	dex-troe-am-FET-a-meen am-FET-a-meen	CNS stimulant, ADHD therapy	Adderall
diazepam	dye-AZ-e-pam	amnestic, antianxiety agent, anticonvulsant, antipanic agent, antitremor agent, sedative-hypnotic, skeletal muscle relaxant adjunct	Valium
digoxin	di-JOX-in	antiarrhythmic, cardiotonic	Lanoxicaps, Lanoxin
diltiazem	dil-TYE-a-zem	antianginal, antiarrhythmic, antihypertensive	Cardizem, Dilacor
divalproex	dye-VAL-pro-ex	anticonvulsant, antimanic, migraine headache prophylactic	Depakote
donepezil	don-EH-pa-zil	dementia symptoms treatment adjunct	Aricept
doxycycline	dox-i-SYE-kleen	systemic antibacterial, antiprotozoal	Vibramycin

Generic Name	Pronunciation	Category	Brand Name
enalapril	e-NAL-a-pril	antihypertensive, vasodilator	Vasotec
escitalopram	es-sye-TAL-oh-pram	antianxiety agent, antidepressant	Lexapro
esomeprazole	es-oh-ME-pray-zole	gastric acid pump inhibitor, antiulcer agent	Nexium
ethinyl estradiol–desogestrel	ETH-in-il es-tra-DYE-ole des-oh-JES-trel	antiendometriotic, systemic contraceptive, gonadotropin inhibitor	Cyclessa, Desogen, Kariva, Mircette, Ortho-Cept
ethinyl estradiol–drospirenone	ETH-in-il es-tra-DYE-ole droh-SPYE-re-none	systemic contraceptive	Yasmin
ethinyl estradiol–levonorgestrel	ETH-in-il es-tra-DYE-ole LEE-voe-nor-jes-trel	antiendometriotic, systemic postcoital contraceptive, systemic contraceptive, estrogen-progestin, gonadotropin inhibitor	Levlen, Nordette, Seasonale, Tri-Levlen, Triphasil, Trivora-28
ethinyl estradiol–norelgestromin	ETH-in-il es-tra-DYE-ole nor-el-JES-troe-min	systemic contraceptive	Ortho Evra
ethinyl estradiol–norethindrone	ETH-in-il es-tra-DYE-ole nor-eth-IN-drone	antiacne agent, antiendometriotic, systemic contraceptive, estrogen-progestin, gonadotropin inhibitor	Estrostep Fe, Femhrt, Loestrin Fe, Ovcon
ethinyl estradiol–norgestimate	ETH-in-il es-tra-DYE-ole nor-JES-ti-mate	antiacne agent, antiendometriotic, systemic contraceptive, estrogen-progestin, gonadotropin inhibitor	Ortho Tri-Cyclen, Ortho Tri-Cyclen Lo
ethinyl estradiol–norgestrel	ETH-in-il es-tra-DYE-ole nor-JES-trel	antiendometriotic, systemic postcoital contraceptive, systemic contraceptive, estrogen-progestin, gonadotropin inhibitor	Lo/Ovral, Low-Ogestrel, Ovral
ezetimibe	e-ZET-e-mibe	antihyperlipidemic	Zetia
felodipine	fe-LOE-di-peen	antianginal, antihypertensive	Plendil
fenofibrate	fen-oh-FYE-brate	antihyperlipidemic	Tricor
fentanyl	FEN-ta-nil	analgesic	Duragesic
		analgesic, anesthesia adjunct	Actiq, Sublimaze
fexofenadine	fex-o-FEN-a-deen	antihistaminic, H_1 receptor	Allegra
fexofenadine-pseudoephedrine	fex-o-FEN-a-deen soo-doe-e-FED-rin	antihistaminic, H_1 receptor–decongestant	Allegra-D
finasteride	fin-AS-tur-ide	benign prostatic hyperplasia therapy agent, hair growth stimulant	Propecia, Proscar
fluconazole	floo-KOE-na-zole	systemic antifungal	Diflucan
fluoxetine	floo-OX-e-teen	antidepressant, antiobsessional agent, antibulemic agent	Prozac, Sarafem
fluticasone	floo-TIK-a-sone	steroidal nasal anti-inflammatory, nasal corticosteroid	Flonase, Flovent

Generic Name	Pronunciation	Category	Brand Name
fluticasone-salmeterol	floo-TIK-a-sone sal-ME-te-role	antiasthmatic, inhalation anti-inflammatory, bronchodilator	Advair Diskus
fluvastatin	FLOO-va-sta-tin	antihyperlipidemic, HMG-CoA reductase inhibitor	Lescol
folic acid	FOE-lik AS-id	diagnostic acid, folate deficiency, nutritional vitamin supplement	many
fosinopril	foe-SIN-oh-pril	antihypertensive, vasodilator	Monopril
furosemide	fur-OH-se-mide	antihypercalcemic, antihypertensive, renal disease diagnostic aid adjunct, diuretic	Lasix
gabapentin	GA-ba-pen-tin	anticonvulsant, antineuralgic	Neurontin
gemfibrozil	jem-FI-broe-zil	antihyperlipidimic	Lopid
glimepiride	GLYE-me-pye-ride	antidiabetic	Amaryl
glipizide	GLIP-i-zide	antidiabetic	Glucotrol
glyburide	GLYE-byoo-ride	antidiabetic	DiaBeta, Glynase, Micronase
glyburide-metformin	GLYE-byoo-ride met-FOR-min	antidiabetic	Glucovance
hydrochlorothiazide	hye-droe-klor-oh-THYE-a-zide	antihypertensive, diuretic, antiurolithic	Esidrix
hydrocodone-acetaminophen	hye-droe-KOE-done a-seat-a-MIN-oh-fen	analgesic	Lortab, Vicodin
hydrocodone-chlorpheniramine	hye-droe-KOE-done klor-fen-EER-a-meen	antihistaminic, H_1 receptor–antitussive	Tussionex
ibuprofen	eye-byoo-PROE-fen	analgesic	Advil, Motrin
insulin glargine	IN-su-lin GLARE-jeen	antidiabetic	Lantus
insulin lispro	IN-su-lin LYE-sproe	antidiabetic	Humalog
ipratropium	i-pra-TROE-pee-um	antiasthmatic	Atrovent
ipratropium-albuterol	i-pra-TROE-pee-um al-BYOO-ter-ole	antiasthmatic-bronchodilator	Combivent
irbesartan	ir-be-SAR-tan	antihypertensive	Avapro
irbesartan-hydrochlorothiazide	ir-be-SAR-tan hye-droe-klor-oh-THYE-a-zide	antihypertensive, diuretic	Avalide
isosorbide mononitrate	eye-soe-SOR-bide mon-oh-NYE-trate	antianginal	Imdur, Ismo
lansoprazole	lan-SOE-pra-zole	gastric acid pump inhibitor, antiulcer agent	Prevacid
latanoprost	la-TA-noe-prost	antiglaucoma agent, ocular antihypertensive	Xalatan
levofloxacin	lee-voe-FLOX-a-sin	systemic antibacterial	Levaquin
levothyroxine	lee-voe-thye-ROX-een	antineoplastic, thyroid function diagnostic aid, thyroid hormone	Levothroid, Synthroid
lisinopril	lyse-IN-oh-pril	antihypertensive, vasodilator	Prinivil, Zestril
lorazepam	lor-AZ-e-pam	amnestic, antianxiety agent, anticonvulsant, antiemetic, antipanic agent, antitremor agent, sedative-hypnotic, skeletal muscle relaxant	Ativan

Generic Name	Pronunciation	Category	Brand Name
losartan	loe-SAR-tan	angiotensin II–receptor antagonist, antihypertensive	Cozaar
losartan-hydrochloro-thiazide	loe-SAR-tan hye-droe-klor-oh-THYE-a-zide	antihypertensive	Hyzaar
meclizine	MEK-li-zeen	antiemetic, antivertigo agent	Antivert
meloxicam	mel-OX-i-kam	antirheumatic (NSAID)	Mobic
metaxalone	me-TAX-a-lone	skeletal muscle relaxant	Skelaxin
metformin	met-FOR-min	antihyperglycemic	Glucophage
methylphenidate	meth-il-FEN-i-date	CNS stimulant, ADHD therapy	Concerta, Metadate, Ritalin
methylprednisolone	meth-il-pred-NIS-oh-lone	steroidal anti-inflammatory, corticoid steroid, immunosuppressant	Medrol
metoprolol	met-oh-PROE-lole	antiadrenergic, antianginal, antianxiety therapy adjunct, antiarrhythmic, antihypertensive, antitremor agent, hypertrophic cardiomyopathy therapy adjunct, myocardial infarction therapy, neuroleptic-induced akathisia therapy, pheochromocytoma therapy adjunct, thyrotoxicosis therapy adjunct, vascular headache prophylactic	Lopressor, Toprol
mirtazapine	mir-TAZ-a-peen	antidepressant	Remeron
mometasone furoate	moe-MET-a-sone FYOOR-oh-ate	nasal steroidal anti-inflammatory, nasal corticosteroid	Nasonex
montelukast	mon-te-LOO-kast	antiasthmatic, leukotriene receptor antagonist	Singulair
moxifloxacin	mox-i-FLOX-a-sin	ophthalmic antibacterial	Vigamox
		systemic antibacterial	Avelox
mupirocin	myoo-PEER-oh-sin	topical antibacterial	Bactroban
naproxen	na-PROX-en	analgesic, nonsteroidal anti-inflammatory, antidysmenorrheal, antigout agent, antipyretic, nonsteroidal anti-inflammatory antirheumatic, vascular headache prophylactic, vascular headache suppressant	Aleve, Naprosyn
niacin	NYE-a-sin	nutritional supplement, vitamin	Niacor, Niaspan
nifedipine	nye-FED-i-peen	antianginal, antihypertensive	Procardia
nitrofurantoin	nye-troe-fyoor-AN-toyn	systemic antibacterial	Macrobid, Macrodantin
nitroglycerin	nye-troe-GLI-ser-in	antianginal, congestive heart failure vasodilator	Minitran, Nitrolingual, Nitrostat

Generic Name	Pronunciation	Category	Brand Name
NPH isophane insulin	NPH EYE-so-fayn IN-su-lin	antidiabetic	Humulin N
NPH regular insulin	NPH REG-u-lar IN-su-lin	antidiabetic	Humulin 70/30
olanzapine	oh-LAN-za-peen	antipsychotic	Zyprexa
olopatadine	oh-loe-pa-TA-deen	ophthalmic antihistaminic, H_1 receptor, ophthalmic mast cell stabilizer, ophthalmic antiallergic	Patanol
omeprazole	oh-ME-pray-zole	gastric acid pump inhibitor, antiulcer agent	Prilosec
oxybutynin	ox-i-BYOO-ti-nin	urinary tract antispasmodic	Ditropan
oxycodone	ox-i-KOE-done	analgesic	OxyContin
oxycodone-acetaminophen	ox-i-KOE-done a-seat-a-MIN-oh-fen	analgesic	Endocet, Percocet, Tylox
pantoprazole	pan-TOE-pray-zole	gastric acid pump inhibitor, antiulcer agent	Protonix
paroxetine	pa-ROX-e-teen	antianxiety agent, antidepressant, antiobsessional agent, antipanic agent, posttraumatic stress disorder agent, social anxiety disorder agent	Paxil
penicillin V	pen-i-SIL-in V	systemic antibacterial	Veetids
phenytoin	FEN-i-toyn	antiarrhythmic, anticonvulsant, trigeminal neuralgic antineuralgic, skeletal muscle relaxant	Dilantin
pimecrolimus	pim-e-KROW-li-mus	immunomodulator	Elidel
pioglitazone	pye-oh-GLI-ta-zone	antidiabetic	Actos
polyethylene glycol	pol-ee-ETH-il-een GLYE-kole	hyperosmotic laxative	Miralax
potassium chloride	poe-tass-EE-um KLOR-ide	antihypokalemic, electrolyte replenisher	Klor-Con
pravastatin	PRA-va-sta-tin	antihyperlipidemic, HMG-CoA reductase inhibitor	Pravachol
prednisone	PRED-ni-sone	steroidal inflammatory, cancer chemotherapy antiemetic, corticosteroid, immunosuppressant	Deltasone
promethazine	proe-METH-a-zeen	antiemetic, antihistaminic, H_1 receptor, antivertigo agent, sedative-hypnotic	Phenergan
promethazine-codeine	proe-METH-a-zeen KOE-deen	antihistaminic, H_1 receptor-antitussive	Promethazine with Codeine
propoxyphene-acetaminophen	proe-POX-i-feen a-seat-a-MIN-oh-fen	analgesic	Darvocet-N 100
propranolol	proe-PRAN-oh-lole	antiadrenergic, antianginal, antianxiety therapy adjunct, antiarrhythmic, antihypertensive, antitremor agent, hypertrophic cardiomyopathy therapy adjunct, myocardial infarction prophylactic, myocardial infarction therapy, neuroleptic-induced akathisia therapy, pheochromocytoma therapy adjunct, thyrotoxicosis therapy adjunct, vascular headache prophylactic	Inderal

Generic Name	Pronunciation	Category	Brand Name
quetiapine	kwe-TYE-a-peen	antipsychotic	Seroquel
quinapril	KWIN-a-pril	antihypertensive, vasodilator	Accupril
rabeprazole	ra-BE-pray-zole	gastric acid pump inhibitor, antiulcer agent	Aciphex
raloxifene	ral-OX-i-feen	selective estrogen receptor modulator, osteoporosis prophylactic	Evista
ramipril	RA-mi-pril	antihypertensive, vasodilator	Altace
ranitidine	ra-NI-ti-deen	histamine H_2–receptor antagonist, antiulcer agent, gastric acid secretion inhibitor	Zantac
risedronate	ris-ED-roe-nate	bone resorption inhibitor	Actonel
risperidone	ris-PER-i-done	antipsychotic	Risperdal
rosiglitazone	ROS-e-glit-a-zone	antidiabetic	Avandia
sertraline	SER-tra-leen	antianxiety agent, antidepressant, antiobsessional agent, antipanic agent, posttraumatic stress disorder therapy agent, premenstrual dysphoric disorder therapy agent	Zoloft
sildenafil	sil-DEN-a-fil	systemic impotence therapy agent	Viagra
simvastatin	SIM-va-sta-tin	antihyperlipidemic, HMG-CoA reductase inhibitor	Zocor
spironolactone	speer-on-oh-LAK-tone	aldosterone antagonist, antihypertensive, antihypokalemic, primary hyperaldosteronism diagnostic aid, diuretic	Aldactone
sulfamethoxazole-trimethoprim	sul-fa-meth-OX-a-zole trye-METH-oh-prim	systemic antibacterial, antiprotozoal	Bactrim, Cotrim, Septra DS
sumatriptan	soo-ma-TRIP-tan	antimigraine agent	Imitrex
tamsulosin	tam-SOO-loh-sin	benign prostatic hyperplasia therapy agent	Flomax
temazepam	tem-AZ-e-pam	sedative-hypnotic	Restoril
terazosin	ter-AYE-zoe-sin	antihypertensive, benign prostatic hyperplasia therapy agent	Hytrin
timolol	TYE-moe-lole	antiadrenergic, antianginal, antianxiety therapy adjunct, antiarrhythmic, systemic antiglaucoma agent, antihypertensive, antitremor agent, hypertrophic cardiomyopathy therapy adjunct, myocardial infarction prophylactic, pheochromocytoma therapy adjunct, thyrotoxicosis therapy adjunct, vascular headache prophylactic	Blocadren
		ophthalmic antiglaucoma agent	Timoptic

Generic Name	Pronunciation	Category	Brand Name
tobramycin-dexamethasone	toe-bra-MYE-sin dex-a-METH-a-sone	ophthalmic corticosteroid, ophthalmic steroidal anti-inflammatory, ophthalmic antibacterial	TobraDex
tolterodine	TOLE-tear-oh-deen	urinary bladder antispasmodic	Detrol
topiramate	toe-PYRE-a-mate	anticonvulsant, antimigraine headache	Topamax
tramadol	TRA-ma-dole	analgesic	Ultram
tramadol-acetaminophen	TRA-ma-dole a-seat-a-MIN-oh-fen	analgesic	Ultracet
trazodone	TRAZ-oh-done	antidepressant, antineuralgic	Desyrel
triamcinolone	trye-am-SIN-oh-lone	inhalation anti-inflammatory, antiasthmatic	Azmacort
		nasal steroidal anti-inflammatory, nasal corticosteroid	Nasacort AQ
triamterene-hydrochlorothiazide	trye-AM-ter-een hye-droe-klor-oh-THYE-a-zide	antihypertensive, antihypokalemic, diuretic	Dyazide, Maxzide
valacyclovir	val-ay-SYE-kloe-veer	systemic antiviral	Valtrex
valsartan	val-SAR-tan	antihypertensive	Diovan
valsartan-hydrochlorothiazide	val-SAR-tan hye-droe-klor-oh-THYE-a-zide	antihypertensive	Diovan HCT
venlafaxine	ven-la-FAX-een	antidepressant, antianxiety agent	Effexor
verapamil	ver-AP-a-mil	antianginal, antiarrhythmic, antihypertensive, hypertrophic cardiomyopathy therapy adjunct, vascular headache prophylactic	Calan, Covera HS, Isoptin, Verelan
warfarin	WAR-far-in	anticoagulant	Coumadin
zolpidem	ZOLE-pi-dem	sedative hypnotic	Ambien

Source: Adapted from RxList, The Top 200 Prescriptions for 2003 by Number of U.S. Prescriptions Dispensed: Generic Name (www.rxlist.com/top200.htm, accessed August 24, 2004). Category information from the U.S. National Library of Medicine and National Institutes of Health MedlinePlus Web site (www.nlm.nih.gov/medlineplus/, accessed December 17, 2004).

Common Drugs That Cannot Be Crushed

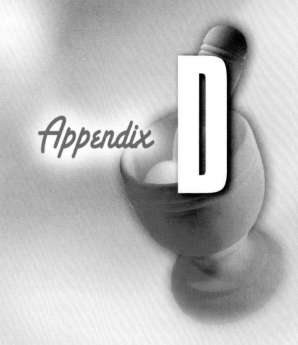

Appendix D

- Adalat CC
- Adderall XR
- Aggrenox
- Allegra D 12/24
- Altoprev 20/60
- Avinza
- Biaxin XL
- Bupropion SR
- Carbidopa/Levodopa ER
- Concerta ER
- Darifenacin XR
- Depakote ER
- Diltia XT/Diltiazem XL
- Ditropan XL
- Effexor XR
- Felodopine XR
- Fosamax
- Glucophage XR
- Glucotrol XL
- Inderal LA
- Indomethacin SR
- Lescol XL
- Methylphenidate LA
- MS Contin
- Niaspan SR
- Nifedipine XL
- Oxycodone XR
- Pentasa
- Pentoxiphylline
- Plendil XR
- potassium chloride
- Procardia XL
- Propranolol LA
- Ritalin LA
- Theophylline XR
- Toprol XL
- Verapamil XR
- Voltaren XR
- Vospire
- Wellbutrin XL

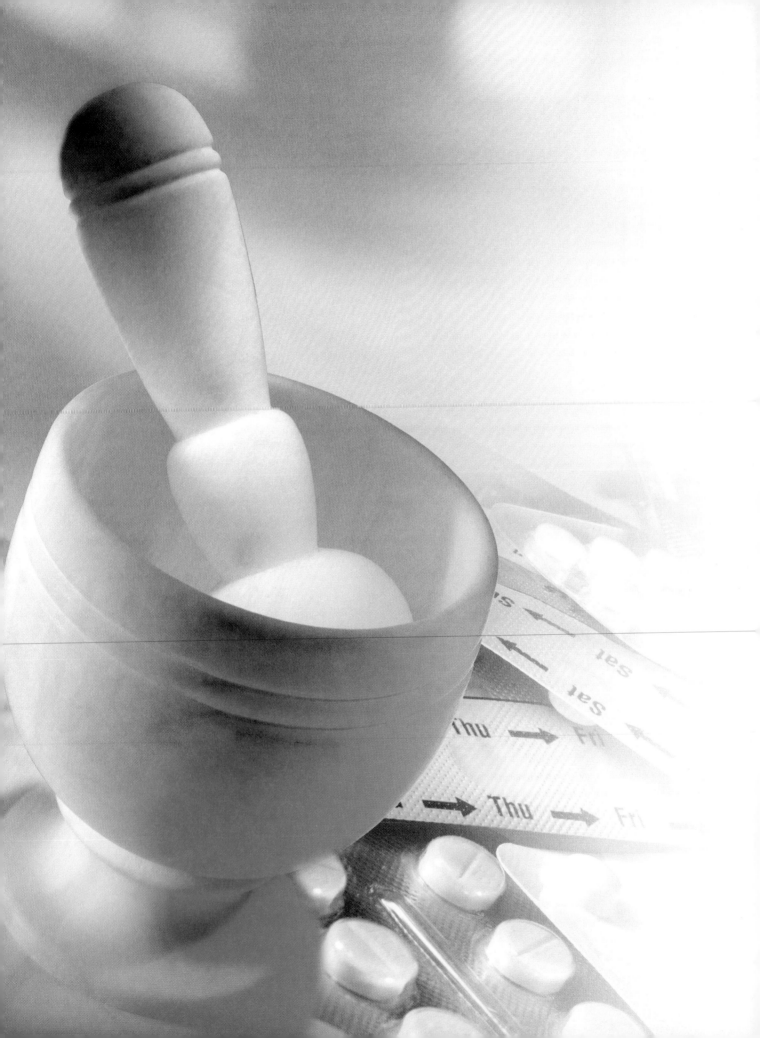

Look-Alike, Sound-Alike Medication Recommendations and Reference Table

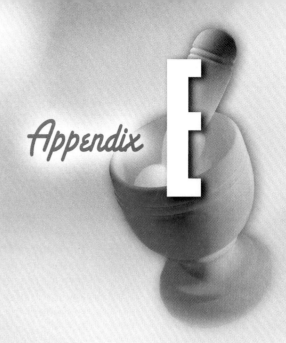

Appendix **E**

While manufacturers have an obligation to review new trademarks for error potential before use, there are some things that prescribers, pharmacists, and pharmacy technicians can do to help prevent errors with products that have look- or sound-alike names. The Institute for Safe Medication Practices (ISMP) (www.ismp.org) has provided the following recommendations designed to prevent dispensing errors.

- **Use electronic prescribing** to prevent confusion with handwritten drug names.
- **Encourage physicians to write prescriptions that clearly specify the dosage form, drug strength, and complete directions.** They should include the product's indication on all outpatient prescriptions and on inpatient *prn* orders. With name pairs known to be problematic, reduce the potential for confusion by writing prescriptions using both the brand and generic name. Listing both names on medication administration records and automated dispensing cabinet computer screens also may be helpful.
- **Whenever possible, determine the purpose of the medication** before dispensing or administering it. Many products with look-alike or sound-alike names are used for different purposes.
- **Accept verbal or telephone orders only when truly necessary.** Require staff to read back all orders, spell the product name, and state its indication. Like medication names, numbers can sound alike, so staff should read the dosage back in numerals (e.g., "one five" for 15 mg) to ensure clear interpretation of dose.
- **When feasible, use magnifying lenses and copyholders** under good lighting to keep prescriptions and orders at eye level during transcription to improve the likelihood of proper interpretation of look-alike product names.
- **Change the appearance of look-alike product names** on computer screens, pharmacy and nursing unit shelf labels, and bins (including automated dispensing cabinets), pharmacy product labels, and medication administration records by highlighting—through boldface, color, and/or tall-man letters—the parts of the names that are different (e.g., hydr**OXY**zine, hydr**ALA**zine).

- **Install a computerized reminder** (also placed on automated dispensing cabinet screens) for the most serious confusing name pairs so that an alert is generated when entering prescriptions for either drug. If possible, make the reminder auditory as well as visual.
- **Affix "name alert" stickers** in areas where look-alike or sound-alike products are stored (available from pharmacy label manufacturers).
- **Store products with look-alike or sound-alike names in different locations**. Avoid storing both products in the fast-mover area. Use a shelf sticker to help locate the product that is moved.
- **Continue to employ an independent check in the dispensing process** (one person interprets and enters the prescription into the computer and another reviews the printed label against the original prescription and the product).
- **Open the prescription bottle or the unit dose package in front of the patient** to confirm the expected product appearance and review the indication. Caution patients about error potential when taking products that have a look-alike or sound-alike counterpart. Take the time to fully investigate the situation if a patient states he or she is taking an unknown medication.
- **Monitor reported errors caused by look-alike and sound-alike medication names** and alert staff to mistakes.
- **Look for the possibility of name confusion when a new product is added to the formulary.** Have a few clinicians handwrite the product name and directions, as they would appear in a typical order. Ask frontline nurses, pharmacists, technicians, unit secretaries, and physicians to view the samples of the written product name as well as pronounce it to determine if it looks or sounds like any other drug product or medical term. It may be helpful to have clinicians first look at the scripted product name to determine how they would interpret it before the actual product name is provided to them for pronunciation. Once the product name is known, clinicians may be less likely to see more familiar product names in the written samples. If the potential for confusion with other products is identified, take steps to avoid errors as listed below.
- **Encourage reporting of errors** and potentially hazardous conditions with look-alike and sound-alike product names and use the information to establish priorities for error reduction. Also maintain awareness of problematic product names and error prevention recommendations provided by the ISMP (www.ismp.org and also listed on the quarterly *Action Agenda*), FDA (www.fda.gov), and USP (www.usp.org).
- **Review Table E.1 for look-alike and sound-alike drug name pairs in use at your practice location**. Decide what actions might be warranted to prevent medication errors. Stay current with alerts from the ISMP, FDA, and USP in case new problematic name pairs emerge.

Table E.1 Look-Alike and Sound-Alike Medications

Abelcet	amphotericin B
Accupril	Aciphex
acetazolamide	acetohexamide
acetohexamide	acetazolamide
Aciphex	Aricept
Aciphex	Accupril
Activase	TNKase
Actonel	Actos

continues

Table E.1 Look-Alike and Sound-Alike Medications—Continued

Actos	Actonel	
Adderall	Inderal	
Advicor	Altocor	
Aggrastat	argatroban	
Aldara	Alora	
Alkeran	Leukeran	Myleran
Allegra	Viagra	
Alora	Aldara	
Altocor	Advicor	
Amaryl	Reminyl	
AmBisome	amphotericin B	
amphotericin B	Abelcet	
amphotericin B	Ambisome	
antacid	Atacand	
Antivert	Axert	
Anzemet	Avandamet	
argatroban	Aggrastat	
Aricept	Aciphex	
aripiprazole	rabeprazole	
Asacol	Os-Cal	
Atacand	antacid	
Atrovent	Natru-Vent	
Avandamet	Anzemet	
Avandia	Prandin	
Avandia	Coumadin	
Avinza	Invanz	
Avinza	Evista	
Axert	Antivert	
BayHep B	BayRab	BayRho-D
BayRab	BayRho-D	BayHep B
BayRho-D	BayHep B	BayRab
Bicillin C-R	Bicillin L-A	
Bicillin L-A	Bicillin C-R	
Brethine	Methergine	
camphorated tincture of opium (paregoric)	opium tincture	
carboplatin	cisplatin	
Cedax	Cidex	
Celexa	Zyprexa	
chlorpromazine	chlorpropamide	
chlorpropamide	chlorpromazine	
Cidex	Cedax	
cisplatin	carboplatin	

continues

Claritin-D	Claritin-D 24
Claritin-D 24	Claritin-D
Clozaril	Colazal
Colace	Cozaar
Colazal	Clozaril
colchicine	Cortrosyn
Comvax	Recombivax HB
Cortrosyn	colchicine
Coumadin	Avandia
Cozaar	Colace
Cozaar	Zocor
dactinomycin	daptomycin
daptomycin	dactinomycin
Darvon	Diovan
daunorubicin	idarubicin
Denavir	Indinavir
Depakote	Depakote ER
Depakote ER	Depakote
Depo-Medrol	Solu-Medrol
Diabenese	Diamox
DiaBeta	Zebeta
Diamox	Diabenese
Diatex (diazepam in Mexico)	Diatx
Diatx	Diatex (diazepam in Mexico)
Dilacor XR	Pilocar
Dilaudid	Dilaudid-5
Dilaudid-5	Dilaudid
Dioval	Diovan
Diovan	Dioval
Diovan	Zyban
Diovan	Darvon
Diprivan	Ditropan
Ditropan	Diprivan
dobutamine	dopamine
dopamine	dobutamine
doxorubicin hydrochloride	liposomal doxorubicin (Doxil)
Duricef	Ultracet
Endocet	Indocin
Engerix-B adult	Engerix-B pediatric/adolescent
Engerix-B pediatric/adolescent	Engerix-B adult
ephedrine	epinephrine
epinephrine	ephedrine

continues

Table E.1 Look-Alike and Sound-Alike Medications—Continued

Estratest	Estratest H.S.
Estratest H.S.	Estratest
ethambutol	Ethmozine
Ethmozine	ethambutol
Evista	Avinza
Femara	Femhrt
Femhrt	Femara
fentanyl	sufentanil
folic acid	folinic acid (leucovorin calcium)
folinic acid (leucovorin calcium)	folic acid
Foradil	Toradol
gentamicin	gentian violet
gentian violet	gentamicin
Granulex	Regranex
Healon	Hyalgan
heparin	Hespan
Hespan	heparin
Humalog	Humulin
Humalog Mix 75/25	Humulin 70/30
Humulin	Humalog
Humulin 70/30	Humalog Mix 75/25
Hyalgan	Healon
hydromorphone	morphine
idarubicin	daunorubicin
Inderal	Adderall
indinavir	Denavir
Indocin	Endocet
infliximab	rituximab
Invanz	Avinza
iodine	Lodine
Isordil	Plendil
isotretinoin	tretinoin
K-Phos Neutral	Neutra-Phos K
Kaletra	Keppra
Keppra	Kaletra
Ketalar	ketorolac
ketorolac	Ketalar
Lamictal	Lamisil
Lamisil	Lamictal
lamivudine	lamotrigine
lamotrigine	lamivudine
Lanoxin	levothyroxine
Lantus	Lente

continues

Lasix	Luvox	
Lente	Lantus	
leucovorin calcium	Leukeran	
Leukeran	Myleran	Alkeran
Levbid	Levisin	
Levisin	Levbid	
levothyroxine	Lanoxin	
Lexapro	Loxitane	
Lipitor	Zyrtec	
liposomal doxorubicin (Doxil)	doxorubicin hydrochloride	
Lodine	iodine	
Lotronex	Protonix	
Loxitane	Lexapro	
Lupron Depot-3 Month	Lupron Depot-Ped	
Lupron Depot-Ped	Lupron Depot-3 Month	
Luvox	Lasix	
Maxzide	Microzide	
Metadate	methadone	
Metadate CD	Metadate ER	
Metadate ER	Metadate CD	
Metadate ER	methadone	
methadone	Metadate ER	
methadone	Metadate	
Methergine	Brethine	
Micronase	Microzide	
Microzide	Maxzide	
Microzide	Micronase	
mifepristone	misoprostol	
Miralax	Mirapex	
Mirapex	Miralax	
misoprostol	mifepristone	
morphine	hydromorphone	
morphine, oral liquid concentrate	morphine, non-concentrated oral liquid	
MS Contin	OxyContin	
Mucinex	Mucomyst	
Mucomyst	Mucinex	
Myleran	Alkeran	Leukeran
Narcan	Norcuron	
Natru-Vent	Atrovent	
Navane	Norvasc	
Neulasta	Neumega	
Neumega	Neupogen	
Neumega	Neulasta	
Neupogen	Neumega	

continues

Table E.1 Look-Alike and Sound-Alike Medications—Continued

Neurontin	Noroxin
Neutra-Phos K	K-Phos Neutral
Norcuron	Narcan
Noroxin	Neurontin
Norvasc	Navane
Novolin 70/30	NovoLog Mix 70/30
NovoLog Mix 70/30	Novolin 70/30
Occlusal-HP	Ocuflox
Ocuflox	Occlusal-HP
opium tincture	camphorated tincture of opium (paregoric)
Os-Cal	Asacol
oxycodone	OxyContin
OxyContin	MS Contin
OxyContin	oxycodone
Pamelor	Panlor DC
Panlor DC	Pamelor
Patanol	Platinol
Paxil	Taxol
Paxil	Plavix
Percocet	Procet
Pilocar	Dilacor XR
Platinol	Patanol
Plavix	Paxil
Plendil	Isordil
pneumococcal 7-valent vaccine	pneumococcal polyvalent vaccine
pneumococcal polyvalent vaccine	pneumococcal 7-valent vaccine
Prandin	Avandia
Precare	Precose
Precose	Precare
Prilosec	Prozac
probenecid	Procanbid
Procanbid	Probenecid
Procardia XL	Protain XL
Procet	Percocet
propylthiouracil	Purinethol
Protain XL	Procardia XL
protamine	Protonix
Protonix	Lotronex
Protonix	protamine
Prozac	Prilosec
Purinethol	propylthiouracil
quinine	quinidine

continues

quinidine	quinine
rabeprazole	aripiprazole
Recombivax HB	Comvax
Regranex	Granulex
Reminyl	Robinul
Reminyl	Amaryl
Retrovir	ritonavir
Rifater	Rifidin
Rifidin	Rifater
Ritalin	ritodrine
Ritalin LA	Ritalin-SR
Ritalin-SR	Ritalin LA
ritodrine	Ritalin
ritonavir	Retrovir
rituximab	infliximab
Robinul	Reminyl
Roxanol	Roxicodone Intensol
Roxanol	Roxicet
Roxicet	Roxanol
Roxicodone Intensol	Roxanol
saquinavir (free base)	saquinavir mesylate
saquinavir mesylate	saquinavir (free base)
Saquinivir	Sinequan
Sarafem	Serophene
Serophene	Sarafem
Seroquel	Serzone
sertraline	Soriatane
Serzone	Seroquel
Sinequan	Saquinivir
Solu-Medrol	Depo-Medrol
Soriatane	sertraline
sufentanil	fentanyl
sumatriptan	zolmitriptan
Taxol	Taxotere
Taxol	Paxil
Taxotere	Taxol
Tegretol	Tequin
Tegretol	Tegretol XR
Tegretol XR	Tegretol
Tequin	Tegretol
Tequin	Ticlid
Testoderm	Testoderm w/ Adhesive
Testoderm w/ Adhesive	Testoderm

continues

tetanus diptheria toxoid (Td)	tuberculin purified protein derivative (PPD)
tiagabine	tizanidine
Tiazac	Ziac
Ticlid	Tequin
tizanidine	tiagabine
TNKase	Activase
TNKase	t-PA
Tobradex	Tobrex
Tobrex	TobraDex
Topamax	Toprol-XL
Toprol-XL	Topamax
Toradol	Foradil
t-PA	TNKase
Tracleer	TriCor
tramadol hydrochloride	trazodone hydrochloride
trazodone hydrochloride	tramadol hydrochloride
tretinoin	isotretinoin
TriCor	Tracleer
tuberculin purified protein derivative (PPD)	tetanus diptheria toxoid (Td)
Tylenol	Tylenol PM
Tylenol PM	Tylenol
Ultracet	Duricef
valacyclovir	valganciclovir
Valcyte	Valtrex
valganciclovir	valacyclovir
Valtrex	Valcyte
Varivax	VZIG
Vexol	VōSol
Viagra	Allegra
vinblastine	vincristine
vincristine	vinblastine
Viokase	Viokase 8
Viokase 8	Viokase
Viracept	Viramune
Viramune	Viracept
VōSol	Vexol
VZIG	Varivax
Wellbutrin SR	Wellbutrin XL
Wellbutrin XL	Wellbutrin SR
Xeloda	Xenical
Xenical	Xeloda
Zantac	Zyrtec
Zebeta	DiaBeta

continues

Zebeta	Zetia
Zestril	Zetia
Zetia	Zebeta
Zetia	Zestril
Ziac	Tiazac
Zocor	Cozaar
zolmitriptan	sumatriptan
Zostrix	Zovirax
Zovirax	Zyvox
Zovirax	Zostrix
Zyban	Diovan
Zyprexa	Zyrtec
Zyprexa	Celexa
Zyrtec	Zyprexa
Zyrtec	Zantac
Zyrtec	Lipitor
Zyvox	Zovirax

Source: This information was reported in the *ISMP Medication Safety Alert! AcuteCare Edition,* January 1996–September 2004. © 2005 Institute for Safe Medication Practices. This material is used with permission of ISMP.

Glossary

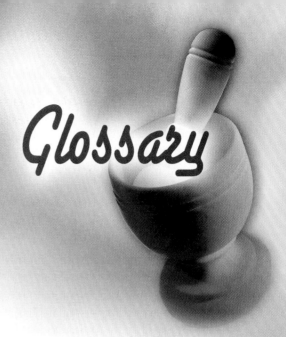

A

accreditation the stamp of approval of the quality of services of a hospital by JCAHO

active ingredient a chemical in the drug product producing the desired therapeutic effect

adverse drug reaction a negative consequence to a patient from taking a particular drug

allergy a state of heightened sensitivity as a result of exposure to a particular substance

alligation the compounding of two or more products to obtain a desired concentration

ampule a single-dose drug container

antibodies the part of the immune system to neutralize antigens or foreign substances in the body

antineoplastic drugs cancer-fighting drugs that are considered cytotoxic materials

appearance the physical look an employee has on the job, including dress and grooming

applications computer software programs that perform particular functions such as word processing, spread sheets, or databases

asepsis the absence of disease-causing microorganisms

aseptic technique the manipulation of sterile products and devices in such a way as to avoid introducing pathogens or disease-causing organisms

assumption error an error that occurs when an essential piece of information cannot be verified and is guessed or presumed

atomic weight the weight of a single atom of that element compared with the weight of one atom of hydrogen

attitude the disposition a worker adopts toward his or her job duties, customers, employer, and coworkers

autoclave a device that generates heat and pressure to sterilize

average inventory the beginning inventory plus the ending inventory divided by two

average wholesale price (AWP) the average price that wholesalers charge the pharmacy for a drug

B

bacteria small, single-celled microorganisms that exist in three main forms: spherical (i.e., cocci), rod shaped (i.e., bacilli), and spiral (i.e., spirilla)

beyond-use dating the date after which a compounded sterile product should not be used

biotechnology the field of study that combines the science of biology, chemistry, and immunology to produce synthetic, unique drugs with specific therapeutic effects

blending the act of combining two substances

brand name the name under which the manufacturer markets a drug; also known as the *trade name*

buccal administration oral administration in which a drug is placed between the gums and the inner lining of the cheek

bulb syringe a device used to irrigate the eyes or ears with water

C

capitation fee a monthly fee paid to the pharmacy by an insurer, whether or not the patient receives any prescriptions during that month

capsule the dose form containing powder, liquid, or granules in a gelatin covering

capture error an error that occurs when focus on a task is diverted elsewhere, and therefore the error goes undetected

catheters devices inserted into veins for direct access to the blood vascular system

Celsius temperature scale the temperature scale that uses zero degrees (i.e., 0° C) as the temperature at which water freezes and 100° C as the temperature at which water boils

central processing unit (CPU) the device used for manipulating computerized data input before output or storage

central venous catheter a catheter placed deep into the body

Certified Pharmacy Technician (CPhT) a pharmacy technician who has passed the PTCE

chain pharmacy a community pharmacy that consists of several similar pharmacies in the region (or nation) that are corporately owned

child-resistant containers special lids attached to prescription vials or bottles to prevent child access and reduce accidental poisonings; by definition, cannot be opened by 80% of children but can be opened by 90% of adults

civil law the areas of the law that concern U.S. citizens and the crimes they commit against one another

Class III prescription balance a two-pan balance used to weigh small amounts of material (120 g or less) with a sensitivity rating of 6 mg

closed questions questions that require a yes or no answer

coinsurance a percentage-based insurance plan whereby the patient must pay a certain percentage of the prescription price

colloidal dispersion the dispersion of ultrafine particles

comminution the act of reducing a substance to small, fine particles

common denominator a number into which each of the unlike denominators of two or more fractions can be divided evenly

community pharmacy any independent or chain pharmacy that dispenses prescription medications to outpatients; also called a *retail pharmacy*

compounded sterile products (CSPs) sterile products that are prepared outside of the pharmaceutical manufacturer's facility

compounding slab a flat, hard, nonabsorbent surface used for mixing compounds; also known as *ointment slab*

computer an electronic device for inputting, storing, processing, and/or outputting information

controlled-release medication a dose form that is formulated to release medication over a long duration of time

controlled substances drugs with potential for abuse; organized into five schedules that specify the way the drug must be stored, dispensed, recorded, and inventoried

copayment the amount the patient is to pay for each prescription, also called copay

coring introducing a small chunk of the rubber closure into the solution while removing medication from a vial

counterbalance a two-pan balance used for weighing material up to 5 kg with a sensitivity rating of 100 mg

creams cosmetically acceptable oil-in-water (O/W) emulsions for topical use on the skin

credentials documented evidence of qualifications

cytotoxic materials hazardous chemicals or drugs that must be handled and prepared with extra precautions

database management system (DBMS) an application that allows one to enter, retrieve, and query records

decimal any number that can be written in decimal notation using the integers 0 through 9 and a point (.) to divide the "ones" place from the "tenths" place (e.g., 10.25 is equal to 10 1/4[piece fraction])

decorum behavior that is in good taste

deductible an amount that must be paid by the insured before the insurance company will consider paying its portion of a medical cost

defendant one who defends against accusations brought forward in the lawsuit

delivery system the device used to deliver the drug; a design feature of the dose form that affects the delivery of the drug; how a medication is formulated to release the active ingredient

denominator the number on the bottom part of the fraction

deoxyribonucleic acid (DNA) the helix-shaped molecule that carries the genetic code

destructive agent a drug that kills bacteria, fungi, viruses, or even normal or cancer cells

diagnostic agent a drug used to diagnose other diseases

diluent a sterile fluid added to a powder to reconstitute, dilute, or dissolve a medication

direct purchasing the ordering of drugs from a pharmaceutical manufacturer

discount a reduced price

discrimination preferential treatment or mistreatment

dispersions liquid dose forms in which undissolved ingredients are mixed throughout a liquid vehicle

dose form how a medication is manufactured (e.g., capsule, tablet)

drug a medical substance or remedy used to change the way a living organism functions; also called a *medication*

Drug Enforcement Administration (DEA) the branch of the U.S. Justice Department that is responsible for regulating the sale and use of drugs with abuse potential

drug tolerance a situation that occurs when the body requires higher doses of a drug to produce the same therapeutic effect

duration of action the length of time a drug gives the desired response or is at the therapeutic level

E

effervescent salts granular salts that release gas and dispense active ingredients into solution when placed in water

electrolytes dissolved mineral salts, commonly found in IV fluids

emulsion the dispersion of a liquid in another liquid

equivalent (Eq) 1 mole divided by its valence, or the number of grams of solute dissolved in 1 mL of solution

ethical dilemma a situation that calls for a judgment between two or more solutions, not all of which are necessarily wrong

ethics the study of standards of conduct and moral judgment that outlines the rightness or wrongness of human conduct or character

etiquette unwritten rules of behavior

extemporaneous compounding the production of medication in an appropriate quantity and dose form from several pharmaceutical ingredients in response to a prescription written by a physician

extra dose error an error in which more doses are received by a patient than were prescribed by the physician

F

Fahrenheit temperature scale the temperature scale that uses 32° F as the temperature at which water freezes and 212° F as the temperature at which water boils

filters devices used to remove contaminants such as glass, paint, fibers, and rubber cores from IV fluids

first-pass effect the extent to which a drug is metabolized by the liver before reaching systemic circulation

floor stock medications stocked on each nursing unit

Food and Drug Administration (FDA) the agency of the federal government that is responsible for ensuring the safety and efficacy of drugs prepared for the market

forceps an instrument used to pick up small objects

formulary a list of drugs that have been preapproved for use by a committee of health professionals; used in hospitals, in managed care, and by many insurance providers

fraction a portion of a whole that is represented as a ratio

franchise pharmacy a member of a small chain of professional community pharmacies that dispense and prepare medications but are independently owned; sometimes called an *apothecary*

fungi parasites that feed on living organisms (or on dead organic material) and reproduce by means of spores

G

gels dispersions containing fine particles for topical use on the skin

generic name a common name that is given to a drug regardless of brand name; sometimes denotes a drug that is not protected by a trademark; also referred to as a USAN (United States Adopted Name); for example, acetaminophen is the generic drug name for Tylenol^R

genetic engineering a hybridization technique for creating monoclonal antibodies (MAbs)

geometric dilution method the combining of drugs using a mortar and pestle

germ theory of disease the idea that microorganisms cause diseases

good manufacturing practice (GMP) laboratory and industry guidelines to ensure a suitable work environment to prepare high-quality medications

graduates flasks used for measuring liquids

gram the metric system's base unit for measuring weight

gross profit the difference between the purchase price and the selling price; also called *markup*

H

harassment mistreatment, sexual or otherwise

health maintenance organizations (HMOs) organizations synonymous with managed care

high-efficiency particulate air (HEPA) filter a device used with laminar flow hoods to filter out most particulate matter (0.3 micron and larger) to prepare parenteral products safely and aseptically

home healthcare pharmacy a pharmacy that dispenses, prepares, and delivers drugs and medical supplies directly to the home of the patient

homeopathic medications very small dilutions of natural drugs claimed to stimulate the immune system

horizontal laminar airflow hood a special biological safety cabinet used to aseptically prepare IV drug admixtures, nutrition solutions, and other parenteral products

hospital pharmacy an institutional pharmacy that dispenses and prepares drugs and provides clinical services in a hospital setting

human failure an error generated by failure that occurs at an individual level

hypertonic solution a parenteral solution with a greater number of particles than blood cells

I

implants medications placed under the skin to deliver the active ingredient slowly

improper fraction a fraction with a value greater than 1 (the numerator's value is larger than the denominator's value)

independent pharmacy a community pharmacy that is privately owned by the pharmacist

inert ingredients inactive chemicals that are added to active ingredients to improve drug formulations; also called inactive ingredients

infection control committee (ICC) a committee of the hospital that provides leadership in relation to infection control techniques

infiltration the breakdown or collapse of a vein that allows the drug to leak into tissues surrounding the catheter site, causing edema or tissue damage or both

informed consent a document written about a study in terms understandable to the lay public

inhalations gases, vapors, solutions, or suspensions intended to be inhaled via the nasal or oral respiratory routes

input devices devices used for getting information into the computer such as a keyboard, mouse, or touch screen

inscription the part of the prescription that lists the medication or medications prescribed, including the drug names, strengths, and amounts

institutional pharmacy pharmacies that are organized under a corporate structure, following specific rules and regulations for accreditation

institutional review board (IRB) a committee of the hospital that ensures the appropriate protection is provided to patients using investigational drugs or procedures

intrarespiratory route the administration of a drug by inhalation into the lungs

intrauterine delivery system a way to deliver medication to prevent conception or treat cancer

intravenous (IV) infusions medications or fluids administered directly into a vein

inventory the entire stock of products on hand for sale at a given time

inventory value the total value of the entire stock of products on hand for sale on a given day

investigational drugs drugs being used in clinical trials that have not yet been approved by the FDA for use in the general population or drugs used for nonapproved indications

isotonic solution a parenteral solution with an equal number of particles as blood cells

IV administration set a sterile, pyrogen-free disposable device used to deliver IV fluids to patients

𝒥

Joint Commission on Accreditation of Healthcare Organizations (JCAHO) an independent, not-for-profit group that sets the standards by which quality of healthcare is measured and accredits hospitals according to those standards

ℒ

large-volume parenterals (LVPs) IV infusions of more than 100 mL

law of agency and contracts the general principle that allows an employee to enter into contracts on the employer's behalf

leading zero a zero that is placed in the one's place in a number that is less than zero and is being represented by a decimal value

least common denominator the smallest number that is evenly divisible by all of the denominators in a group of fractions

levigation the process reducing the particle size of a solid during the preparation of an ointment

liter the metric system's base unit for measuring volume

local use the site-specific application of a drug

long-term care facility an institution that provides care for geriatric and disabled patients; includes extended-care facility (ECF) and skilled-care facility (SCF)

lotion a liquid for topical application containing insoluble dispersed solids or immiscible liquids

lozenges medications in a sweet-taste formulation that is absorbed in the mouth

𝓜

mail-order pharmacy a large-volume centralized pharmacy operation that uses automation to fill and mail prescriptions to the patient

malpractice a form of negligence in which the standard of care was not met and was a direct cause of injury

managed care a type of health insurance system that emphasizes keeping the patient healthy or diseases controlled to reduce healthcare costs

markup *see* gross profit

master formula sheet the list of ingredients needed and procedures to follow when compounding; also called a *compounding log*

medical error any circumstance, action, inaction, or decision related to healthcare that contributes to an unintended health result

Medicare Prescription Drug, Improvement, and Modernization Act (MMA) of 2003 a voluntary insurance program started in January 2006 that provides partial coverage of prescriptions for patients eligible for Medicare

medication errors medical errors in which the source of error or harm includes a medication

medication fill list a complete list of all current medications for all hospital patients; used to create a unit dose profile

MEDMARX an Internet-based program for use by hospitals and healthcare systems for documenting, tracking, and trending medication errors

MedWatch a voluntary program run by the FDA for reporting serious adverse events, product problems, or medication errors; serves as a clearinghouse to provide information on safety alerts for drugs, biologics, diet supplements, and medical devices including drug recalls

meniscus the moon-shaped or concave appearance of a liquid in a graduated cylinder used in measurement

meter the metric system's base unit for measuring length

metered-dose inhaler (MDI) a device used to administer a drug in the form of compressed gas through inhalation into the lungs

metric system the measurement system based on subdivisions and multiples of 10; made up of three basic units: meter, gram, and liter

milliequivalent (mEq) a millimole divided by its valence

millimole (mM) a molecular weight, expressed as milligrams

mixed number a whole number and a fraction

modem a device for connecting a computer to a remote computer via telephone lines

mole (M) the measurement of an element equal to its atomic weight in grams

molecular weight the sum of the atomic weights of all the atoms in one molecule of a compound

monitor a display screen that provides a visual representation of data that have been input and/or processed

monoclonal antibodies (MAbs) single-cell antibodies produced in a laboratory to produce a pure antibody against a known specific antigen; used in cancer immunotherapy

mortar and pestle instruments used for mixing and grinding pharmaceutical ingredients

multiple-lumen catheter a catheter used to separately administer potentially physically incompatible drugs

𝒩

National Association of Boards of Pharmacy (NABP) an organization that represents the practice of pharmacy in each state and develops pharmacist licensure exams

National Drug Code (NDC) number a unique number assigned to a product to identify the manufacturer, drug, packaging size, and type

nebulizers devices used to deliver medication in a fine-mist form to the lung; often used in treating asthma

new drug application (NDA) the process through which drug sponsors formally propose that the FDA approve a new pharmaceutical for sale and marketing in the United States

nonverbal communication communication without words through facial expression, body contact, body position, and tone of voice

nosocomial infection an infection acquired by patients when they are in the hospital

nuclear pharmacist a certified pharmacist specializing in procuring, storing, compounding, dispensing, and providing information about radioactive pharmaceuticals used for diagnostic and therapeutic purposes

nuclear pharmacy a pharmacy that prepares and distributes radioactive pharmaceuticals to treat and diagnose disease

numerator the number on the upper part of the fraction

𝒪

ocular inserts a type of contact lens device with active medication for administration in the eye

oil-in-water (O/W) emulsion an emulsion containing a small amount of oil dispersed in water; like a cream

ointments semisolid emulsions for topical use on the skin

omission error an error in which a prescribed dose is not given

open-ended questions questions that require a descriptive answer, not yes or no

operating system a software program that performs essential functions such as maintaining a list of file names, issuing processing instructions, and controlling output

oral administration medication administration (through swallowing) for absorption along the GI tract into systemic circulation; can also refer to topical administration such as local treatment on the lips or mouth

oral syringe a device without a needle to administer medication to pediatric or elderly patients unable to swallow tablets or capsules

organizational failure errors generated by failure because of organizational rules, policies, or procedures

orphan drug a medication approved by the FDA to treat rare diseases

osmolality the amount of particulate per unit volume of a liquid preparation, measured in milliosmoles (mOsm)

osmotic pressure the osmotic pressure of red blood cells is 285 mOsm/L

over-the-counter (OTC) drug a drug sold without a prescription

package insert an information sheet required by the FDA and provided by a drug manufacturer that includes information on the product's indication and uses, dose, contraindications and warnings, as well as side effects and adverse reactions

paraprofessional a trained person who assists a professional person

parenteral solutions products that are prepared in a sterile environment for administration by injection

pastes water-in-oil (W/O) emulsions containing more solid material than an ointment

pathophysiology the study of diseases and illnesses affecting the normal function of the body

patient-controlled analgesia (PCA) infusion devices devices used by a patient to deliver small doses of medication to the patient for chronic pain

patient identifiers any demographic information that can identify the patient such as name, address, phone number, social security number, or medical identification number

patient profile a record kept by the pharmacy that lists a patient's identifying information, insurance information, medical history, prescription history, and prescription preferences

percent the number or ratio per 100

percentage of error the acceptable range of variation above and below the target measurement; used in compounding and manufacturing

peripherally inserted central (PIC) line a very fine catheter that is threaded through the peripheral vein into the subclavian vein; can be inserted by a skilled nurse

peripheral venous catheter a catheter inserted into a vein close to the surface of the skin

pharmaceutical care a philosophy of care that expanded the pharmacist's role to include appropriate medication use to achieve positive outcomes with prescribed drug therapy

pharmaceutics the study of the release characteristics of specific drug dose forms

pharmacist one who is licensed to prepare and dispense medications, counsel patients, and monitor outcomes pursuant to a prescription from a licensed health professional

pharmacodynamic agent a drug that alters body functions in a desired way

pharmacognosy the study of medicinal functions of natural products of animal, plant, or mineral origins

pharmacokinetics the activity of a drug within the body over a period of time; includes absorption, distribution, metabolism, and elimination

pharmacology the science of drugs and their interactions with the systems of living animals

pharmacy and therapeutics (P&T) committee a committee of the hospital that reviews, approves, and revises the hospital's formulary

pharmacy technician an individual working in a pharmacy who, under the supervision of a licensed pharmacist, assists in activities not requiring the professional judgment of a pharmacist; also called the *pharmacy tech* or *tech*

Pharmacy Technician Certification Examination (PTCE) an examination developed by the Pharmacy Technician Certification Board (PTCB) that technicians must pass to be certified and receive the title of CPhT

pH value the degree of acidity or alkalinity of a solution; less than 7 is acidic and more than 7 is alkaline

piggyback a small-volume parenteral (SVP) admixture often containing a medication that is attached to an existing IV line

pipette a long, thin, calibrated hollow tube used for measuring liquids less than 1.5 mL

plaintiff one who files a lawsuit for the courts to decide

plasters solid or semisolid, medicated or nonmedicated preparations that adhere to the skin

policy and procedure manual a book that outlines activities in the pharmacy, defines the roles of individuals, and lists guidelines

powder a finely divided combination or admixture of drugs and/or chemicals ranging in size from extremely fine (1 micron or less) to very coarse (about 10 mm)

powder volume (pv) the amount of space occupied by a freeze-dried medication in a sterile vial, used for reconstitution; equal to the difference between the final volume and the volume of the diluting ingredient or the diluent volume

prescription benefits manager (PBM) a company that administers drug benefits from many different insurance companies

prime vendor purchasing an agreement made by a pharmacy for a specified percentage or dollar volume of purchases

printer a device for creating hard copy or paper output

professional someone with recognized expertise in a field where expectations are that they use their knowledge and skills to benefit others and to operate with some autonomy in an ethical manner

profit the amount of revenue received that exceeds the expense of the sold product

proper fraction a fraction with a value of less than 1 (the numerator's value is smaller than the denominator's value)

prophylactic agent a drug used to prevent disease

proportion a comparison of equal ratios

protected health information (PHI) medical information that is protected by HIPAA such as medical diagnoses, medication profiles, and results of laboratory tests

protocol a list of drugs and doses developed and approved by a physician for use by a nurse or pharmacist in the absence of the physician; similar to "standing orders"

protozoa single-cell organisms that inhabit water and soil

pulverization a process to reduce a solid tablet into a fine powder

punch method a method for filling capsules in which the body of a capsule is repeatedly punched into a cake of medication until the capsule is full

purchasing the ordering of products for use or sale by the pharmacy

quality assurance (QA) program a feedback system to improve care

radiopharmaceuticals drugs containing radioactive ingredients often used for diagnostic or therapeutic purposes

random-access memory (RAM) the temporary, nonpermanent memory of the computer in which information is held while it is being input and processed

ratio a comparison of numeric values

read-only memory (ROM) permanent memory containing essential operating instructions for the computer

receiving a series of procedures for delivery of products

recertification the periodic updating of certification

recombinant DNA a technique that uses living organisms or parts of organisms for specific purposes such as creating a synthetic drug like insulin

ribonucleic acid (RNA) an important component of genetic code that arranges amino acids into proteins

root cause analysis a logical and systematic process used to help identify what, how, and why something happened to prevent recurrence

route of administration a way of getting a drug onto or into the body

satellite pharmacy a minipharmacy located on a nursing unit of the hospital

scanner a device for inputting images into the computer

selection error an error that occurs when two or more options exist and the wrong option is chosen

semisynthetic drugs drugs that contain both natural and synthetic components

sentinel event an unexpected occurrence involving death or serious physical or psychologic injury or the potential for occurrences to happen

sharps used needles; a potential source of infection

signa the part of the prescription that indicates the directions for the patient to follow

small-volume parenterals (SVPs) an IV infusion of 100 mL or less commonly used to administer drugs

solute an ingredient dissolved in a solution or dispersed in a suspension

solutions liquid dose forms commonly containing carbohydrates, proteins, electrolytes, minerals, or medications

solvent the vehicle that makes up the greater part of a solution

spatulas stainless steel, plastic, or hard rubber instruments used for transferring or mixing solid pharmaceutical ingredients

spatulation a process used to blend ingredients, often used in the preparation of creams and ointments

spray the dose form that consists of a container with a valve assembly that, when activated, emits a fine dispersion of liquid, solid, or gaseous material

standard of care the usual and customary level of practice in the community

stat medications medications that are to be administered immediately

sterilization a process that destroys the microorganisms in a substance, resulting in asepsis

storage devices devices used to store information that has been input into the computer such as floppy disk drive, hard drive, tape drive, CD drive, or removable disk drive

subclavian vein a vein in the neck, lying below the clavicle and jugular vein

sublingual administration oral administration where a drug is placed under the tongue and is rapidly absorbed into the bloodstream

subscription the part of the prescription that lists instructions to the pharmacist about dispensing the medication, including information about compounding or packaging instructions, labeling instructions, refill information, and information about the appropriateness of dispensing drug equivalencies

suppositories solid formulations containing a drug for rectal or vaginal administration

suspension the dispersion of a solid in a liquid

synthesized drug a drug that is artificially created

synthetic drug a drug that is artificially created but in imitation of natural-occurring substances

systemic use the application of a drug by means of absorption into the bloodstream

T

tablet the solid dose form produced by compression and containing one or more active ingredients

technical failure an error generated by failure because of location or equipment

therapeutic agent a drug that prevents, cures, diagnoses, or relieves symptoms of a disease

therapeutic effect the desired pharmacological action of a drug on the body

third-party administration (TPA) direct billing by the pharmacy to the customer's insurer

topical administration administration of a drug to the skin or any mucous membrane such as eye, nose, ears, lungs, vagina, urethra, and colon; usually administration of a drug directly to the surface of the skin

tort the legal term for personal injuries in a lawsuit

total parenteral nutrition (TPN) a specially formulated parenteral solution that provides for the nutritional needs intravenously (IV) when a patient cannot or will not eat; also known as hyperalimentation solutions

toxicology the study of the toxic effects of drugs or other substances in the body

transdermal delivery system (TDS) the method of delivering medication via the skin; like a patch

triage the ranking of patients for treatment or customer care by the priority of their needs

trituration the process of rubbing, grinding, or pulverizing a substance to create fine particles, generally by means of a mortar and pestle

turnover rate the number of times the entire stock is used and replaced each year, calculated by the annual dollar purchases divided by the average inventory

unit dose an amount of a drug prepackaged for a single administration to a particular patient at a particular time

unit dose profile the documentation that provides the information necessary to prepare the unit doses and includes patient name and location, medication and strength, frequency or schedule of administration, and quantity for each order

unit of use a fixed number of dose units in a drug stock container, usually consisting of a month's supply, or 30 tablets or capsules.

United States Pharmacopeia (USP) the independent scientific organization responsible for setting official quality standards for all prescription drugs, OTC drugs, and dietary supplements sold in the United States

United States Pharmacopeia–National Formulary (USP–NF) a book that contains U.S. standards for medicines, dose forms, drug substances, excipients or inactive substances, medical devices, and dietary supplements

universal claim form (UCF) a form used for requesting an insurance company to provide coverage for a prescription

universal precautions procedures followed in healthcare settings to prevent infection as a result of exposure to blood or other bodily fluids

urethral route administration of a drug by insertion into the urethra

USP Chapter 797 guidelines on parenteral product preparation developed by the United States Pharmacopeia (USP) that have become standards for hospital accreditation

Vaccine Adverse Event Reporting System (VAERS) a postmarketing surveillance system operated by the FDA and CDC that collects information on adverse events that occur after immunization

vaginal route administration of a drug by application of a cream or insertion of a tablet into the vagina

valence the number that represents an element's capacity to combine to form a molecule of a stable compound

vertical laminar airflow hood a special biological safety cabinet used to aseptically prepare hazardous drugs, especially cytotoxic drugs

viruses minute infectious agents that do not have all of the components of a cell and thus can replicate only within a living host cell

water-in-oil (W/O) emulsion an emulsion containing a small amount of water dispersed in an oil; like an ointment

wholesaler purchasing the ordering of drugs and supplies from a local vendor who delivers the product to the pharmacy on a daily basis

wrong dose error an error in which the dose is either above or below the correct dose by more than 5%

wrong dose form error an error in which the dose form or formulation is not the accepted interpretation of the physician order

wrong time error a medication error in which any drug is given 30 minutes or more before or after it was prescribed, up to the time of the next dose, not including as needed orders

$\mathcal{Y}$

Y-site an injection port found on most IV administration sets

Note: Italicized page locators denote figures or photos; t denotes tables.

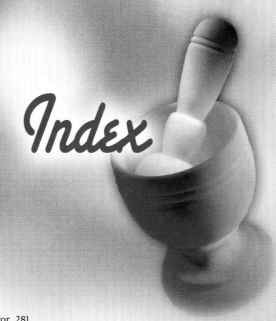

Index

Cultural differences, sensitivity to, 306–307
Cytotoxic drugs, 235
    aseptic technique and preparation, 238
    commonly used, 236t
    exposure incident report, *237*
    technique for handling, 236–238

U

V

W

Y

Z

Photo Credits